Pinch OF Nom
ENJOY

First published 2022 by Bluebird
an imprint of Pan Macmillan
The Smithson, 6 Briset Street, London EC1M 5NR
EU representative: Macmillan Publishers Ireland Ltd, 1st Floor,
The Liffey Trust Centre, 117–126 Sheriff Street Upper,
Dublin 1, D01 YC43

Associated companies throughout the world
www.panmacmillan.com

ISBN 978-1-5290-6226-7

1 3 5 7 9 8 6 4 2
A CIP catalogue record for this book is available from the British Library.
Printed and bound in China.

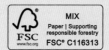

Publisher Carole Tonkinson
Managing Editor Martha Burley
Production Manager Sarah Badhan
Art Direction Nikki Dupin and Emma Wells, Studio Nic&Lou
Design Emma Wells and Beth Free, Studio Nic&Lou
Illustrations Shutterstock / Emma Wells and Beth Free
Food Styling Kate Wesson and Octavia Squire
Prop Styling Max Robinson

Visit www.panmacmillan.com to read more about all our books
and to buy them. You will also find features, author interviews and
news of any author events, and you can sign up for e-newsletters
so that you're always first to hear about our new releases.

& Kay Allinson

Pinch OF Nom
ENJOY

GREAT-TASTING FOOD
FOR EVERY DAY

bluebird
books for life

CONTENTS

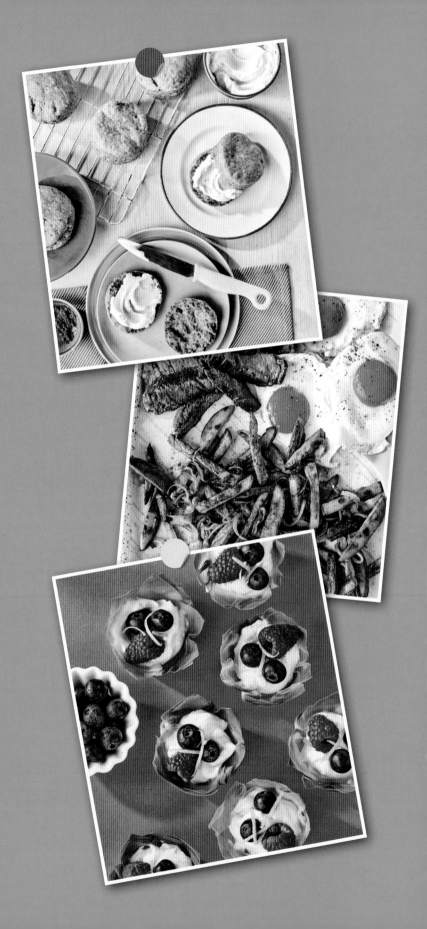

WELCOME to Pinch OF Nom

ENJOY

HELLO

We're completely over the moon to be sharing cookbook number FIVE with you! This book simply wouldn't have been possible without the Pinch of Nom community, and it means the world to us that we can carry on sharing our love of food with you all. YOU have played a huge role in bringing this book to life – whether you know it or not! Your photos, comments and messages constantly inspire us, and they're what sparked the whole theme of the book: 'Enjoy'. More than ever before, this is a collection of properly healthy, hearty dishes that you'll love making as much as you love eating them.

SO, WHAT CAN I EXPECT FROM ENJOY?

We love food and we know you do too – it brings us all together. It's not just about the eating of it either, there's so much joy to be found in preparing, cooking and sharing food, and that's what these recipes are all about.

In writing this book we've taken on board everything we've heard from our readers over the years, listening to you telling us about the kinds of recipes that you truly enjoy making. We hope that you'll find exciting new flavours and memorable old favourites inside these pages – recipes that you'll want to get stuck into and share with all of your loved ones.

From simple yet satisfying midweek dinners to decadent puds that taste way more indulgent than they really are, these 100 brand-new recipes are made to be enjoyed. We're talking tempting dishes such as Pork and Pineapple Kebabs (page 62), Pizza Nachos (page 84) and irresistible Chocolate Toffee Puddings (page 260).

And don't worry, we haven't forgotten to give some more takeaway classics a Pinch of Nom makeover! You'll find fresh fakeaways to spice up your meal plan each week. We've packed so much love and flavour into each one, that you won't even realise just how slimming-friendly they are.

Enjoying cooking means being able to cook the recipes in a way that suits you, so we've made sure that loads of these recipes include more than one method. Turn on your slow cooker or crack out the air fryer – we've got you covered!

Plus, we've dropped plenty of handy tips and swaps on the pages, so keep your eyes peeled if you're looking for easy ways to make any of the recipes vegan, vegetarian, gluten-free or dairy-free. This is food for everyone, and we hope you enjoy every recipe as much as we enjoyed creating it for you.

Kay x Kate

THE FOOD

As a classically trained chef, Kate has always loved recreating dishes and putting an original spin on classic recipes. This is how the very first Pinch of Nom recipes came to be, and it's this passion that means we can continue to bring fresh new flavours to you today. Kate and her small team love nothing more than getting into the kitchen and experimenting with ingredients until some Pinch of Nom magic is created!

It's so important to us that every single one of our recipes uses simple, budget-friendly ingredients that you can use across multiple dishes. To help you keep costs down, we'll only ever use an item that seems less common if it adds something really special to a dish – and even then, we'll try to make sure it's an ingredient that you can use more than once.

These recipes are designed to suit any level of cooking skill, so if you're a beginner in the kitchen, you'll still be able to make a tasty plate of food. As you cook through the book, we hope you'll discover a whole new love and enjoyment of cooking meals at home.

This book is about food that everyone can enjoy, so a whopping 49 of the 100 recipes are vegetarian. Almost all of the other dishes can be made veggie-friendly (and vegan too) with a couple of simple swaps, such as using a protein replacement of your choice. We've even flagged vegetarian and vegan recipes to make them nice and easy to spot.

SLIMMING-FRIENDLY FOOD, MADE to be Enjoyed

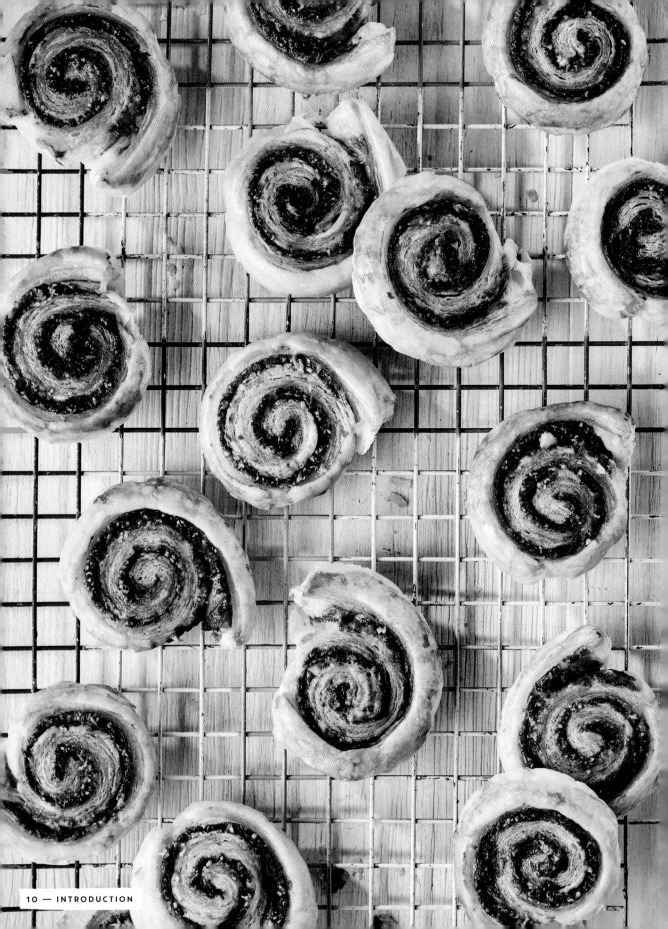

RECIPE TAGS

EVERYDAY LIGHT

These recipes can be used freely throughout the week. All the meals, including accompaniments, are under 400 calories. Or, in the case of sides, snacks and sweet treats, under 200 calories. Of course, if you're counting calories, you still need to keep an eye on the values, but these recipes should help you stay under your allowance.

WEEKLY INDULGENCE

These recipes are still low in calories at between 400 and 500 calories including accompaniments, or 200–300 for sides, snacks and sweet treats, but should be saved for once or twice a week. Mix them into your Everyday Light recipes for variety.

SPECIAL OCCASION

These recipes are often lower in calories than their full-fat counterparts, but they need to be saved for a special occasion. This tag indicates any main meals that are over 500 calories, or over 300 for sides, snacks and sweet treats.

All of these calculations and dietary indicators are for guidance only and are not to be taken as complete fact without checking ingredients and product labelling yourself.

KCAL *and* CARB VALUES

All of our recipes have been worked out as complete meals, using standardised portion sizes for any accompaniments, as advised by the British Nutrition Foundation. Carb values are included for those who need to measure their intake.

GLUTEN-FREE RECIPES

For gluten-free recipes, look out for the handy icon. All these recipes are either free of gluten or we have suggested gluten-free ingredient swaps of common ingredients, such as stock cubes and Worcestershire sauce. Please check labelling to ensure the product you buy is gluten-free.

FREEZABLE RECIPES

Look out for the 'Freeze Me' icon to indicate freezer-friendly dishes. The icon applies to the main dish only, not the suggested accompaniments.

OUR RECIPE ICONS

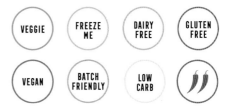

BATCH COOKING

We know how much our community loves getting organised with a good batch-cooking session! There are plenty of recipes in the book that you can batch cook simply by making a bigger portion (look out for the Batch Friendly icon). For instance, try doubling the quantities for the Poultryman's Pie (page 168) and freezing it for a rainy day. It's important to freeze food safely, so we've included the latest NHS food-safety guidelines (correct at the time of writing).

- **Divide up your portions** so you don't have to refrigerate or freeze leftovers in bulk. There's nothing worse than chiselling away at a huge, frozen block of food! Individual portions also cool, freeze and defrost loads quicker.

- **Check you've got space** in your fridge or freezer before you start cooking!

- **Use airtight containers** or freezer bags. If you invest in some decent, microwave-safe containers, they won't crack or melt. Make sure they are properly sealed to avoid 'freezer burn' (uninvited air damaging your food).

- **Use refrigerated foods within 2 days.** Many recipes like curries and chillies taste even better after 24 hours in the fridge, but they won't keep for much longer than that.

- **Label your batch-cooked meals.** Extra portions can be stored away for busier days, but be sure to write the date you made it (and what it is!) on a freezer-proof sticker. Meals can be frozen for 3-6 months. Beyond 6 months is still safe, but the food may not taste as good.

- **Only ever reheat food once.**

- **Defrost thoroughly** in the fridge or microwave before reheating food.

- **Reheat and eat food within 24 hours** of defrosting it. NHS guidelines (correct at the time of writing) state that you should reheat food until it reaches 70°C/158°F and holds that temperature for 2 minutes. Make sure it's piping hot throughout. Stir while reheating to ensure this.

- **Rice and pasta are best cooked fresh.** You can freeze the sauce or meat for some recipes, but in most cases it'll be best to cook the accompaniments right before serving. Some foods can't be reheated or just taste a lot nicer when they're freshly cooked.

- **Store rice carefully** if you plan to batch cook it. Rice is safe to freeze and reheat, but only if it's stored in the right way. Cool it as quickly as possible (ideally within 1 hour) by putting it in a wide, shallow container. The longer rice is left at room temperature, the greater the risk that it could grow harmful bacteria. Keep cooked rice in the fridge no longer than 1 day before reheating it, or you can freeze it and defrost thoroughly in the fridge before reheating. Always make sure you reheat rice until it is piping hot, and never reheat it more than once.

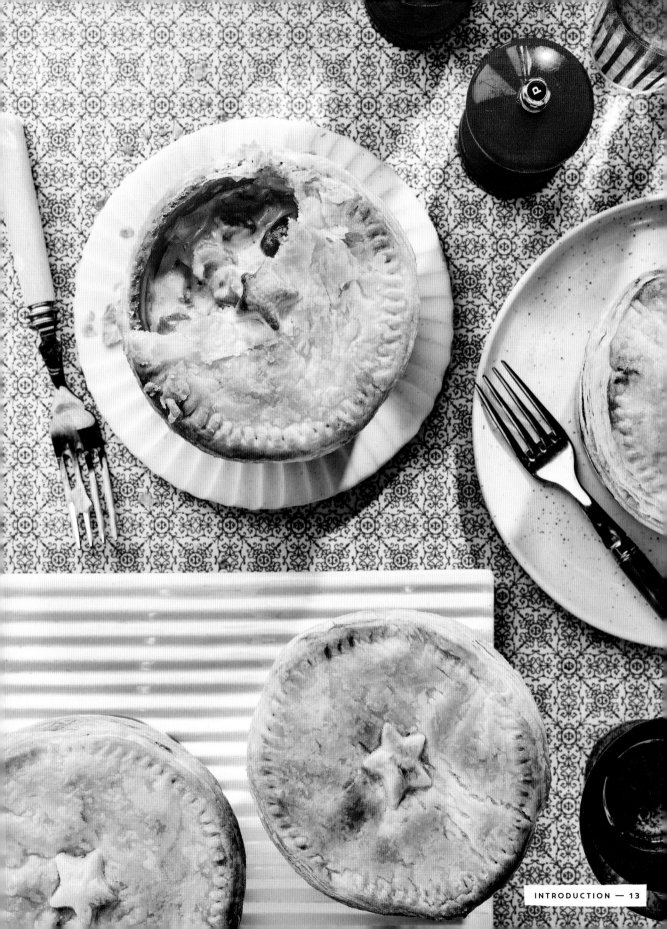

KEY INGREDIENTS

PROTEIN

Lean meats are a great source of protein, providing essential nutrients and keeping you feeling full between meals. Use the leanest possible cuts and trim off all visible fat when cooking the recipes in this book. In many of our recipes you'll find that you can switch the type of protein for whatever meat you prefer. This especially applies to any mince recipes; turkey, beef or pork mince are easily interchangeable. Fish is also a great source of protein, and it's naturally low in fat. Pinch of Nom's favourite phrase? If it swims, it slims! Fish provides nutrients that the body struggles to produce naturally, making it perfect for lots of our super-slimming recipes. And don't forget, veggie protein options can always be used instead of meat in all of the recipes in this book.

HERBS *and* SPICES

We love a bit of spice! One of the best ways to keep your food interesting when changing ingredients for lower fat/sugar/calorie versions is to season it well with herbs and spices. In particular, mixed spice blends, either shop-bought or homemade, taste fantastic – see our aromatic Chana Masala (page 44). Don't be shy with spices! We've added a spice-level icon to the recipes in this book, so you know what to expect. The beauty of cooking dishes yourself is you can always adjust the heat to your liking – add more or less chilli to suit. Always taste your food before adding extra spicing; this is particularly important if you're planning to double up. You'll often find that you don't need to double the amount of all the ingredients to achieve the right flavour – spices, vinegars, mustard and hot sauces should be added gradually, to taste.

STOCKS, SAUCES *and* THICKENERS

When you remove fat from a dish, flavours can dwindle. Adding spices is one way to boost flavours, but often the acidity in a recipe is much more important. When it comes to balancing and boosting flavours in our dishes, we love to use vinegar, soy sauce, fish sauce, Worcestershire sauce or Henderson's relish. One of Pinch of Nom's essential ingredients is the humble stock cube or pot; they add instant flavour and they're so versatile. We use various flavoured stock cubes and pots throughout this book, they are easily substituted. White wine stock pots, for example, can be tricky to find, but you can use 100ml of dry white wine and reduce the amount of water used in the recipe by 100ml instead (bear in mind this will add extra calories). It's worth noting that sauces, stock cubes and pots are often high in salt, so you may want to swap for reduced-salt versions.

We're often asked for tips on how to thicken soups, sauces and gravies. In the pre-slimming days, we wouldn't have thought twice about using a few tablespoons of flour to thicken liquids, but now we're always looking for alternatives. Letting liquids reduce is a good way of thickening sauces without adding anything extra. As the moisture evaporates, the flavours get more concentrated too, so the end result will taste even better.

You can also thicken recipes with potatoes. They're super starchy so they can be blitzed or mashed into your sauce or soup to soak up extra liquid. Bear in mind that this method will add extra calories (1 large potato, approx. 369g, is about 311 kcal). A tomato-based dish can be thickened slightly using tomato puree. This will add about 50 kcal per 51g tablespoon.

You can use egg yolks or whole beaten eggs to thicken some soups and sauces. Drizzle a little of the hot liquid onto the egg, whisking vigorously, then stir the egg into the pan and heat gently until it thickens. 1 medium (57g) egg is about 76 kcal and 1 medium (18g) egg yolk is about 55 kcal.

If making a roux-style sauce you can cut down on calories by making a slurry rather than using loads of butter. Mix your flour with a little water, then stir it into boiling liquid and simmer for a few minutes to cook the flour. 1 level tablespoon (20g) of plain flour is about 71 kcal. Another option is using cornflour, made into a slurry in the same way as above. Be sure to cook it until the starchy taste has gone. 1 level tablespoon of cornflour (20g) is about 69 kcal.

It can be tempting to thicken stews or chillies with gravy granules, but this can add quite a few calories. 1 teaspoon (5g) of gravy granules is about 21 kcal (depending on the brand). It's worth bearing in mind that gravy granules can also be high in salt.

LEMONS *and* LIMES

Lemons and limes pack a punch when it comes to flavour. They're perfect for adding a zing to our Carne Asada recipe (page 59).

REDUCED-FAT DAIRY

Substituting high-fat dairy products with clever alternatives can make a dish instantly lower in calories. You'll find that we'll often use low-fat cream cheese or spreadable cheese rather than the higher-fat versions. The same applies to any recipes that may traditionally contain heavy, high-calorie cream. We have swapped this out for a light double cream alternative such as Elmlea.

PLANT-BASED ALTERNATIVES

We often use plant-based alternatives to dairy milk because they're low in fat and bring added flavour to a dish. Coconut dairy-free milk alternative is a great substitute for high-fat tinned coconut milk, and almond milk adds a lovely nutty flavour to recipes. Make sure you pick up the unsweetened coconut or almond milk alternatives rather than any tinned versions; these will normally be found in a carton container.

TINS

Tinned beans, tomatoes and sweetcorn all come in handy time and time again. We often use them to add texture and flavour to stews, soups and salads. Using tinned ingredients can help to keep costs down, and you'll never know the difference – used in these sorts of recipes they'll taste just as good as their fresh counterparts.

FROZEN FRUIT *and* VEG

Frozen fruit and veg make great filler ingredients and are perfect low-cost alternatives for recipes such as stews, where fresh ingredients aren't always necessary. Most of the time they're already peeled and chopped too, so they save time as well as money.

PULSES, RICE *and* BEANS

High in both protein and fibre, keeping a few tins of beans and pulses in the cupboard is never going to do any harm! Rice is a great accompaniment to so many Pinch of Nom recipes.

BREAD

A great source of fibre, wholemeal bread is filling and versatile too – you can use slices to make Viking Toast (page 34), or whizz it into breadcrumbs to coat our Mini Chicken Kyiv Balls (page 116). We often use gluten-free breads as they tend to contain fewer calories and less sugar, making them an easy swap when you want to shave off a few calories.

EGGS

Eggs are protein-rich, tasty and versatile! The humble egg can be used in so many different ways. From baking and binding ingredients together, to having a starring role in our Fry-Up Frittata (page 33) you'll never go wrong if you have a box of eggs in the house.

LOW-CALORIE SPRAY

One of the best ways to cut down on cooking with oils and fats is to use a low-calorie cooking spray. A spritz of this will make little difference to the end result of your food, but it can make a huge difference to the calories consumed.

READY-MADE PASTRY

We have a few recipes using pastry in this book. There's no need to become a pastry chef overnight – just buy it ready-made! Not only can you usually find a light version with reduced calories, but ain't nobody got the time to be making filo pastry for our Steak and Kidney Pie (page 120)!

TORTILLA WRAPS *and* SANDWICH THINS

Pinch of Nom is well known for creating magic with wraps! Wholegrain or wholewheat wraps provide fibre and fill you up too. You can use them in a traditional way, like in our Peri-Peri Chicken Wraps (page 53) or bake them until they're crispy in our Chipotle Chicken Taquitos recipe (page 46). We also do some magic things with a sandwich thin – check out our Apple and Cherry Bakes on page 256.

SUGAR-FREE TOFFEES

Using sugar-free toffees is a clever way to get caramel flavours into a recipe without needing to use loads of butter and sugar. A couple of our dessert recipes in this book call for sugar-free creamy toffees. It's important to make sure you pick up the 'creamy' version – hard butter toffees or candies won't give the same results.

SWEETENER

There are so many sweeteners out there, it can be tricky to know which is the best substitute for regular sugar. Sweeteners vary in sweetness and swapping them weight-for-weight with regular sugar can give you different results. In our recipes we use granulated sweetener, not powdered sweetener, as it has larger 'crystals'. This can be used weight-for-weight anywhere that you're replacing sugar.

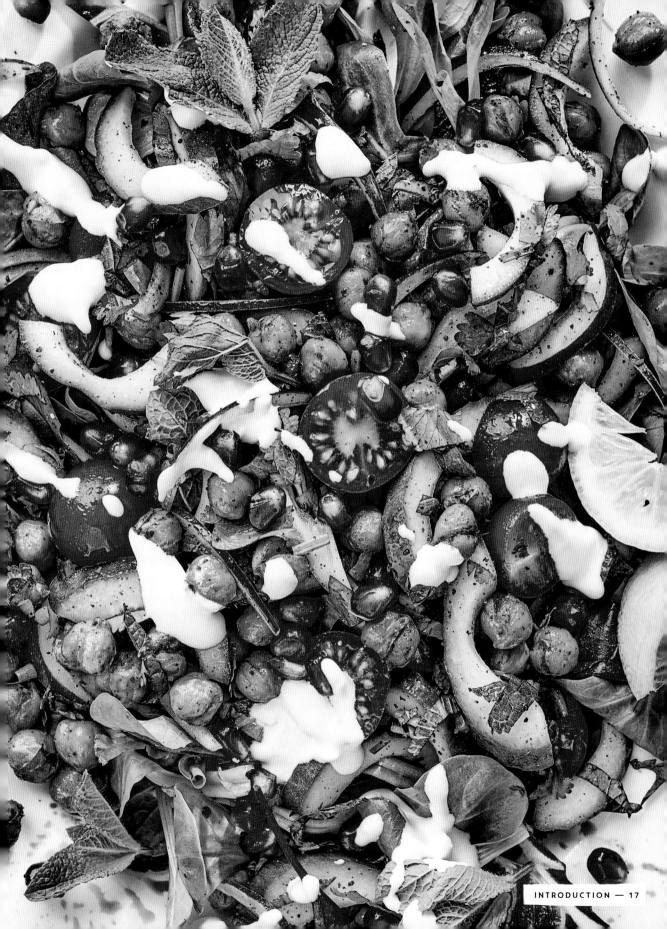

OUR FAVOURITE KIT

NON-STICK PANS

If there's one bit of kit that Pinch of Nom would advise as an investment kitchen piece, it would be a decent set of non-stick pans. The better the non-stick quality of your pans, the fewer cooking oils and fats you'll need to use in order to stop food sticking and burning. Keep your pans in good health by cleaning them properly and gently with soapy water. We recommend picking up a good set of saucepans, a small and a large frying pan.

MIXING BOWLS

A couple of mixing bowls will come in handy time and time again. We'd suggest getting at least two, a smaller one and a large one will see you through most kinds of recipes. Smaller bowls give you more control when you're whisking ingredients and larger bowls mean more room to mix it up.

KITCHEN KNIVES

Every kitchen needs a good set of knives. If you can, invest in some good quality, super-sharp knives –

blunt knives have a habit of bouncing off ingredients, which can make them more dangerous than sharper ones. You'll need to mind your fingers with super-sharp knives too, but you'll be glad you invested when you've got knives that glide through veg, saving you so much time and effort. For slicing ingredients really thinly, you can also pick up a mandoline; it's not essential but it will make our Herby Quiche with Potato Crust (page 136) so much speedier.

KNIFE SHARPENER

Once you've invested in your sharp knives, you'll want to keep them that way! Keep those babies nice and sharp so you can carry on slicing and dicing like a pro.

CHOPPING BOARDS

As well as protecting your surfaces, a good set of chopping boards are the key to a safe and hygienic kitchen. We'd suggest picking up a full set of colour-coordinated chopping boards, with separate boards for veg, meat, fish and dairy. They'll make it so much easier to keep your ingredients separate and most sets are easy to clean and tidy away once your meal prep is sorted.

POTATO MASHER

Used in a number of recipes, you'll need a decent masher to make sure you've got smooth, creamy mash to spoon onto your dishes.

SLOW COOKER

We're big fans of slow cookers. Throw in some ingredients, go out, enjoy your day and return to a home-cooked meal, ready and waiting for you. They're a relatively inexpensive bit of kit that will save you a lot of time. We use a 3.5-litre slow cooker – please don't attempt to make dishes in a slow cooker that is any smaller than this.

FOOD PROCESSOR / BLENDER / STICK BLENDER

These are essential pieces of kit for a lot of Pinch of Nom recipes. We like to make sauces from scratch, so a decent blender or food processor is a lifesaver. A stick blender can be used on most occasions if you're looking for something cheaper or more compact. It's well worth the investment for the flavour of all those homemade sauces.

TUPPERWARE *and* PLASTIC TUBS

Many of the Pinch of Nom recipes in the book are freezable and ideal for batch cooking. It's a good idea to invest in some freezer-proof tubs – and they don't have to be plastic. For a more eco-friendly solution, choose glass storage containers; just remember to check they're freezer-safe.

Note on plastic: We have made a conscious effort to reduce the amount of non-reusable plastic such as cling film when making our recipes. There are great alternatives to cling film now available, such as silicone stretch lids, beeswax food covers, fabric food covers and biodegradable food and freezer bags.

RAMEKIN DISHES

One of the best ways to handle portion control on sweet treats or desserts is to serve up your puddings in individual portions. By making dishes in small ramekins, you not only give yourself a set portion (which makes calorie counting so much easier), but it also makes the food look super faaaaancy!

OVENWARE

For lots of our recipes, you'll need either an oven tray, roasting tin or oven dish. We'd recommend making sure you've got some baking trays, square and round cake tins, a loaf tin, a large, heavy-based casserole dish with a lid, a pie dish, quiche dish and lasagne dish as essential items. Keep your ovenware in tip-top condition for longer by lining them with non-stick baking paper before cooking. If a specific size of dish is essential to the success of a recipe, we've listed this as 'Special Equipment'.

HOB

We cook on an induction hob. If you have a ceramic/hot-plate hob you may have to cook dishes for a little longer.

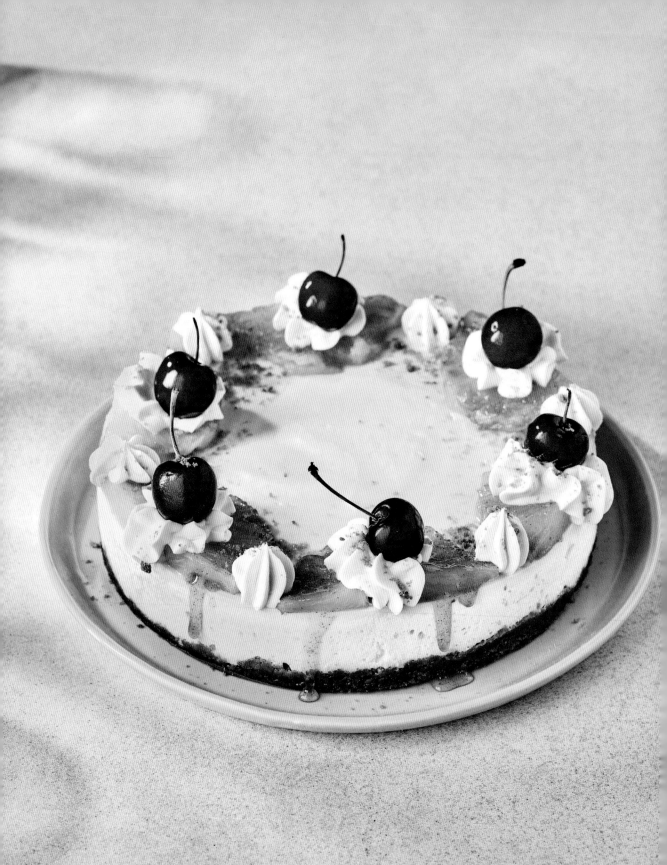

FINE GRATER

Using a fine grater is one of those surprising revelations. You won't believe the difference between grating cheese with a fine grater versus a standard grater. 45g of cheese, for example, can easily cover an oven dish when using a fine grater. You can also use it for citrus zest, garlic and ginger – it helps a little go a long, long way.

HEATPROOF JUG

A measuring jug is essential for measuring out wet ingredients. We recommend getting a heatproof version that you can stick in the microwave when needed.

AIR FRYER

Air fryers have become a slimming staple in recent years. The ultimate in convenience, they give you crispy, deep-fried textures and flavours without having to plunge your food into high-calorie oils. Food cooks more quickly in an air fryer, and any excess cooking oils drain away for a lighter, crispier finish. They're great for chips, breaded meats and so much more. If your air fryer doesn't have a preheat function, heat it at cooking temperature for a few minutes before air-frying your food.

MEASURING SPOONS

Want to make sure you never get muddled between a tsp and tbsp? Pinch of Nom has absolutely, definitely never made this mistake. Honest. But these days we're never without a trusty set of measuring spoons, which help make sure it's not a tablespoon of chilli when it should have been a teaspoon. Just make sure you use a butter knife to level off the spoon – you'll be surprised how much extra you add when the spoonful is heaped.

GARLIC CRUSHER

You'll never miss the faff of finely chopping garlic once you've invested in a garlic crusher. Relatively cheap to pick up, you won't go back after you've squeezed that first clove into a perfect paste. It'll save you so much time and it helps your garlic spread evenly throughout the dish.

ELECTRIC PRESSURE COOKER

A pressure cooker is a great investment if you're looking to save time. The high-pressure cooking process creates perfectly tender meat and makes stews taste as though they've been bubbling away for hours. We recommend electric models for safety and ease of use.

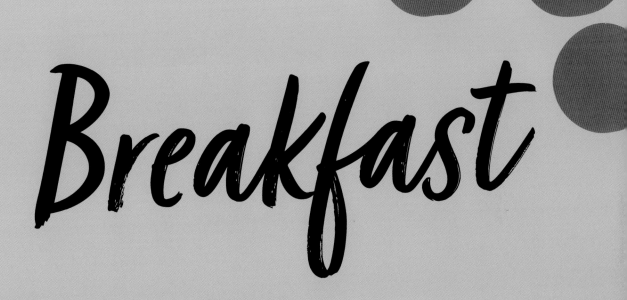

Breakfast

VEGGIE

DAIRY FREE

USE DF ALTERNATIVE FOR CREAM CHEESE

GLUTEN FREE

USE GF BREAD

CREAMY STRAWBERRY FRENCH TOAST

🕐 **10 MINS**   🍲 **6 MINS**   ✗ **SERVES 4**

PER SERVING:
196 KCAL / 28G CARBS

100g low-fat cream cheese
4 tsp white granulated sweetener
¼ tsp vanilla extract
4 slices medium-thick white bread (about 36g each)
4 medium strawberries, stalks removed and thinly sliced
2 medium eggs
good pinch of ground cinnamon
low-calorie cooking spray

FOR THE TOP
¼ tsp icing sugar
4 tsp maple syrup

TO ACCOMPANY *(optional)*
50g extra strawberries per person (+ 21 kcal per serving)

French toast for breakfast always feels like such a treat, but our healthy twist means that this recipe is much lighter than you'd expect! We've filled these golden toasted sandwiches with sweetened cream cheese and a layer of fresh strawberries, and they're just as irresistible as they look. Drizzle with maple syrup, grab your cuppa and tuck in.

Everyday Light ───────────────

Place the cream cheese, sweetener and vanilla extract in a small bowl and mix with a spoon until completely blended.

Spread the cream cheese mixture over two slices of bread. Place the sliced strawberries in a single layer over the cream cheese mixture and pop one of the plain slices of bread on top of each, to make two sandwiches.

Crack the eggs onto a large plate and add the cinnamon. Beat with a fork until the eggs and cinnamon are completely mixed.

Dip the sandwiches in the egg on both sides, allowing all the egg to be soaked up into the bread.

While the sandwiches are soaking, spray a large frying pan with low-calorie cooking spray and place over a medium heat. When the frying pan is hot, carefully transfer the sandwiches to the frying pan using a fish slice. The sandwiches may be fragile after soaking, so lift them carefully.

Fry the sandwiches for 2–3 minutes on each side, using a fish slice to turn them once, until golden brown and a little crisp.

Remove from the frying pan using a fish slice and cut each sandwich in half diagonally, to make a total of four triangles.

Place on a plate, dust with a little icing sugar and drizzle with maple syrup. Serve while hot, either alone or with a few extra strawberries if you like.

TIP: Using a fish slice is the best way to lift the sandwiches in and out of the frying pan as it will support them well. Depending on the size of your frying pan you may need to cook one toasted sandwich at a time.

SWAP THIS: You could swap the strawberries for the same weight of raspberries.

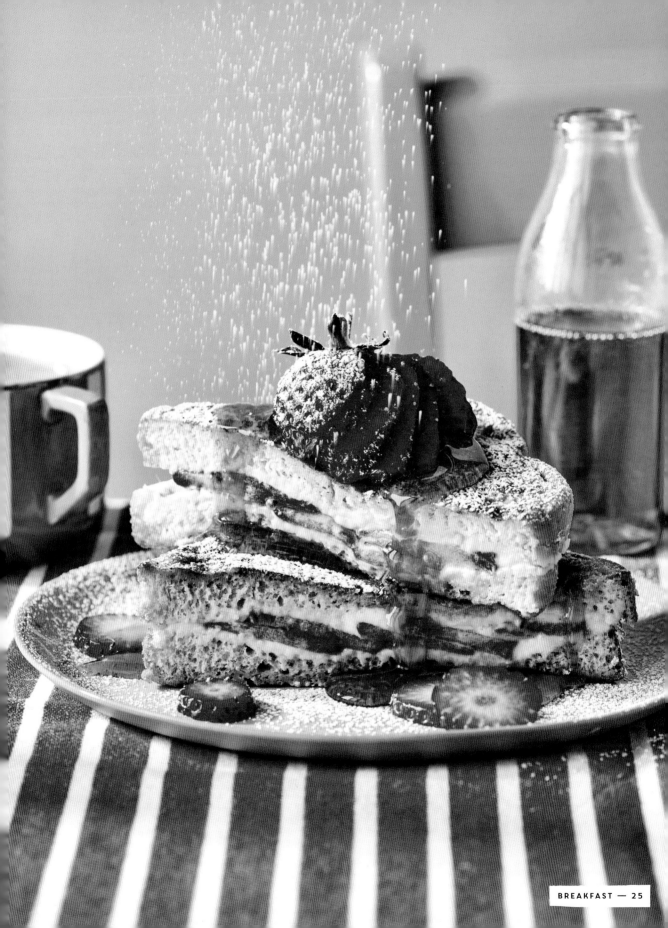

USE VEGETARIAN MOZZARELLA

HASSELBACK TOMATOES

🕐 **10 MINS**   🗑 **VARIABLE** (SEE BELOW)   ✕ **SERVES 2**

PER SERVING:
172 KCAL / 9.8G CARBS

low-calorie cooking spray
2 medium beef tomatoes, stalks removed
2 garlic cloves, peeled and crushed
sea salt and freshly ground black pepper
150g reduced-fat mozzarella, well drained and cut into 10 thin slices
10 fresh large basil leaves, stalks removed

TO ACCOMPANY *(optional)*
1 slice of wholemeal toast (+ 93 kcal per serving) or 75g mixed salad (+ 15 kcal per serving)

We've sliced these juicy tomatoes hasselback style, before stuffing them with melty mozzarella and fragrant basil, so you get all those Italian-inspired flavours in every bite. Serve as a starter before a tasty pasta dish, or add one on the side of grilled meat or fish. We especially love them with toast or a crunchy green salad for a light, refreshing brunch.

Everyday Light ——————————————————

OVEN METHOD
🗑 **20 MINS**

Preheat the oven to 180°C (fan 160°C/gas mark 4). Grease a small ovenproof dish with low-calorie cooking spray.

Place the tomatoes stalk side down on a chopping board. Make five deep cuts in each tomato, being careful not to cut right through, then place stalk side down in the greased ovenproof dish.

Gently ease the cuts open, rub the garlic inside each cut and season well with salt and black pepper. Push a slice of mozzarella and a basil leaf into each cut.

Spray with low-calorie cooking spray and place the dish in the oven for about 20 minutes until the tomatoes are tender and the mozzarella is melting.

AIR-FRYER METHOD
🗑 **15 MINS**

SPECIAL EQUIPMENT
Air fryer

Preheat the air fryer to 160°C. Grease a small ovenproof dish with low-calorie cooking spray. If your air fryer isn't big enough for an ovenproof dish, place a sheet of foil into the bottom of the basket and grease that instead.

Place the tomatoes stalk side down on a chopping board. Make five deep cuts in each tomato, being careful not to cut right through, then place stalk side down in the greased ovenproof dish or on the foil.

TIP: Placing the tomatoes stalk side down in the dish helps to keep them stable.

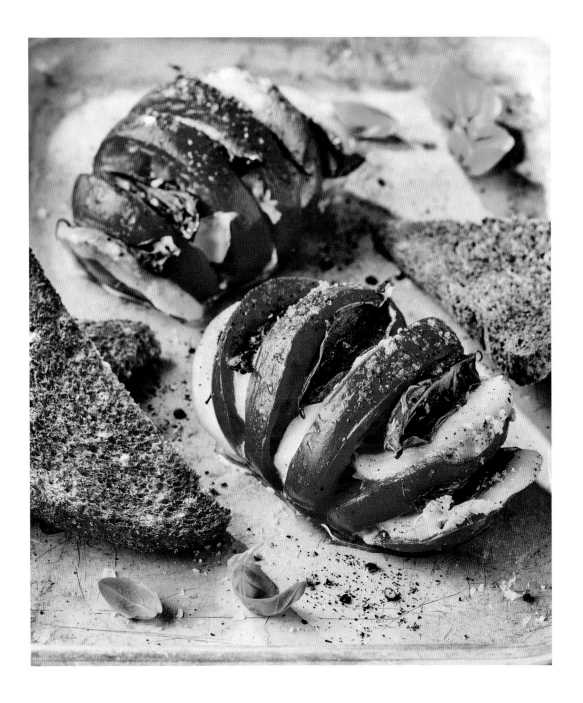

Gently ease the cuts open, rub the garlic inside each cut and season well with salt and black pepper. Push a slice of mozzarella and a basil leaf into each cut.

Spray with low-calorie cooking spray and place into the air fryer for 12–15 minutes until the tomatoes are tender and the mozzarella is melting.

CREAMY BACON *and* MUSHROOM PANCAKES

🕐 **10 MINS**   🪣 **20 MINS**   ✕ **SERVES 4**

*PLUS 10 MINS RESTING

PER SERVING:
282 KCAL /30G CARBS

FOR THE PANCAKES
125g plain flour
¼ tsp salt
1 medium egg, beaten
300ml skimmed milk
low-calorie cooking spray

FOR THE FILLING
low-calorie cooking spray
200g large flat mushrooms,
   sliced
4 smoked bacon medallions,
   cut into large dice
½ tsp garlic granules
180g low-fat cream cheese
80g baby spinach leaves
sea salt and freshly ground
   black pepper
10g Parmesan cheese, finely
   grated

Who said pancakes always have to be sweet? If you're looking for a new breakfast idea, these savoury pancakes will get your morning off to a flipping good start! Nice and quick to make, we've loaded them up with bacon and mushrooms cooked in a creamy, garlicky sauce. Whip up a batch for a tasty weekend brunch.

Everyday Light ─────────────────────────

To make the pancakes, sift the flour and salt into a medium mixing bowl and make a well in the centre. Whisk together the egg and milk in a small bowl. Pour the egg and milk mixture into the well, a little at a time, and beat with a balloon whisk until just smooth.

Cover and place in the fridge to rest for about 10 minutes.

Preheat the oven to 150°C (fan 130°C/gas mark 2).

Spray a large non-stick frying pan with low-calorie cooking spray and spread around the pan using a piece of kitchen paper. Place the frying pan over a medium heat. When the pan is hot, pour in a small ladleful of the batter. Tilt the pan to swirl the batter quickly to coat the bottom of the pan and make a thin pancake.

Cook for about 1 minute until golden on the underside. You can check by gently lifting one edge of the pancake with a palette knife to see if the pancake is golden.

Flip the pancake over gently using a palette knife, or if you're feeling brave you can toss it! Cook for about a minute on the second side until golden, then transfer to a plate and cover with a square of non-stick baking paper.

Grease the frying pan again and repeat cooking until you've made another three pancakes; stacking them up with non-stick baking paper between each one. Cover tightly with kitchen foil and place in the preheated oven to keep warm while you make the filling.

TIP: Rest the pancake batter in the fridge for at least 10 minutes before cooking, as this allows the flour to hydrate, resulting in better pancakes.

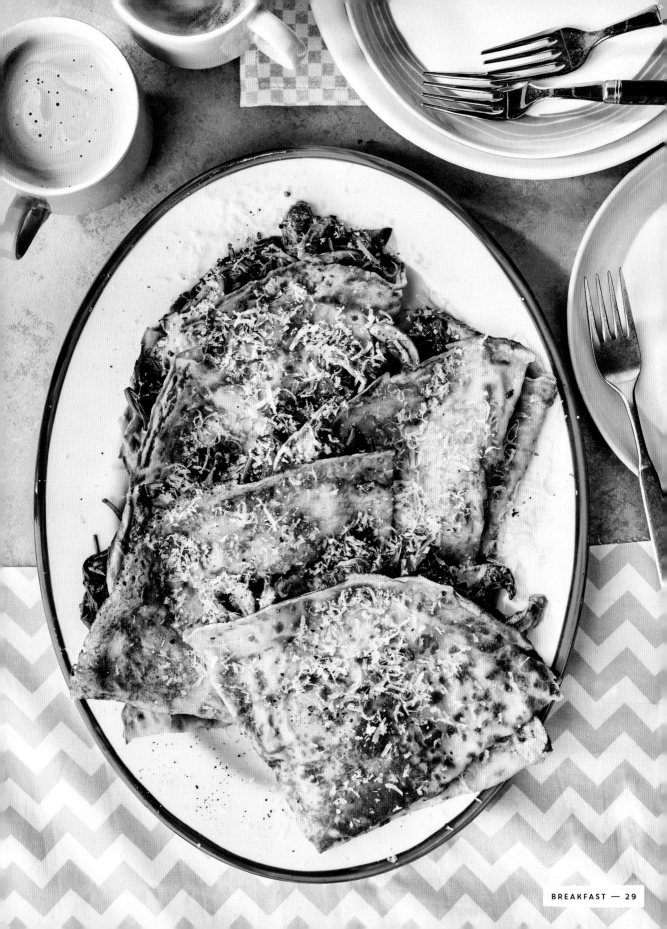

To make the filling, spray the same frying pan with low-calorie cooking spray and place over a medium heat. Add the mushrooms and fry for 3 minutes. Add the bacon and garlic granules and cook for 4–5 minutes until the bacon is cooked through.

Remove the frying pan from the heat and stir in the cream cheese until completely mixed with the mushrooms and bacon. The heat from the pan will melt the cream cheese.

Lower the heat and return the frying pan to the stove. Add the spinach and stir in until just wilted; this should take about 2–3 minutes. Season to taste with salt and black pepper.

Remove the pancakes from the oven. Place a quarter of the hot filling on one half of the first pancake. Fold the pancake over the filling and then fold again – you should now have a triangle-shaped, folded pancake.

Repeat until you have four stuffed pancakes. Place on plates and sprinkle with a little Parmesan cheese. Serve at once.

"

Thank you Kay and Kate for giving me the confidence to cook healthy and delicious meals.

—— TRACEY

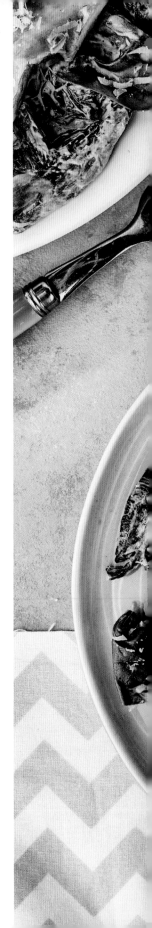

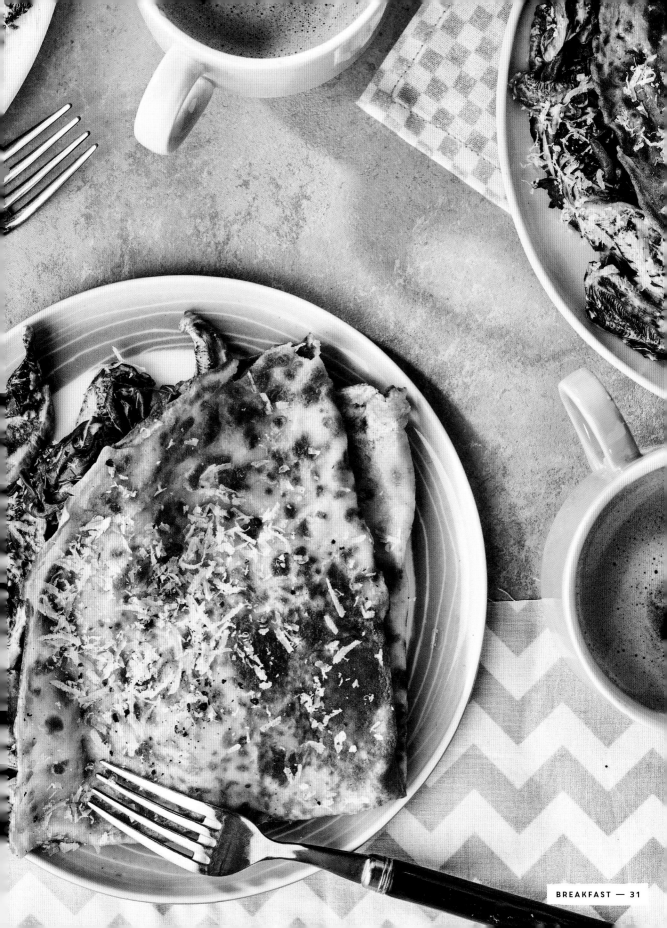

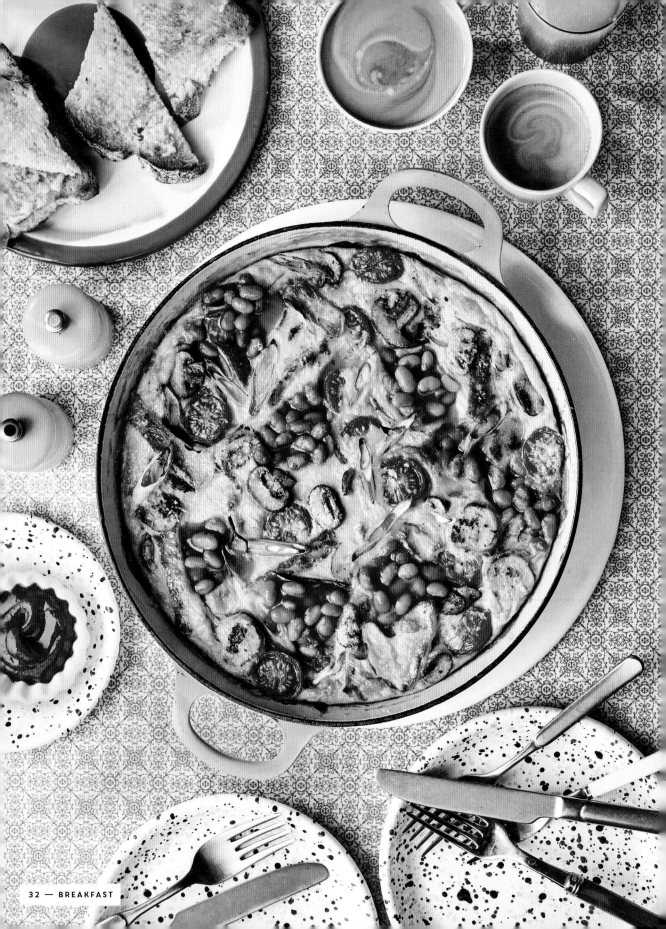

FRY-UP FRITTATA

🕐 **10 MINS**　🗑 **35 MINS**　✗ **SERVES 4**

GLUTEN FREE

USE GF SAUSAGES

LOW CARB

PER SERVING:
323 KCAL / 9.2G CARBS

low-calorie cooking spray
2 reduced-fat sausages, sliced
3 smoked bacon medallions, sliced
5 mushrooms, sliced
10 cherry tomatoes, sliced in half
10 medium eggs
10g Parmesan cheese, finely grated
100g tinned baked beans
2 spring onions, trimmed and sliced
sea salt and freshly ground black pepper

TO ACCOMPANY *(optional)*
1 slice of white toast (42g) (+ 104 kcal per serving)

> **MAKE IT VEGGIE:**
> For a vegetarian frittata, swap the meat for your favourite meat-free sausage and bacon alternative.

Fancy all the best bits of a fry up crammed into a frittata that you can pack up for later? Load it up with bacon, sausage, beans and mushrooms, before baking in the oven until it's perfect. Make this super-filling brekkie ahead of time and keep it in the fridge, or slice it up and pack it into a picnic for later in the day.

Weekly Indulgence ————————————————

Preheat the oven to 180°C (fan 160°C/gas mark 4).

Spray an ovenproof frying pan with low-calorie cooking spray and place over a medium heat. Add the sliced sausage and bacon and cook for 4 minutes until browned. Place on a plate and put to one side.

Add the mushrooms and tomatoes to the pan and cook for 2 minutes until coloured and soft. Place on a plate and put to one side.

Put the eggs, 100ml of water and grated Parmesan into a mixing jug and whisk until combined. Season with salt and pepper.

Spray the pan with a little more low-calorie cooking spray and pour in three-quarters of the beaten egg. Cook for 4 minutes, stirring the egg gently and creating ripples in the egg mixture as it begins to set.

Once the egg has begun to set, scatter the sausages, bacon, tomatoes and mushrooms on top of the egg.

Sprinkle over the sliced spring onions and add spoonfuls of beans. Pour over the remaining egg mix and cook for 5 minutes.

Once the frittata has set underneath, pop the pan into the oven for 20 minutes until the top is golden brown and the egg is cooked through.

Slice into quarters and serve.

VEGGIE

DAIRY
FREE

USE DF MILK
ALTERNATIVE
AND CHEESE

GLUTEN
FREE

USE GF
BREAD AND
HENDERSON'S
RELISH

VIKING TOAST

 5 MINS   **10 MINS**   ✕ **SERVES 1**

PER SERVING:
294 KCAL / 17G CARBS

SPECIAL EQUIPMENT
Grill pan and rack

low-calorie cooking spray
½ small onion, peeled and
  thinly sliced
40g reduced-fat mature
  Cheddar cheese, grated
½ tsp Henderson's relish or
  Worcestershire sauce
small pinch of mustard
  powder
1 medium egg yolk
1 tsp skimmed milk
sea salt and freshly ground
  black pepper
1 medium slice of wholemeal
  bread, about 37g

Looking for a speedy brunch with bold flavours? This Viking Toast is the one! Inspired by the melty cheese and onion from our Viking Pork recipe, we thought we'd try out the same golden, tangy topping on toast (and it works a treat!). Forget about plain old cheese on toast, mornings don't come much tastier than this.

Everyday Light ───────────────────

Spray a small frying pan with low-calorie cooking spray and place over a medium heat. Add the onion and fry for 2–3 minutes, until softened and beginning to brown.

Place the cooked onion in a small bowl and add the cheese, Henderson's relish or Worcestershire sauce, mustard powder, egg yolk and milk and season well with salt and black pepper. Mix well.

Preheat the grill to a medium heat. Place the bread on the grill-pan rack and place under the grill until just beginning to colour. Remove from under the grill.

Turn the toast over and evenly spread the cheese and onion mixture over the untoasted side. Place back under the grill for about 3–4 minutes or until the cheese has melted and is golden brown. Serve at once.

TIP: To have your lunch with a little more heat, add a small pinch of mild chilli powder, chilli flakes or a few drops of hot pepper sauce to the cheese and onion mixture.

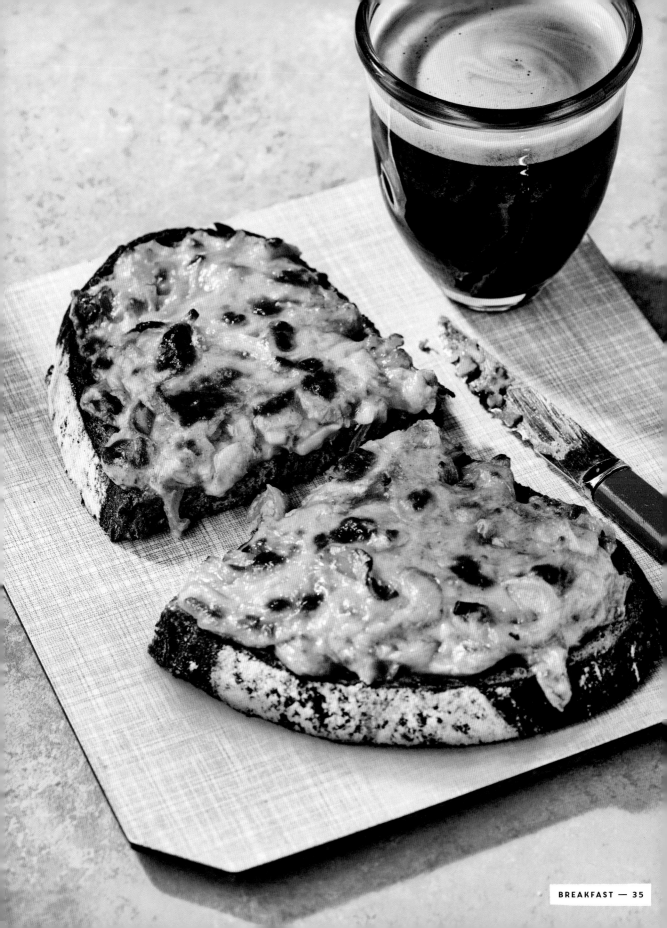

PUMPKIN SPICE SCONES

🕐 **10 MINS**   🗑 **18 MINS**   ✕ **MAKES 6 SCONES**

PER SCONE:
244 KCAL / 35G CARBS

SPECIAL EQUIPMENT
7cm (3in) round cutter

200g pumpkin, peeled and
chopped into chunks
220g self-raising flour, plus
extra for dusting
¼ tsp ground nutmeg
¼ tsp ground cinnamon
¼ tsp ground ginger
pinch of mixed spice
½ tsp baking powder
50g reduced-fat spread
2 tbsp white granulated
sweetener
50–80ml skimmed milk
150g low-fat cream cheese
1 tsp honey

If you're someone who can't wait for pumpkin spice flavours to come into season, you need to try these fluffy scones! Filled with classic autumnal flavours, they're perfect with a cuppa at any time of year. Don't forget the spread! They're best enjoyed slightly warm with our yummy homemade cream cheese and honey mix.

Everyday Light

Preheat the oven to 200°C (fan 180°C/gas mark 6) and line a baking tray with non-stick baking paper.

Add the pumpkin to a saucepan, and cover with water and bring to the boil. Lower the heat and cook for 8 minutes until the pumpkin is soft. Drain and mash well. Leave to cool completely.

Add the flour, nutmeg, cinnamon, ginger, mixed spice and baking powder to a mixing bowl and stir. Add the reduced-fat spread and rub into the flour with your fingers until the mix looks like breadcrumbs. Add the sweetener and stir again.

Add the pumpkin mash and 50ml of milk to the bowl and stir quickly. If the mixture looks too dry add an extra splash of milk until it comes loosely together.

Tip the dough out onto a floured surface and bring it together so that it starts to smooth out (try not to handle too much as it will make your scones tough once baked). Pat or lightly roll out the dough until it's about 2cm (½in) thick.

Using the round cutter, cut your scones into shape. Press the leftover dough together and re-cut until you have six scones.

Place the scones onto the lined baking tray and brush the tops with the remaining milk. Bake for 10 minutes until risen and golden on top. Leave to cool on a wire rack.

Add the cream cheese to a small bowl and stir the honey through. When the scones have cooled to just warm, slice and spread with the cream cheese mixture to serve.

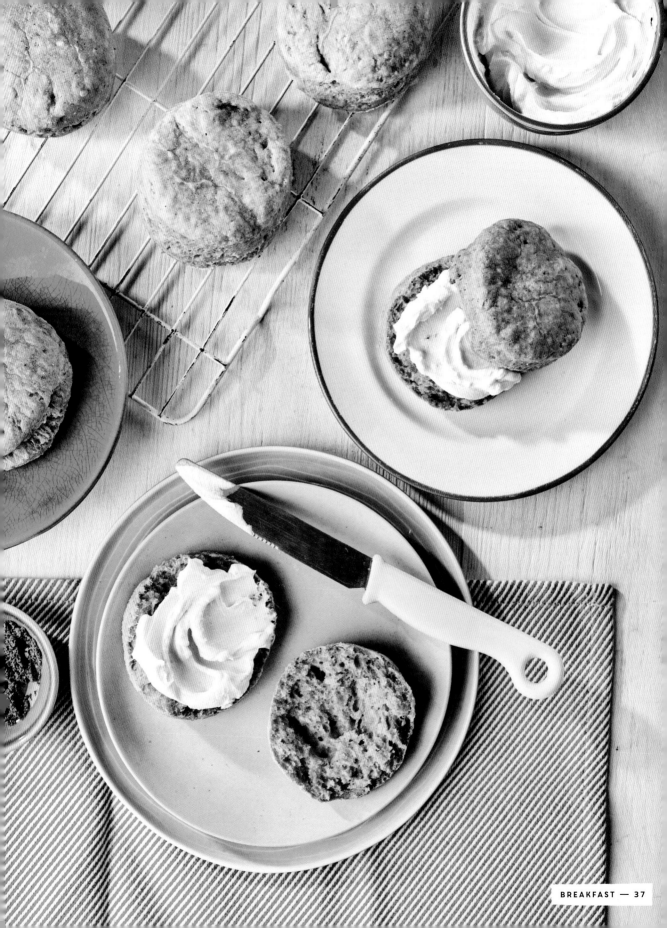

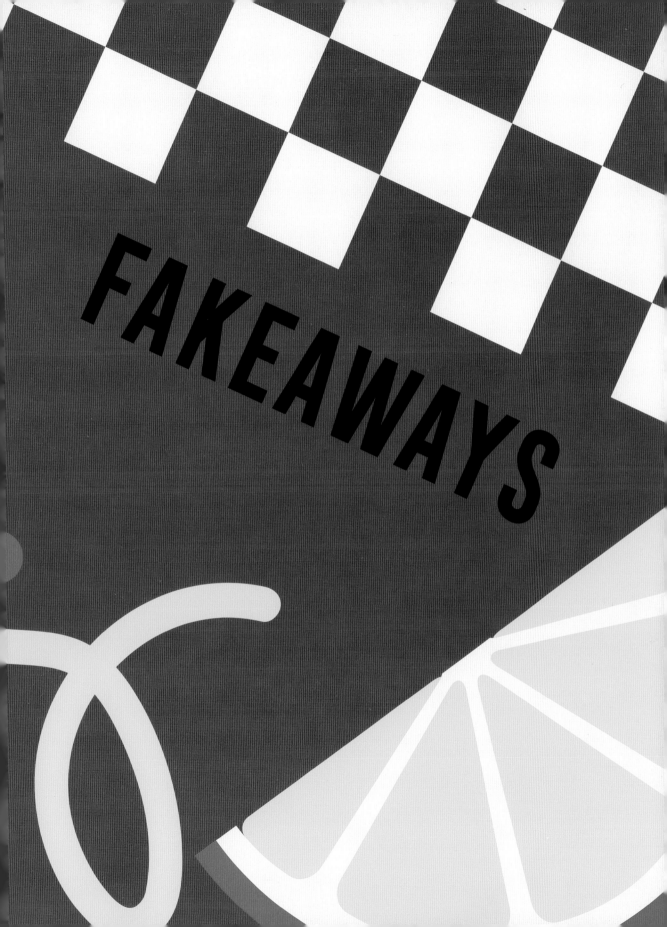

FAKEAWAYS

FREEZE
ME

DAIRY
FREE

GLUTEN
FREE

USE GF
SPAGHETTI
AND GF STOCK
POT

CHICKEN PICCATA

 15 MINS   **VARIABLE** (SEE BELOW)   ✗ **SERVES 4**

PER SERVING:
265 KCAL / 31G CARBS

4 skinless chicken breasts,
  about 150g each
4 tbsp cornflour
sea salt and freshly ground
  black pepper
low-calorie cooking spray

FOR THE SAUCE
2 onions, peeled and thinly
  sliced
2 garlic cloves, peeled and
  crushed
1 chicken stock pot, made up
  with 450ml boiling water
1 white wine stock pot
juice of 1 lemon
1 lemon, skin left on, thinly
  sliced, any large pips
  removed
sea salt and freshly ground
  black pepper
2 tsp cornflour
2 tbsp capers in brine,
  drained
handful of flat-leafed
  parsley, stalks removed and
  roughly chopped (optional)

TO ACCOMPANY
50g spaghetti or linguine
  (+ 177 kcal per serving)

SWAP THIS: You can use
white wine instead of a white
wine stock pot. Replace the
white wine stock pot with
100ml of medium or dry
white wine and use 350ml
of boiling water instead of
450ml to make up the chicken
stock pot. If you do this, you'll
need to adjust the calories
accordingly.

Inspired by a classic Italian dish, this lemony chicken was
an instant favourite in our house. The traditional recipe
usually has a rich butter sauce, but we've pulled out a few
slimming-friendly swaps to make our version nice and
light. If you love citrusy sauces, this one's for you – the
lemons become so soft you can eat them, and add so
much flavour!

Weekly Indulgence ───────────────────────────

HOB-TOP METHOD
🗑 **55 MINS**

Cut each chicken breast vertically into four thin slices along
its length.

Place the 4 tablespoons of cornflour on a plate and season
with salt and black pepper. Dip the chicken pieces in the
cornflour mixture to lightly coat each piece all over.

Spray a large frying pan (for which you have a lid) with
low-calorie cooking spray and place over a medium heat.
When the pan is hot, add the chicken pieces and fry for
15–20 minutes until slightly crispy and lightly golden in
places. Turn the chicken occasionally to cook evenly. Place
onto a sheet of kitchen paper and set aside.

To make the sauce: spray the frying pan with a little more
low-calorie cooking spray. Place over a medium heat
and add the onion. Cook slowly for 10–15 minutes, stirring
occasionally, until golden brown and softened. Add the
garlic and fry for a further 2–3 minutes, stirring occasionally.

Lower the heat and add the chicken stock, white wine
stock pot, lemon juice and lemon slices and season well
with salt and black pepper to taste. Stir until the white
wine stock pot dissolves.

In a small bowl, blend the 2 teaspoons of cornflour with
2 teaspoons of cold water until the mixture is smooth. Add
to the sauce in the frying pan and stir in. Lower the heat
and simmer, uncovered, for 4–5 minutes, until the sauce
thickens slightly.

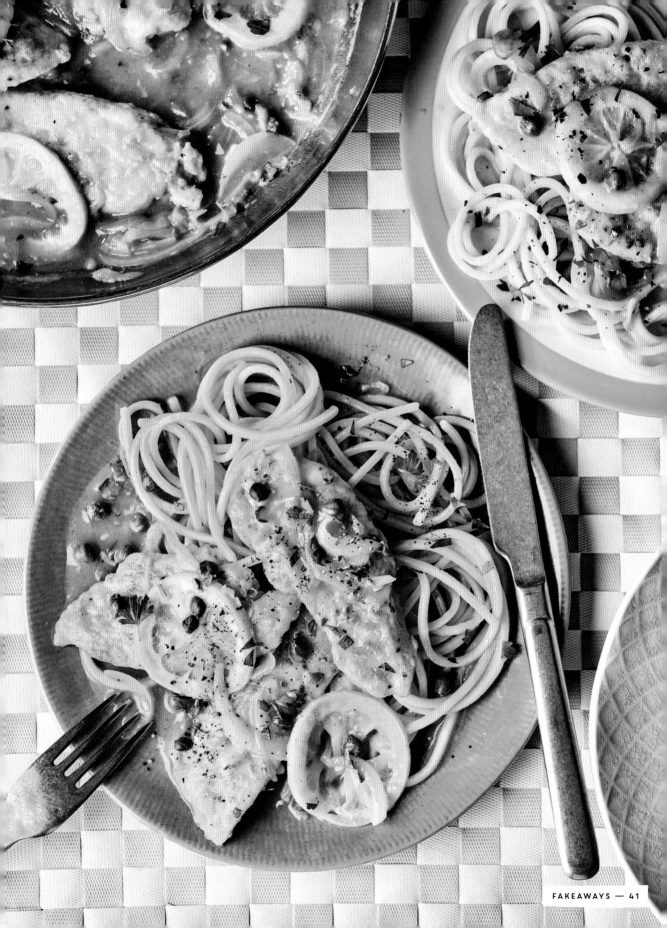

Add the reserved cooked chicken and the capers to the frying pan and stir. Cover with a tight-fitting lid and simmer over a low heat for about 10 minutes or until the chicken is piping hot right through, the lemon slices are soft, and the sauce is thickened and glossy.

Sprinkle with roughly chopped flat-leafed parsley to garnish if you like, and serve with pasta or an accompaniment of choice.

AIR-FRYER METHOD
🔲 20 MINS

SPECIAL EQUIPMENT
Air fryer

Cut each chicken breast vertically into four thin slices along its length.

Place the 4 tablespoons of cornflour on a plate and season with salt and black pepper. Dip the chicken pieces in the cornflour mixture to lightly coat each piece all over.

Preheat the air fryer to 170°C. Spray a little low-calorie cooking spray over the air fryer basket, then add the coated chicken slices in an even, single layer.

Depending on the size of your air fryer you may have to cook the coated chicken in batches.

Spray a little more low-calorie cooking spray over the top of the coated chicken and air-fry for 15–20 minutes, turning halfway through. The coated chicken should be slightly crispy and lightly golden in places, the juices should run clear and there should be no sign of pinkness.

To make the sauce: spray the frying pan with a little more low-calorie cooking spray. Place over a medium heat and add the onion. Cook slowly for 10–15 minutes, stirring occasionally, until golden brown and softened. Add the garlic and fry for a

further 2–3 minutes, stirring occasionally. Lower the heat and add the chicken stock, white wine stock pot, lemon juice and lemon slices and season well with salt and black pepper to taste. Stir until the white wine stock pot dissolves.

In a small bowl, blend the 2 teaspoons of cornflour with 2 teaspoons of cold water until the mixture is smooth. Add to the sauce in the frying pan and stir in. Lower the heat and simmer, uncovered, for 4–5 minutes, until the sauce thickens slightly.

Add the reserved cooked chicken and the capers to the frying pan and stir. Cover with a tight-fitting lid and simmer over a low heat for about 10 minutes or until the chicken is piping hot right through, the lemon slices are soft, and the sauce is thickened and glossy.

Sprinkle with roughly chopped flat-leafed parsley to garnish if you like, and serve with pasta or an accompaniment of choice.

OVEN METHOD
🔲 30 MINS

Preheat the oven to 190°C (fan 170°C/gas mark 5) and line a large baking tray with a sheet of non-stick baking paper.

Cut each chicken breast vertically into four thin slices along its length.

Place the 4 tablespoons of cornflour on a plate and season with salt and black pepper. Dip the chicken pieces in the cornflour mixture to lightly coat each piece all over.

Place the coated chicken on the lined baking tray in a single layer.

Spray the top of the coated chicken slices with low-calorie cooking spray and place in the preheated oven for 20–25 minutes. Turn over halfway through and spray with a little more low-calorie cooking spray.

The coated chicken should be slightly crispy and lightly golden in places, the juices should run clear and there should be no sign of pinkness.

To make the sauce: spray the frying pan with a little more low-calorie cooking spray. Place over a medium heat and add the onion. Cook slowly for 10–15 minutes, stirring occasionally, until golden brown and softened. Add the garlic and fry for a further 2–3 minutes, stirring occasionally.

Lower the heat and add the chicken stock, white wine stock pot, lemon juice and lemon slices and season well with salt and black pepper to taste. Stir until the white wine stock pot dissolves.

In a small bowl, blend the 2 teaspoons of cornflour with 2 teaspoons of cold water until the mixture is smooth. Add to the sauce in the frying pan and stir in. Lower the heat and simmer, uncovered, for 4–5 minutes, until the sauce thickens slightly.

Add the reserved cooked chicken and the capers to the frying pan and stir. Cover with a tight-fitting lid and simmer over a low heat for about 10 minutes or until the chicken is piping hot right through, the lemon slices are soft, and the sauce is thickened and glossy.

Sprinkle with roughly chopped flat-leafed parsley to garnish if you like, and serve with pasta or an accompaniment of choice.

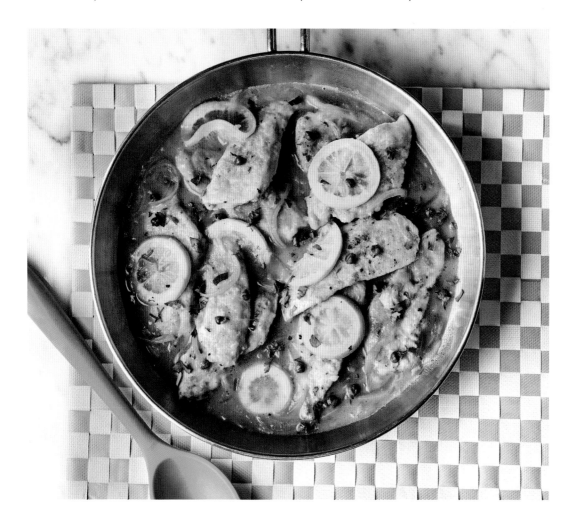

VEGAN

FREEZE ME

DAIRY FREE

GLUTEN FREE

CHANA MASALA

🕐 **5 MINS**   🗑 **VARIABLE** (SEE BELOW)   ✕ **SERVES 4**

PER SERVING:
225 KCAL / 29G CARBS

low-calorie cooking spray
2 tsp garam masala
1 tsp paprika
1 tsp ground turmeric
1 tsp ground coriander
4 garlic cloves, peeled and minced
1 large onion, peeled and finely diced
1 x 400g tin chopped tomatoes
1 tbsp lemon juice
2 x 400g tins chickpeas, drained and rinsed
1 tbsp tomato puree
sea salt and freshly ground black pepper
pinch of white granulated sweetener, to taste
1 large handful of fresh coriander leaves (about 12g), stalks removed and roughly chopped

TO ACCOMPANY (optional)
4 wholemeal pitta breads (+ 184 kcal per serving)

TIP: This dish is mild but if you want some heat, you can add some dried chilli powder, to taste, with the other spices in the first step.

All the clues you need are in the name for this one: chickpeas (chana) in sauce (masala). All the warm-coloured spices make these saucy chickpeas a bright addition to any plate! You can even pop it in the slow cooker for extra convenience.

Weekly Indulgence

HOB-TOP METHOD
🗑 **20 MINS**

Spray a large frying pan with low-calorie cooking spray and place over a medium heat. Add the dried spices, garlic and onion and cook for 5 minutes, until the spices are gently toasted and the onions have begun to soften.

Add the tomatoes, lemon juice, chickpeas and stir well. Simmer for 10 minutes until the sauce has started to thicken.

Stir in the tomato puree and simmer for another 5 minutes until you have a thick, rich sauce. Season with salt, black pepper and sweetener, to taste. Stir through the fresh coriander before serving, with pitta bread if you like.

SLOW-COOKER METHOD
🗑 **6 HOURS**

SPECIAL EQUIPMENT
Slow cooker

Spray a large frying pan with low-calorie cooking spray and place over a medium heat. Add the dried spices, garlic and onion and cook for 5 minutes, until the spices are gently toasted and the onions have begun to soften.

Transfer to the slow cooker. Add the tomatoes, lemon juice and chickpeas and stir well. Cover and cook on low for 5 hours 30 minutes.

Stir in the tomato puree and cook for another 20–30 minutes without the lid, so the sauce starts to thicken. Season with salt, black pepper and sweetener, to taste. Stir through the fresh coriander before serving, with pitta bread if you like.

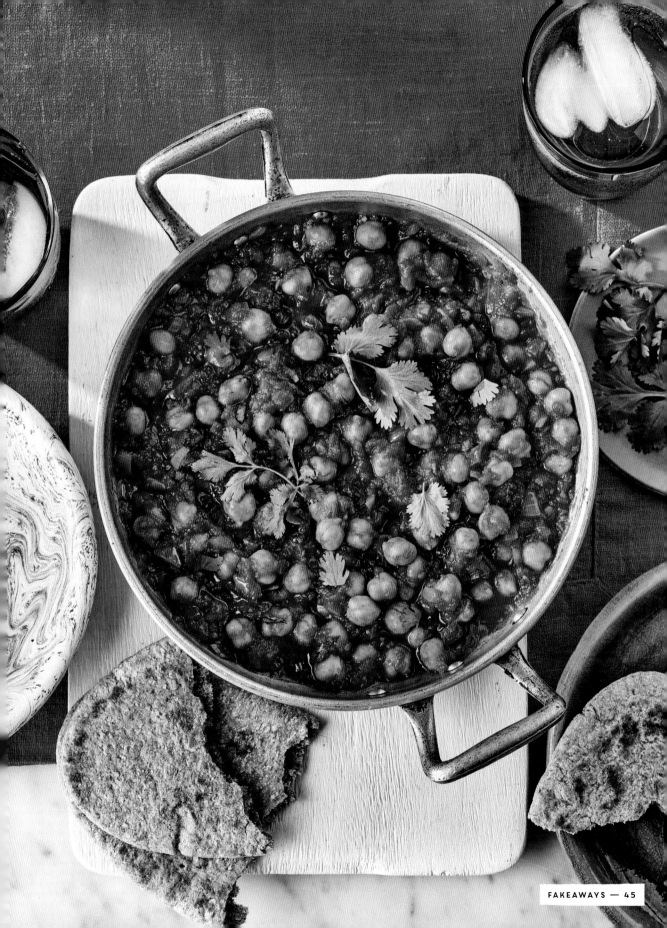

DAIRY FREE

USE DF CHEESE AND YOGHURT

GLUTEN FREE

USE GF TORTILLA WRAPS

CHIPOTLE CHICKEN TAQUITOS

🕐 **15 MINS**   🗑 **VARIABLE** (SEE BELOW)   ✕ **SERVES 4**

PER SERVING:
464 KCAL / 52G CARBS

SPECIAL EQUIPMENT
Stick blender or mini chopper
8 cocktail sticks

FOR THE TAQUITOS
low-calorie cooking spray
1 red onion, peeled and diced
2 garlic cloves, peeled and
   crushed
½ medium red pepper,
   deseeded and diced
1 tbsp tomato puree
1½ tbsp chipotle paste
250g cooked chicken,
   shredded
200g tinned chopped tomatoes
1 tbsp low-fat cream cheese
sea salt and freshly ground
   black pepper
8 soft mini tortilla wraps,
   about 33g each
60g reduced-fat Cheddar
   cheese, finely grated

FOR THE SALSA
2 salad tomatoes, deseeded
   and finely diced
2 spring onions, finely sliced
10g fresh coriander leaves, stalks
   removed and finely chopped
juice of ½ lime
¼ tsp sriracha sauce
sea salt and freshly ground
   black pepper

**FOR THE CREAMY
AVOCADO SAUCE**
½ medium avocado, stoned
   and peeled
3 tbsp fat-free natural yoghurt
4g fresh coriander leaves,
   stalks removed

These Taquitos are inspired by the popular Mexican dish. Traditionally, taquitos are tacos that have been filled with meat and deep-fried until they're golden and delicious. We've saved a few calories by baking our smoky chicken-filled tortilla wraps in the oven or the air fryer. With creamy avocado sauce and vibrant salsa, they are the perfect bite.

Weekly Indulgence ——————————————

OVEN METHOD
🍳 **25 MINS**

Preheat the oven to 200°C (fan 180°C/gas mark 6) and line a roasting tray with a sheet of non-stick baking paper.

Spray a large frying pan with low-calorie cooking spray and place over a medium heat. Add the red onion and fry for 3 minutes, until softening and coloured.

Add the garlic and red pepper and cook for a further 2 minutes. Add the tomato puree and chipotle paste and stir to combine with the onion and pepper.

Add the cooked, shredded chicken to the frying pan and stir to coat.

Pour in the chopped tomatoes, lower the heat and simmer for 4–5 minutes, until the chicken is heated through. Remove from the heat and stir in the cream cheese until fully incorporated. Season to taste with salt and black pepper.

Place the tortilla wraps on a microwave-safe plate and heat in the microwave for 60 seconds on high, so they soften and become easier to work with. Add some of the chicken mixture, in a sausage shape, along one edge of the tortilla wrap and sprinkle over most of the cheese.

Roll the wrap up tightly to create a sausage-shaped taco, encasing the filling. Use a cocktail stick to secure the seam and repeat to make eight taquitos.

Spray the lined baking tray with low-calorie cooking spray and place the taquitos seam side down. Spray the tops with low-calorie cooking spray.

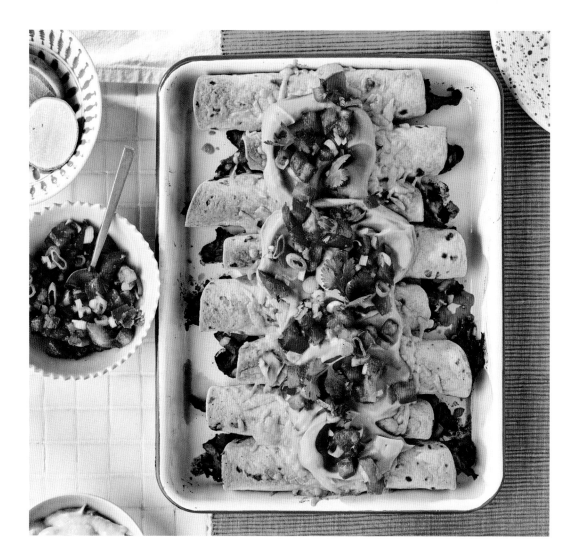

¼ tsp garlic powder
juice of ½ lime
sea salt and freshly
  ground black pepper

TO ACCOMPANY *(optional)*
75g mixed salad (+ 15
  kcal per serving)

> **TIP:** If you don't have any cooked chicken, you can poach a chicken breast to use in this recipe. Add the chicken breast to a saucepan and cover with boiling water. Cook over a medium heat for 20 minutes.

Pop in the oven for 15 minutes, until lightly golden and crispy. While the taquitos are cooking, add all the salsa ingredients to a small bowl, stir until combined and pop in the fridge until ready to serve.

For the creamy avocado sauce, place all the ingredients into a mini chopper – or use a stick blender and blitz until smooth. If it's a little thick, add a splash of water until it's the right consistency for drizzling.

Remove the taquitos from the oven, pull out the cocktail sticks and discard. Serve the taquitos with a drizzle of the creamy avocado sauce, a little of the salsa, the remaining grated cheese and a mixed salad if you like.

AIR-FRYER METHOD
🍚 20 MINS

SPECIAL EQUIPMENT
Air fryer

Spray a large frying pan with low-calorie cooking spray and place over a medium heat.

Add the red onion and fry for 3 minutes, until softening and coloured.

Add the garlic and red pepper and cook for a further 2 minutes. Add the tomato puree and chipotle paste and stir to combine with the onion and pepper. Add the cooked, shredded chicken to the frying pan and stir to coat.

Pour in the chopped tomatoes, lower the heat and simmer for 4–5 minutes, until the chicken is heated through. Remove from the heat and stir in the cream cheese, until fully incorporated. Season to taste with salt and black pepper.

Place the tortilla wraps on a microwave-safe plate and heat in the microwave for 60 seconds on high, so they soften and become easier to work with. Add some of the chicken mixture, in a sausage shape, along one edge of a tortilla wrap and sprinkle over most of the cheese.

Preheat the air fryer to 180°C. Roll the wrap up tightly to create a sausage-shaped taco, encasing the filling. Use a cocktail stick to secure the seam and repeat to make eight taquitos.

Line the base of the air fryer basket with a sheet of non-stick baking paper. Place the taquitos seam-side down into the lined air fryer basket. Spray the tops with low-calorie cooking spray.

Cook for 8–10 minutes until lightly golden and crispy. Depending on the size of your air fryer, you may need to do this in batches.

While the taquitos are cooking, add all the salsa ingredients to a small bowl. Stir until combined and pop in the fridge until ready to serve.

For the creamy avocado sauce, place all the ingredients into a mini chopper – or use a stick blender and blitz until smooth. If it's a little thick, add a splash of water until it's the right consistency for drizzling.

Remove the taquitos from the air fryer, pull out the cocktail sticks and discard. Serve the taquitos with a drizzle of the creamy avocado sauce, the remaining cheese, a little of the salsa and a mixed salad if you like.

SWAP THIS: Swap the chicken for shredded cooked turkey breast.

TIPS: If your air fryer doesn't have a preheat function, we suggest heating at cooking temperature for a few minutes before cooking your food.

TIKKA MASALA SALMON

🕐 **10 MINS***   🗑 **VARIABLE** (SEE BELOW)   ✕ **SERVES 6**

*PLUS 10 MINS MARINATING

FREEZE ME

GLUTEN FREE
USE GF STOCK CUBE

LOW CARB

PER SERVING:
254 KCAL / 10G CARBS

FOR THE SALMON MARINADE
50g fat-free Greek yoghurt
½ tsp each turmeric, garam masala, ground coriander and paprika
sea salt and black pepper
4 salmon fillets, skin removed (about 120g each)

FOR THE TIKKA MASALA
low-calorie cooking spray
1 onion, peeled and diced
1 yellow pepper, deseeded and diced
100g courgette, diced
2 garlic cloves, peeled and crushed
5cm (2in) piece of ginger, peeled and finely grated
1 tsp each chilli pepper, ground coriander, ground cumin and garam masala
1 x 400g tin chopped tomatoes
100g passata
1 tbsp tomato puree
50ml vegetable stock (1 stock cube dissolved in 50ml boiling water)
handful of fresh coriander leaves and lemon wedges, to serve (optional)

TO ACCOMPANY *(optional)*
4 wholemeal folded flatbread (+ 114 kcal per 35g serving) or 50g uncooked basmati rice per portion, cooked according to packet instructions (+ 173 kcal per 125g cooked serving)

Fish and curry might sound like an unusual combo, but trust us – it really works! We've swapped out chicken for protein-packed salmon chunks, and we love how well the salmon fillets soak up the tikka flavouring. We've used peppers and courgettes, but this curry will repurpose any leftover veggies. Try bulking yours out with aubergine, green beans or cauliflower.

Everyday Light ————————————————————————

HOB-TOP METHOD
🗑 **25 MINS**

In a bowl, add the yoghurt and spices and stir until combined. Taste and season with salt and pepper, if required. Chop each salmon fillet into chunks and add to the marinade and toss to coat. Cover and leave to marinate for 10 minutes.

Spray a frying pan with low-calorie cooking spray and place over a medium heat. Add the salmon pieces to the pan and cook for 5 minutes, turning until all sides are lightly browned and slightly crispy. Remove the salmon and put on a plate to one side.

Spray the pan with a little more low-calorie cooking spray, add the onion and pepper and cook for 4 minutes over a medium heat. Add the courgette, garlic and ginger and cook for a further 2 minutes.

When the vegetables are soft, add in the spices and stir until the vegetables are coated. Pour in the chopped tomatoes, passata, tomato puree and vegetable stock and give the pan a good stir.

Bring the pan to the boil then lower the heat and simmer for 5 minutes until the vegetables are soft. Add the salmon pieces back to the pan and stir lightly, trying not to break up the salmon. Heat for 5 minutes until the salmon is hot throughout, then sprinkle with the coriander leaves.

Serve with lemon wedges, if liked, and flatbread or your choice of accompaniment.

ELECTRIC PRESSURE COOKER METHOD
🍲 25 MINS

SPECIAL EQUIPMENT
Electric pressure cooker

In a bowl, add the yoghurt and spices and stir until combined. Taste and season with salt and pepper, if required. Chop each salmon fillet into chunks and add to the marinade and toss to coat. Cover and leave to marinate for 10 minutes.

Spray the pressure cooker with low-calorie cooking spray and set to sauté. Add the salmon pieces to the pressure cooker and cook for 5 minutes, turning until all sides are lightly browned and slightly crispy.

Remove the salmon from the pressure cooker to a plate and put to one side. Spray the pressure cooker with a little low-calorie cooking spray and use a wooden spoon to scrape any crispy bits from the bottom of the pot.

Add the onion and pepper and cook for 4 minutes. Add the courgette, garlic and ginger, and cook for a further 2 minutes. When the vegetables are soft, add in the spices and stir until the vegetables are coated. Pour in the chopped tomatoes, passata, tomato puree and vegetable stock and give the pan a good stir.

Press cancel on the pressure cooker and secure the lid. Set the pressure release to 'sealing', then select the manual setting programme and set a timer for 4 minutes.

Once the programme has finished, and the pressure cooker has beeped, use the quick-release function by moving the pressure release to 'venting'. Once the pressure has released, press cancel and remove the lid.

Stir the mixture and set the pressure cooker to 'sauté'. Add the salmon to the tikka masala sauce and allow the pot to bubble for 4 minutes until the salmon is heated through. Try not to stir the pot too much as it will break up the salmon chunks.

Press cancel on the pressure cooker and serve the curry with fresh coriander and lemon wedges, if liked, and flatbread or your choice of accompaniment.

> **TIPS:** It's important to deglaze the pressure cooker with low-calorie cooking spray in the second step as this will remove any crispy bits from the bottom of the pot; this will avoid the burn message later on in cooking. Stir the pan only lightly when you add the salmon back to the sauce – you want the salmon to hold its chunky shape without breaking up too much!

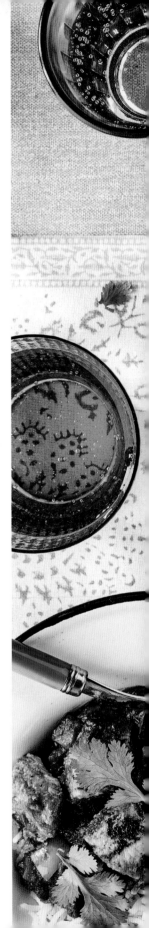

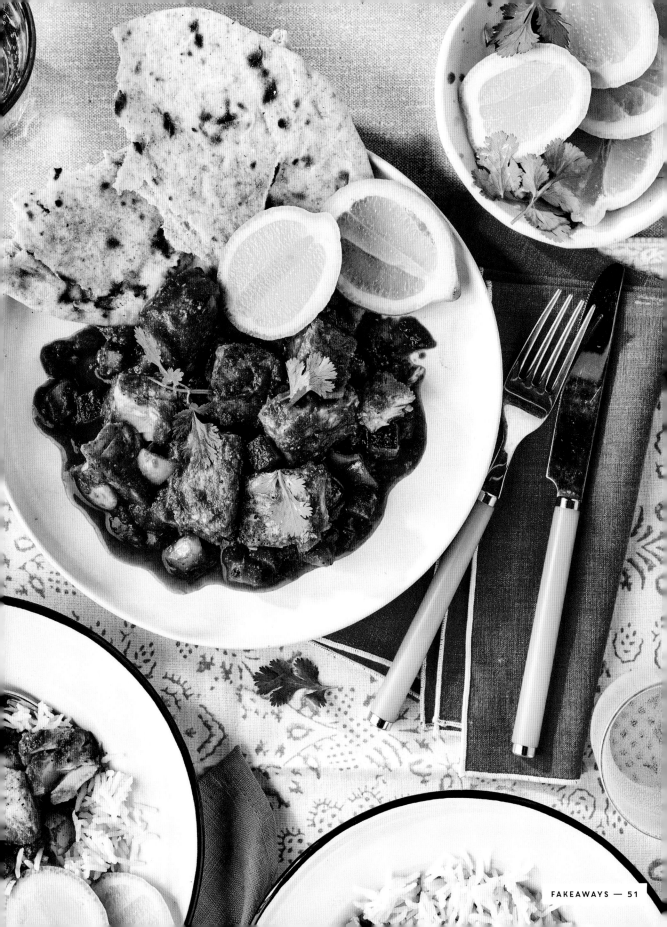

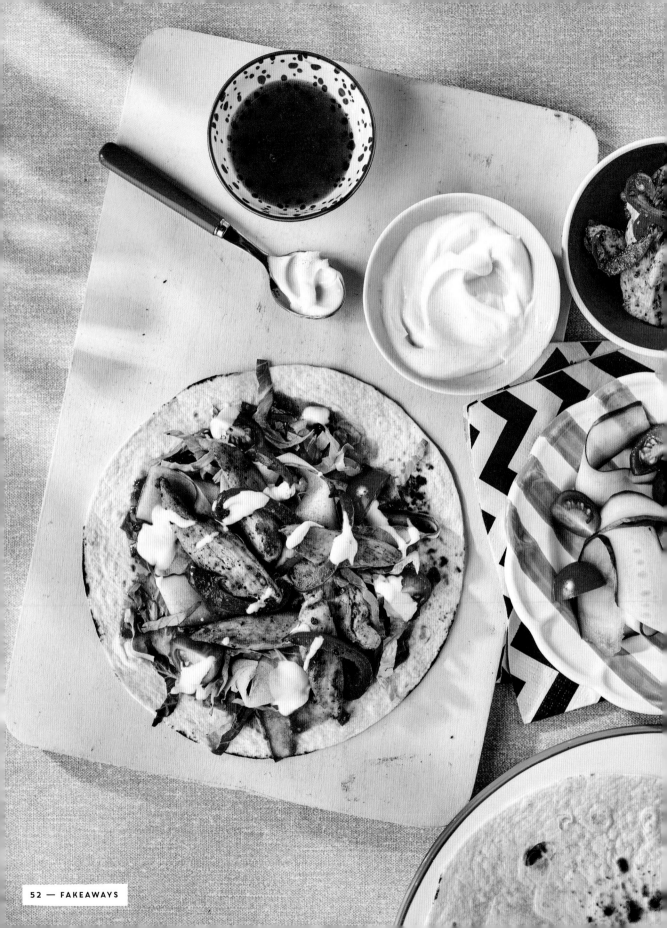

PERI-PERI CHICKEN WRAP

🕐 **10 MINS**   🍳 **10 MINS**   ✕ **SERVES 2**

PER SERVING:
284 KCAL / 42G CARBS

FOR THE WRAP
low-calorie cooking spray
1 medium chicken breast,
  sliced
2 tsp peri-peri seasoning
20g red pepper, deseeded
  and finely sliced
2 low-calorie soft tortilla
  wraps
50g lettuce, shredded
half a cucumber, sliced into
  ribbons
2 cherry tomatoes, quartered
2 tsp light mayonnaise

FOR THE CHILLI JAM
½ red chilli, seeds removed
  and finely diced
2 tbsp honey
2 tsp reduced-sugar ketchup
1 tsp cider vinegar
1 tsp granulated sweetener
¼ tsp chilli powder
¼ tsp smoked paprika

We absolutely love a cheeky Nando's, and the Peri-Peri Chicken Wrap is one of our go-to orders! Better for your budget and your calorie count, this fakeaway gives the restaurant favourite a run for its money. We've wrapped up fresh peri-peri seasoned chicken breast and homemade sweet-and-spicy chilli jam, so you can enjoy the best bits in comfort at home.

Everyday Light ——————————————————

Add the chilli jam ingredients to a small saucepan and place over a very low heat. Heat for 4 minutes, until just bubbling and thick. Leave it to one side to cool and thicken.

Spray a frying pan with low-calorie cooking spray and place over a medium heat. Add the chicken and sprinkle over the peri-peri seasoning.

Fry the chicken for 5 minutes, then add the sliced pepper and fry for a further 3 minutes. Check the chicken by slicing into a piece and checking there is no pinkness.

Heat the tortilla wraps for 60 seconds in the microwave and spread the chilli jam over the two tortillas.

Spoon the chicken into the centre of the wrap and add the lettuce, cucumber and tomatoes. Drizzle over the mayonnaise.

Fold the top and bottom of the wrap into the centre of the wrap, and then roll up from one edge to enclose the filling.

TIP: Heating the tortillas makes it easier to fold and roll the finished wrap.

CHILEAN-STYLE STEAK *and* FRIES

🕐 **15 MINS***   🗑 **VARIABLE** (SEE BELOW)   ✗ **SERVES 4**

*PLUS 10 MINS MARINATING

PER SERVING:
453 KCAL / 53G CARBS

low-calorie cooking spray
1kg potatoes, skin left on and
   sliced into 5mm thick fries
½ tsp sweet smoked paprika
2 extra-lean medallion
   steaks, about 170g each
   (visible fat removed)
2 tbsp light or dark soy sauce
2 tbsp Henderson's relish or
   Worcestershire sauce
3 garlic cloves, peeled and
   minced
1 large onion, peeled and
   finely sliced
4 medium eggs
sea salt and black pepper,
   to taste

TO ACCOMPANY *(optional)*
75g mixed salad (+ 15 kcal
   per serving)

Friday night dinner or weekend brunch? We're always in the mood for these crispy fries topped with sticky onions, juicy steak and a fried egg. This meal feels like such a treat, but our homemade chips and a lean cut of meat help keep the calories down. Cook your steak just how you like it, then cut into that runny yolk: perfection!

Weekly Indulgence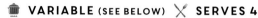

OVEN METHOD
🗑 **40 MINS**

FOR THE FRIES: Preheat the oven to 220°C (fan 200°C/gas mark 7). Line a large baking tray with foil and spray with low-calorie cooking spray. Place the fries onto the tray.

Spray the fries with low-calorie cooking spray and sprinkle on the paprika. Toss until evenly coated. Spread the fries out on the tray, using a second baking tray if there isn't enough room.

Place the fries in the middle of the oven for 30 minutes. Carefully flip and respray with low-calorie cooking spray before placing back into the oven for another 10 minutes, or until crispy on the outside and soft inside.

FOR THE STEAK: While the fries are in the oven, place the steaks into a medium bowl. Pour over the soy sauce, Henderson's relish and add the garlic. Give it a stir and leave to marinate for around 10 minutes.

Spray a frying pan with low-calorie cooking spray and place over a medium heat. Add the onion and cook gently for 5 minutes until it begins to soften. Push the onions around the edge of the pan to make room for the steaks (flip your fries at this point if you haven't already!).

Place the steaks into the hot pan and pour the rest of the marinade on top. Cook the steaks to your preference. The exact times will vary depending on the thickness of your steak; it will be around 2 minutes each side for rare, 3 minutes each side for medium and 4 minutes each side for well done. You can check how done it is by pressing

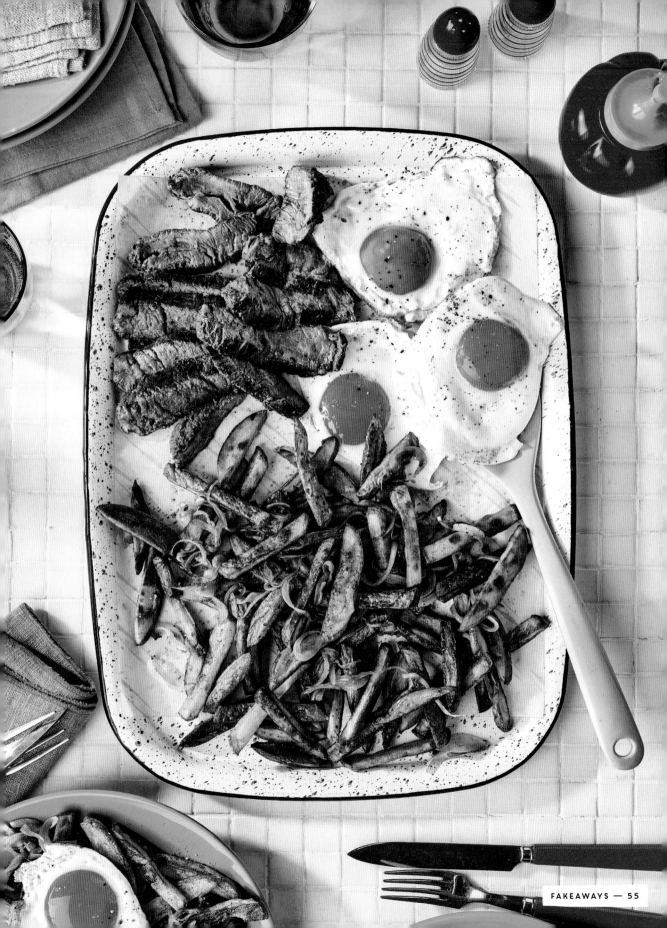

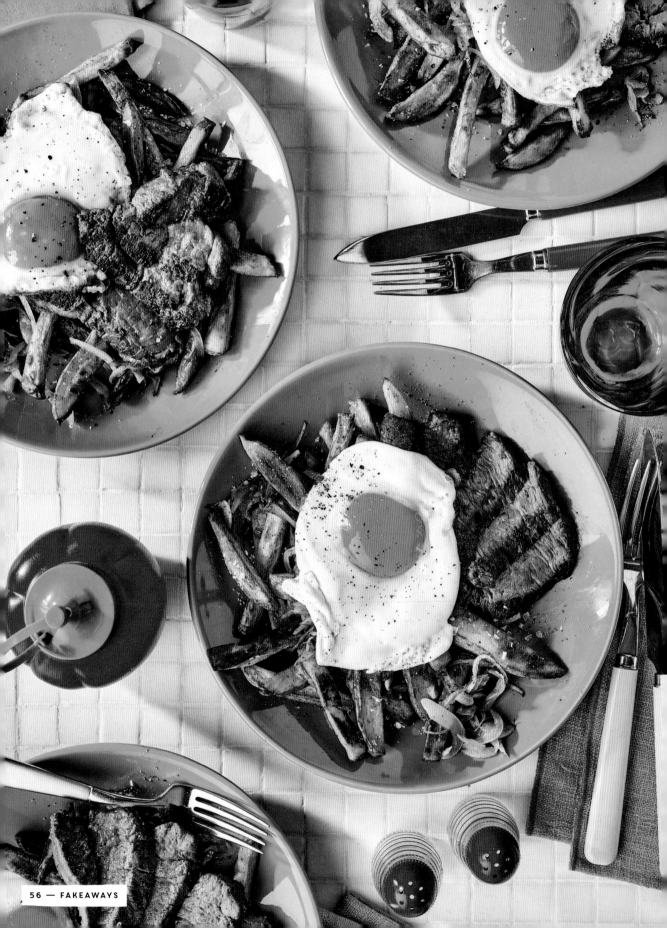

the steak with your finger. When you press down a rare steak will be quite spongy with little resistance, a medium steak will only have a little resistance and a well-done steak will be quite firm.

Once cooked, take the steak and onions out of the pan and leave to rest, with some foil loosely placed over them, for a few minutes before slicing it into thin slices.

FOR THE EGG: While the steak is resting, spray the pan you used for the meat with some low-calorie cooking spray. Place it over a medium heat and, when hot, crack your eggs in. Cover with a lid and cook for 3 minutes. When done, the white will be opaque and the yolk will be slightly set on top. Cook with the lid on for a minute longer if you like your eggs fully set.

Lay your fries out on a plate and top with the onion, sliced steak and fried egg. Season with salt and black pepper to taste.

AIR-FRYER METHOD
30 MINS

SPECIAL EQUIPMENT
Air fryer

FOR THE FRIES: Preheat the air fryer to 190°C. Place the fries into a bowl and spray with low-calorie cooking spray. Sprinkle on the paprika and toss until coated evenly.

Place the fries into the air fryer basket and cook for 20–30 minutes, shaking the basket occasionally. Air fryers can vary, so check regularly to make sure they don't burn. When cooked through they will be crispy on the outside and soft inside. Depending on the size of your air fryer you may need to do this in batches.

FOR THE STEAK: While the fries are in the air fryer, place the steaks into a medium bowl. Pour over the soy sauce, Henderson's relish and garlic. Give it a stir and leave to marinate for around 10 minutes.

Spray a frying pan with low-calorie cooking spray and place over a medium heat. Add the onion and cook gently for 5 minutes, until it begins to soften. Push the onions around the edge of the pan to make room for the steaks.

Place the steaks into the hot pan and pour the rest of the marinade on top. Cook the steaks to your preference. The exact times will vary depending on the thickness of your steak; it will be around 2 minutes each side for rare, 3 minutes each side for medium and 4 minutes each side for well done. You can check how done it is by pressing the steak with your finger. When you press down, a rare steak will be quite spongy with little resistance, a medium steak will only have a little resistance and a well-done steak will be quite firm.

Once cooked, take the steak and onions out of the pan and leave to rest, with some foil loosely placed over them, for a few minutes before slicing it into thin slices.

FOR THE EGG: While the steak is resting, spray the pan you used for the meat with some low-calorie cooking spray. Place it over a medium heat and, once it is hot, crack your eggs in. Cover with a lid cook for 3 minutes. When done, the white will be opaque and the yolk will be slightly set on top. Cook with the lid on for 1 minute longer if you like your eggs fully set.

Lay your fries out on a plate and top with the onion, sliced steak and fried egg. Season with salt and black pepper to taste.

TIP: If your air fryer doesn't have a preheat function, we suggest heating at cooking temperature for a few minutes before air-frying your food.

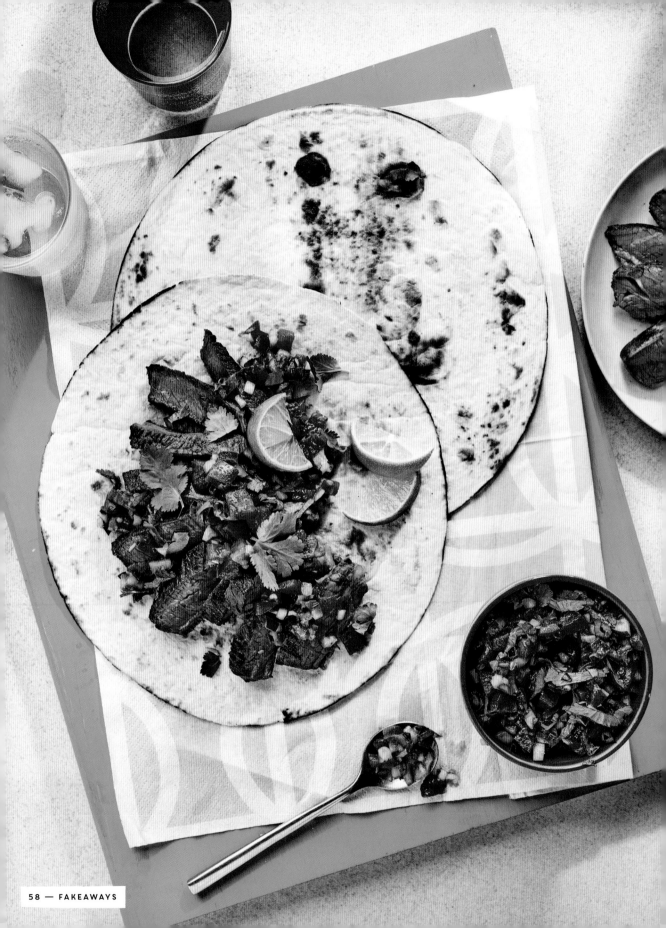

CARNE ASADA

🕐 **15 MINS***   🗑 **10 MINS**   ✕ **SERVES 4**

*PLUS 1 HOUR MARINATING

PER SERVING:
266 KCAL / 26G CARBS

2 beef rump steaks, 200g
  each, visible fat removed
low-calorie cooking spray
4 low-calorie soft tortilla
  wraps
8 lime wedges, to garnish
  (optional)

FOR THE MARINADE
juice of 1 large orange
juice of 2 limes
1 green chilli, deseeded and
  finely chopped
4 garlic cloves, peeled and
  crushed
1 tbsp chopped fresh
  coriander (stalks removed)
pinch of mild chilli powder
¼ tsp salt
¼ tsp ground black pepper

FOR THE PICO DE GALLO-STYLE SALSA
2 salad tomatoes, deseeded
  and finely diced
¼ onion, peeled and finely
  diced
2 tbsp chopped fresh
  coriander (stalks removed)
juice of ½ lime
pinch of dried chilli flakes
pinch of white granulated
  sweetener or sugar

TO ACCOMPANY *(optional)*
50g uncooked basmati
  rice per portion, cooked
  according to packet
  instructions (+ 173 kcal per
  125g cooked serving)

Our take on a Mexican-style grilled steak dish that's popularly served in tacos or burritos is served inside a soft, low-calorie tortilla wrap, with a punchy, fresh pico de gallo-inspired salsa. Balancing zesty citrus and chilli spice with tender beef, this dish is a treat for lunch, or add rice for a really filling dinner the whole family will love.

Weekly Indulgence

Place the marinade ingredients in a shallow dish and stir to combine. Place the steaks in the dish and spoon the marinade over. Cover and place in the fridge for about 1 hour to marinate, turning over halfway through.

Meanwhile, make the salsa. Place all the ingredients in a small bowl, stir to combine and set aside.

Spray a large frying pan with low-calorie cooking spray and place over a medium to high heat. When the frying pan is hot, add the steaks, discarding the marinade, and fry for about 5 minutes on each side for medium-rare. The steaks should be well browned and starting to char a little on the outside and slightly pink inside. If you prefer steak well done, fry for a couple of minutes longer. If you prefer it rare, fry for a couple of minutes less. Timings are a guide only and will depend on the thickness of the steaks you are frying.

Remove the steaks from the frying pan and place on a chopping board. Leave to stand for 5 minutes before slicing into wafer-thin strips.

Place a tortilla wrap on each of four plates, divide the strips of beef and some of the salsa among them. Squeeze over a wedge or two of lime per wrap (optional) and fold the wraps around the filling.

Serve alone or with a small portion of basmati rice or other accompaniment of your choice.

TIP: This dish has a mild to medium chilli heat. If you prefer things spicy, add a little more chilli powder or reduce if you prefer things mildly spiced.

FREEZE ME

BURGERS ONLY

GLUTEN FREE

USE GF ROLLS

CHEESY NACHO BURGER

🕐 **20 MINS**  **12 MINS** ✕ **SERVES 4**

PER SERVING:
458 KCAL / 39G CARBS

FOR THE BURGERS
250g 5%-fat minced beef
½ tsp smoked paprika
½ tsp chilli powder
¼ tsp garlic granules
¼ tsp onion granules
¼ tsp ground cumin
¼ tsp dried oregano

FOR THE GUACAMOLE
½ avocado, stone and skin
  removed, mashed with a fork
3 cherry tomatoes, diced
1 spring onion, trimmed and
  finely sliced
1 tsp lime juice
¼ tsp sriracha sauce
sea salt and freshly ground
  black pepper

TO ASSEMBLE
40g lightly salted tortilla chips
40g reduced-fat Cheddar
  cheese, finely grated
low-calorie cooking spray
½ red pepper, deseeded and
  finely sliced
½ green pepper, deseeded
  and finely sliced
4 reduced-fat processed
  cheese slices
4 wholemeal rolls, about
  60g each, sliced in half
30g sliced jalapeño peppers,
  drained from a jar
2 tbsp light mayonnaise
½ tsp sriracha sauce

SWAP THIS: Swap the
beef for 5%-fat minced
lamb or turkey.

There's no need to pick up the takeaway menu – these Cheesy Nacho Burgers have got everything you're craving! They're seriously fully loaded, stacked with all your favourite Mexican-style toppings. We're talking peppers, cheesy tortilla chips, guacamole, spicy mayo... do we need to say more?

Weekly Indulgence

In a large mixing bowl add all the burger ingredients and mix together with your hands until the herbs and spices are fully incorporated. Divide the mixture into four, shape into burger patties and leave to one side.

Line a baking tray with greaseproof paper and make four small stacks of tortilla chips. Top with the grated cheese and pop under a hot grill for 1 minute until the cheese is melted. Leave to one side.

Spray a small frying pan with low-calorie cooking spray and place over a medium heat. Add the peppers and cook for 8 minutes until softened and starting to brown.

While the peppers are cooking, spray a large frying pan with low-calorie cooking spray and place over a medium heat. Add the burger patties and fry for 4–5 minutes on each side. Turn off the heat and add a slice of cheese to the top of each burger. Leave to one side to melt a little.

In a small bowl combine the guacamole ingredients, mix until smooth and season with salt and pepper.

Spread a little of the guacamole onto the bottom half of each roll. Add a burger patty and top with a few of the peppers. Add a stack of the tortilla chips on top of the peppers, and finish with a few jalapeños.

Mix the mayonnaise and sriracha sauce together, drizzle over the top of the burger stack and place the top of the roll on the top. Serve.

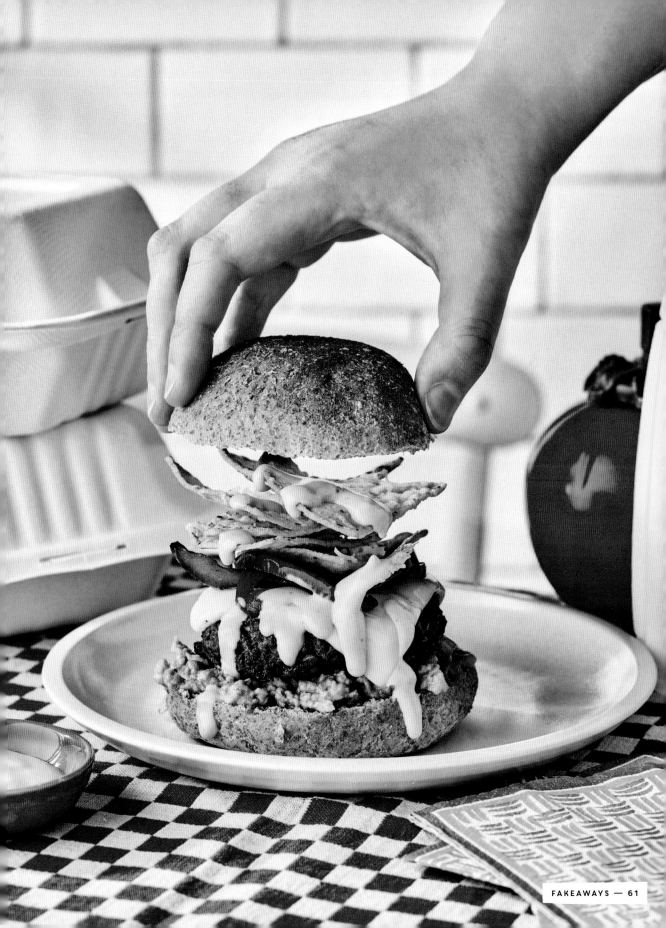

PORK *and* PINEAPPLE KEBABS

🕐 **15 MINS**   🗑 **VARIABLE** (SEE BELOW)   ✕ **SERVES 4**

*PLUS 1 HOUR MARINATING

PER SERVING:
220 KCAL /24G CARBS

SPECIAL EQUIPMENT
8 skewers

2 tbsp honey
1 tbsp light soy sauce
1 tsp lime juice
¼ tsp smoked paprika
¼ tsp garlic granules
¼ tsp onion granules
¼ tsp ground ginger
¼ tsp Chinese five-spice
300g diced pork (visible fat removed)
16 cherry tomatoes
400g fresh pineapple, skinned, cored, eyes removed and cut into chunks (prepared weight)
½ red onion, peeled and cut into chunks
½ red pepper, deseeded and chopped into chunks
½ green pepper, deseeded and chopped into chunks
½ yellow pepper, deseeded and chopped into chunks

TO ACCOMPANY (*optional*)
4 low-calorie soft tortilla wraps (+ 120 kcal per serving)
75g mixed salad (+ 15 kcal per serving)

TIP: If you are using bamboo skewers, be sure to soak them in water before cooking to stop them from burning.

This baked sweet and sour recipe really puts your store cupboard ingredients to good use. With a bit of spice, a bit of sweetness and a bit of tang, there's something for everyone here. The key is in marinating the pork: the longer, the better.

Everyday Light ———————————————————

OVEN METHOD
🗑 **20 MINS**

Combine the honey, soy sauce, lime juice and all the spices in a mixing bowl. Add the pork and toss to coat well. Cover and pop into the fridge for 1 hour. Preheat the oven to 190°C (fan 170°C/gas mark 5).

Thread a cherry tomato onto the end of each skewer, then thread with alternating pork, pineapple and vegetables, finishing with another cherry tomato. Repeat for all eight skewers, then brush the finished kebabs with a little of the leftover marinade and pop into the oven for 10 minutes.

Turn the kebabs over and brush with a little more of the marinade. Cook for a further 10 minutes. Serve with wraps and salad.

AIR-FRYER METHOD
🗑 **12 MINS**

SPECIAL EQUIPMENT
Air fryer

Combine the honey, soy sauce, lime juice and all the spices in a mixing bowl. Add the pork and toss to coat well. Cover and pop into the fridge for 1 hour. Preheat the air fryer to 190°C.

Thread a cherry tomato onto the end of each skewer, then thread with alternating pork, pineapple and vegetables, finishing with another cherry tomato. Repeat for all eight skewers, then brush the finished kebabs with a little of the leftover marinade and pop into the air fryer for 6 minutes.

Turn the kebabs over and brush with a little more of the marinade. Cook for a further 6 minutes. Serve with wraps and salad.

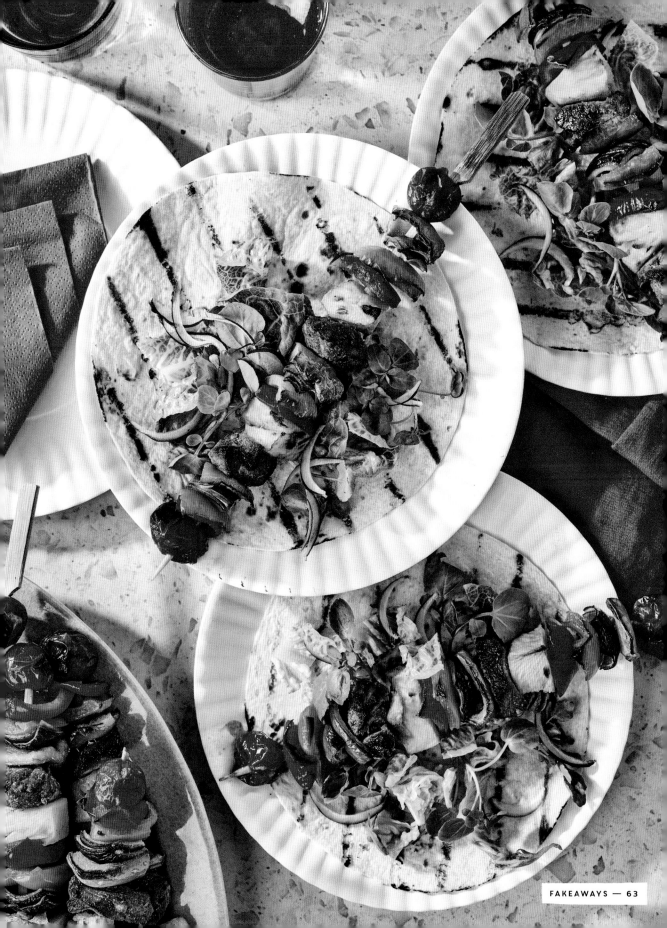

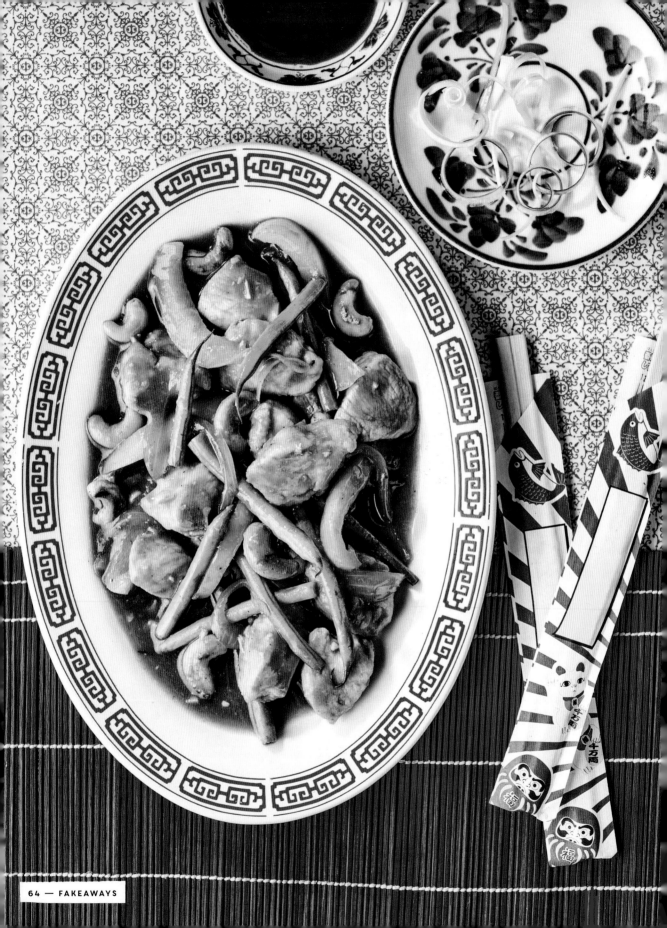

CHICKEN *with* YELLOW BEAN SAUCE

🕐 **15 MINS**   🗑 **15 MINS**   ✕ **SERVES 4**

FREEZE ME

DAIRY FREE

GLUTEN FREE

USE GF STOCK CUBE AND SOY SAUCE

PER SERVING:
400 KCAL / 26G CARBS

520g diced chicken breast
2 tbsp cornflour
low-calorie cooking spray
2 onions, peeled and sliced
4 garlic cloves, peeled and crushed
2 medium yellow peppers, deseeded and sliced
100g fine green beans, trimmed and halved
4 tbsp Chinese yellow bean sauce
200ml chicken stock (½ chicken stock cube dissolved in 200ml boiling water)
2 tbsp light soy sauce
25g unsalted cashew nuts
sea salt and freshly ground black pepper
1 spring onion, trimmed and cut into long strips (optional)

TO ACCOMPANY *(optional)*
50g uncooked basmati rice per portion, cooked according to packet instructions (+ 173 kcal per 125g cooked serving)

We've given one of our favourite takeaways a Pinch of Nom twist. Salty and a bit sweet, this Chinese-inspired recipe is on your table in under half an hour – no way a delivery could beat that! Plenty of fresh veggies give a satisfying crunch, and fill you up without adding calories.

Weekly Indulgence ─────────────

Place the chicken in a medium mixing bowl and add the cornflour. Toss to coat all over.

Spray a large frying pan or wok with low-calorie cooking spray and place over a medium to high heat. When the frying pan or wok is really hot, add the chicken and stir-fry for 4–5 minutes, until lightly browned and sealed on all sides.

Add the onions, garlic and peppers and stir-fry for 3–4 minutes. Next, add the green beans and continue to stir-fry for a further 2–3 minutes, until the vegetables are tender but still retain a little crispness, then add the yellow bean sauce and stir evenly.

Add the stock, soy sauce and cashew nuts. Simmer, uncovered, for 1–2 minutes until the sauce has thickened slightly, the chicken is no longer pink inside, and the juices run clear.

Taste and season with salt and black pepper if needed.

Garnish with spring onion, if using, and serve with basmati rice or an accompaniment of your choice.

MAKE IT VEGGIE: For a vegetarian meal, swap the chicken for Quorn fillets.

TIP: Leaving out the cashew nuts will reduce the calories in a portion of this dish to 266 kcal and 21g of carbohydrates.

USE GF SOY SAUCE

STEAK *and* PEPPER SKEWERS

🕐 **10 MINS**   🗑 **VARIABLE** (SEE BELOW)   ✕ **SERVES 2**

***PLUS 45 MINS MARINATING**

PER SERVING:
294 KCAL / 28G CARBS

SPECIAL EQUIPMENT
4 skewers

FOR THE MARINADE
1 tbsp balsamic vinegar
1 tbsp dark soy sauce
1 tbsp lime juice
1 tbsp honey
¼ tsp sriracha sauce
¼ tsp smoked paprika
¼ tsp garlic granules
¼ tsp onion granules
1 rump steak, about 225g in total, visible fat removed and steak cut into chunks

FOR THE SKEWERS
1 red pepper, deseeded and cut into chunks
1 green pepper, deseeded and cut into chunks
1 red onion, peeled and quartered
8 cherry tomatoes
low-calorie cooking spray

FOR THE DRESSING
5g fresh basil, finely chopped
5g fresh parsley, finely chopped
2 tsp balsamic vinegar
1 tsp lime juice
1 tsp honey

TO ACCOMPANY *(optional)*
75g mixed salad (+ 15 kcal per serving)

Bring barbecue flavours indoors with these meaty, veg-filled skewers! We've combined lean rump steak pieces with chunky peppers, red onion and cherry tomatoes to make colourful, slimming-friendly skewers you can either oven bake or air fry. They taste so good, you won't believe they're only 294 calories per serving – even with a drizzle of herby dressing included!

Everyday Light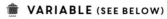

OVEN METHOD
🗑 **15 MINS**

Combine the marinade ingredients together in a bowl and add the rump steak, stirring to combine and coat the steak. Cover and leave for 45 minutes to marinate.

Preheat the oven to 200°C (fan 180°C/gas mark 6).

Thread your skewers with alternating steak, red pepper, green pepper, red onion and cherry tomatoes.

Add the skewers to a baking tray, spray with a little low-calorie cooking spray and cook for 15 minutes.

While the skewers are cooking, combine the basil, parsley, balsamic vinegar, lime juice and honey in a small bowl.

When the skewers are cooked, drizzle them with the herb dressing and serve with a mixed salad if you like.

AIR-FRYER METHOD
🗑 **10 MINS**

SPECIAL EQUIPMENT
Air fryer

Combine the marinade ingredients together in a bowl and add the rump steak, stirring to combine and coat the steak. Cover and leave for 45 minutes to marinate.

Preheat the air fryer to 200°C.

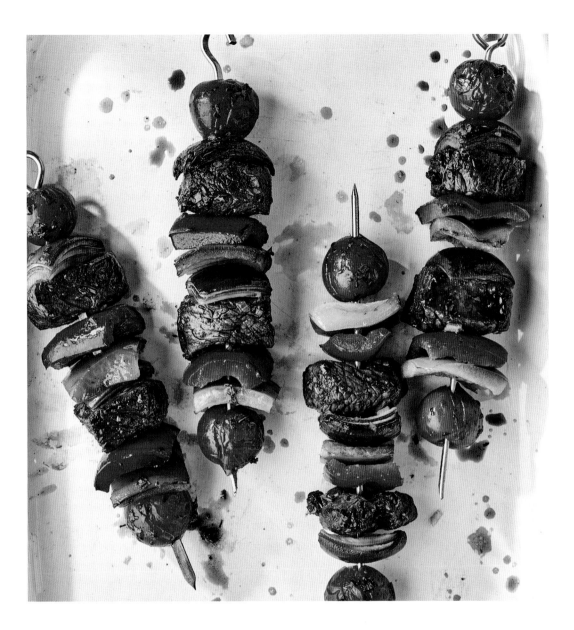

TIP: **TIP:** If you are using bamboo skewers, be sure to soak them in water before cooking to stop them from burning.

TIP: If your air fryer doesn't have a preheat function, we suggest heating at cooking temperature for a few minutes before adding your food.

Thread your skewers with alternating steak, red pepper, green pepper, red onion and cherry tomatoes.

Add the skewers to your air fryer, spray with a little low-calorie cooking spray and cook for 10 minutes. Depending on the size of your air fryer, you may need to cook in batches.

While the skewers are cooking combine the basil, parsley, balsamic vinegar, lime juice and honey in a bowl.

When the skewers are cooked, drizzle them with the herb dressing and serve with a mixed salad if you like.

FREEZE ME

CHILLI ONLY

DAIRY FREE

USE DF CHEESE

GLUTEN FREE

USE A GF STOCK CUBE

HARISSA CHILLI
with CRISPY POTATOES

🕐 **15 MINS** 🗑 **25 MINS** ✕ **SERVES 4**

PER SERVING:
392 KCAL / 38G CARBS

400g potatoes, no need to peel
low-calorie cooking spray
½ tsp smoked paprika
1 onion, peeled and diced
1 medium carrot, peeled and diced
1 garlic clove, peeled and crushed
500g 2%-fat minced turkey
3 tbsp harissa paste
1 tbsp tomato puree
1 tbsp Henderson's relish or Worcestershire sauce
1 x 400g tin chopped tomatoes
1 x 400g tin kidney beans, drained rinsed
1 beef stock cube
¼ tsp ground cumin
20g reduced-fat feta cheese, crumbled
4g fresh coriander leaves, stalks removed and chopped

TO ACCOMPANY *(optional)*
Portion of pickled red onion (see Tip; + 16 kcal per serving)

If you find some leftover harissa paste in the back of your fridge, show it some love by turning it into this quick, low-calorie chilli. Because harissa is made from a blend of red chillies, it has a lovely smoky flavour. We love that you can let the potatoes do their thing in the oven while you whip up the turkey-mince chilli.

Weekly Indulgence

Preheat the oven to 200°C (fan 180°C/gas mark 6). Chop the potatoes into 1cm (½in)-thick slices and place in a bowl of cold water to rinse off the starch. Drain the potato slices in a colander, then dry them using some kitchen towel.

Spread out in a single layer on a baking tray. Spray with low-calorie cooking spray, sprinkle over the paprika and toss to coat.

Place into the oven for 25 minutes, turning halfway through, until soft inside and crispy on the outside. While the potatoes are cooking, spray a large frying pan with low-calorie cooking spray and place over a medium heat. Add the onion and carrot and fry for 5 minutes until softening.

Add the garlic and fry for a further 2 minutes. Add the turkey mince and continue to fry until browned on all sides. Stir in the harissa paste, tomato puree, Henderson's relish, chopped tomatoes and kidney beans.

Crumble in the stock cube and stir through the ground cumin. Lower the heat and simmer the chilli for 10 minutes, while the potatoes finish cooking.

Remove the potatoes from the oven and serve with the chilli. Sprinkle with the feta and chopped coriander and serve with pickled red onion if you wish.

SWAP THIS: You could swap the potatoes for peeled and sliced sweet potatoes, and use other types of mince if you prefer.

TIP: We serve this chilli with a side of pickled red onion. Peel and thinly slice a red onion and add to a small bowl with 3 tbsp white wine vinegar, a pinch of salt and pinch of white granulated sweetener. Toss to coat and leave to one side while you make the chilli.

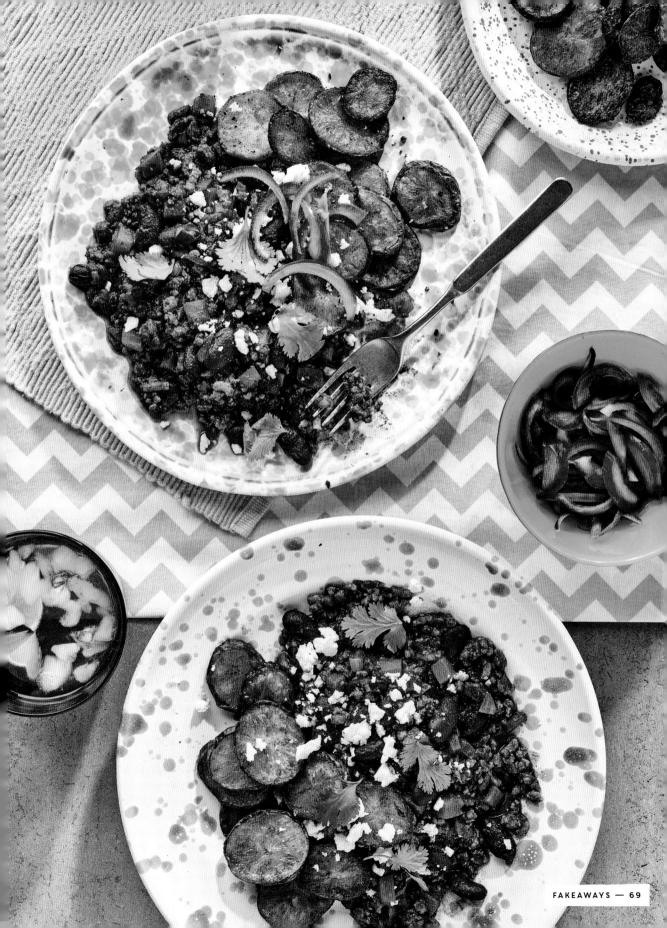

CHICKEN *and* CHEESE CURRY PIE

🕐 **35 MINS***   🗑 **1 HOUR 20 MINS**   ✗ **SERVES 4**

***PLUS 1 HOUR MARINATING**

PER SERVING:
501 KCAL / 49G CARBS

SPECIAL EQUIPMENT
18 x 27cm (7 x 10½in)
ovenproof dish
Food processor or
handheld stick blender

650g diced chicken breast
low-calorie cooking spray
handful of coriander leaves,
  to serve

FOR THE TIKKA MARINADE
2 tsp hot paprika
1 tsp ground coriander
1 tsp ground cumin
1 tsp garam masala
½ tsp ground turmeric
½ tsp ground ginger
½ tsp garlic granules
½ tsp salt
pinch of ground black pepper
pinch of cayenne pepper
3 tbsp fat-free Greek-style
  yoghurt
juice of 1 lemon

FOR THE CURRY SAUCE
low-calorie cooking spray
1 onion, peeled and finely
  chopped
1 medium carrot, peeled and
  finely chopped
1 garlic clove, peeled and
  crushed
1 tbsp mild curry powder
400ml coconut dairy-free
  milk alternative
1 tbsp white wine vinegar
150g low-fat cream cheese
100g reduced-fat mature
  Cheddar, finely grated
sea salt and black pepper

This twist on a comfort food favourite might sound unusual, but cheese, curry and mashed potatoes all in one dish means that this is pretty much the dream dinner when you want something warm and comforting. The smell when it's bubbling in the oven is too good to be true! Don't skip the marinating as it really bumps up the flavour.

Special Occasion

First make the tikka marinade: place the paprika, coriander, cumin, garam masala, turmeric, ginger, garlic granules, salt, pepper and cayenne pepper in a small bowl and mix well.

Place the chicken in a medium non-metallic bowl and add the Greek yoghurt and the lemon juice. Stir until the chicken is coated. Add the marinade spices and mix until thoroughly coated. Cover and place in the fridge to marinate for 1 hour.

Meantime, make the curry sauce. Spray a medium saucepan with low-calorie cooking spray and place over a medium heat. Add the onion and carrot and cook, stirring well, for 10 minutes until starting to soften. Add the garlic and curry powder and cook, stirring, for 1–2 minutes.

Lower the heat and add the coconut dairy-free milk alternative and the vinegar, stirring well. Cover with a lid and simmer gently on the lowest heat for about 20 minutes, until the onion and carrot are just tender. Don't worry if the mixture appears a little curdled at this stage, it will become smooth once blitzed.

While the curry sauce is cooking, place a large saucepan of cold water over a high heat. Add the potatoes, cover and bring to the boil. Once boiling, lower the heat and simmer, partially covered, for 20 minutes until tender.

Drain the potatoes well and return to the saucepan. Add the milk and garlic granules and season with salt and black pepper. Mash the potatoes until smooth, cover and set aside.

Preheat the oven to 200°C (fan 180°C/gas mark 6).

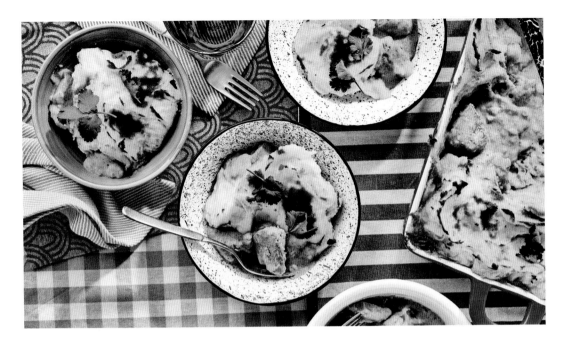

FOR THE TOP

800g potatoes, peeled and
  cut into large chunks
75ml skimmed milk
½ tsp garlic granules
sea salt and freshly ground
  black pepper

TO ACCOMPANY *(optional)*

80g steamed vegetables
  (+ 38 kcal per serving)

MAKE IT VEGGIE: For a
vegetarian curry pie, swap
the chicken for Quorn fillets.

TIPS: Avoid using a metal
bowl and utensils when
preparing the marinated
chicken. The marinade may
cause a reaction with the
metal and give the chicken a
metallic taste. Use a low-fat
cream cheese rather than
a fat-free one, as the sauce
will freeze and reheat better
if you are planning to batch
cook the pie.

After the curry sauce has cooked, carefully pour into a food
processor or use a handheld stick blender to blitz until smooth
and return to the saucepan. Cover with a lid and set aside.

To make the chicken tikka, spray a large frying pan with
low-calorie cooking spray and place over a high heat.
When the frying pan is hot, add the marinated chicken and
fry for 3–4 minutes to seal on all sides.

Transfer the sealed chicken and juices to the ovenproof
dish and place in the oven for 15 minutes or until there is
no sign of pinkness inside. Tip the cooked chicken and
any juices into the saucepan of curry sauce and stir. Place
over a low heat and simmer gently, uncovered, for about
5 minutes to heat through.

Remove from the heat and stir in the cream cheese
and Cheddar cheese until melted and until the sauce is
completely blended and smooth. Taste and season with
salt and black pepper if needed.

Transfer the mixture into the ovenproof dish and spread
out evenly. Place spoonfuls of mashed potato on top and
carefully spread a thin layer of potato over the top of the
filling. Use a fork to create lines, swirls or other decoration
that you like. Place on a baking tray and place in the oven
for 20–25 minutes until golden.

Top the pie with coriander leaves and serve with steamed
vegetables or other accompaniment of your choice.

SLOPPY JOE PIZZA

🕐 **5 MINS**   🗑 **20 MINS**   ✕ **SERVES 4**

PER SERVING:

295 KCAL / 30G CARBS

1 small red onion, peeled and diced

½ red pepper, deseeded and diced

1 chicken stock cube

100ml boiling water

250g 5%-fat minced pork

½ tsp garlic granules

½ tsp onion granules

½ tsp smoked paprika

2 tsp Henderson's relish

2 tsp balsamic vinegar

200g tinned chopped tomatoes

8 tsp tomato puree

4 low-calorie soft tortilla wraps

2 spring onions, trimmed and finely sliced

½ orange pepper, deseeded and sliced

60g reduced-fat Cheddar cheese, finely grated

If you love our Sloppy Dogs recipe, you'll love this Sloppy Joe Pizza. We've used the same signature 'sloppy' flavours to make this scrumptious, super simple recipe. How good does a tomatoey base, paprika-seasoned pork mince, onions, veggies and a melty cheese topping sound? To keep that good stuff slimming friendly, we've used a thin and crispy, low-calorie tortilla wrap base.

Everyday Light

Preheat the oven to 190°C (fan 170°C/gas mark 5) and line a baking tray with baking parchment.

Add the onion and diced red pepper to a frying pan and place over a medium heat. Crumble the stock cube into the boiling water and pour into the pan. Cook for 5 minutes until the onions are softened and the stock has turned glossy.

Add the minced pork, garlic granules, onion granules, paprika, Henderson's relish and 1 teaspoon balsamic vinegar. Fry for 4 minutes, breaking up the minced pork with a wooden spoon, until it has browned all over.

Pour in the chopped tomatoes and add 4 teaspoons of tomato puree; stir and simmer for 5 minutes, until the sauce has become thick and reduced. You don't want the sauce to be too thin when spreading onto your pizza.

In a bowl, combine the remaining 4 teaspoons tomato puree and 1 teaspoon balsamic vinegar. Place the tortilla wraps onto the lined baking tray and spread the tomato puree mixture onto the wraps.

Spoon the pork onto the wraps, add the spring onions and sliced orange pepper. Top with the grated cheese and pop into the oven for 6 minutes, until the cheese has melted, and the tortilla wraps have started to go a little crispy round the edges. These cook quickly, so be careful not to burn them.

SWAP THIS: You can swap the pork for 5%-fat minced beef or turkey. You could also swap the chicken stock cube for a beef or pork one.

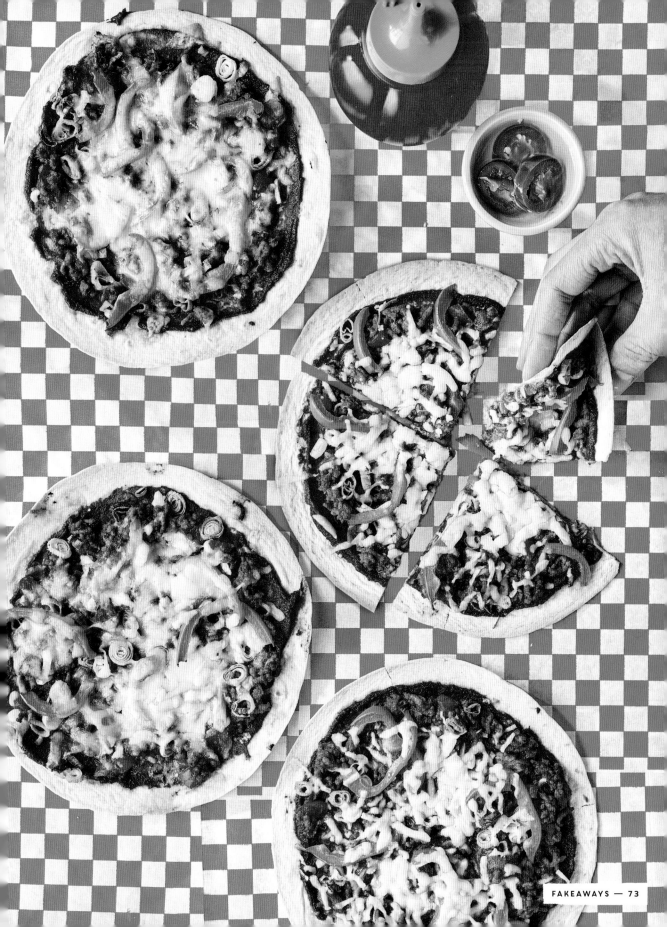

FREEZE ME
FISHCAKES ONLY

GLUTEN FREE
USE GF WRAPS

TIKKA FISHCAKE WRAP

🕐 **5 MINS***   🗑 **VARIABLE** (SEE BELOW)   ✕ **SERVES 4**

*PLUS 30 MINS CHILLING

PER SERVING:
243 KCAL / 29G CARBS

FOR THE FISHCAKES
100g peeled and diced
 potato (around ½ large
 potato)
sea salt and freshly ground
 black pepper
260g tinned tuna in brine,
 drained
½ tsp ground coriander
½ tsp ground cumin
½ tsp garlic granules
½ tsp smoked paprika
½ tsp garam masala
¼ tsp ground ginger
¼ tsp dried mint
¼ tsp chilli powder
1 tsp lime juice
1 medium egg, beaten
low-calorie cooking spray

TO SERVE
4 low-calorie soft tortilla wraps
2 tbsp light mayonnaise
2 tsp mint sauce
1 little gem lettuce, thinly
 sliced
4 cherry tomatoes, quartered

TO ACCOMPANY (optional)
75g mixed salad (+ 15 kcal
 per serving)

TIP: If you want to
make the fishcakes in
advance, you can leave
them for a few hours in
the fridge until you are
ready to cook.

Most of the ingredients for this tasty, tikka-spiced lunch are probably in your cupboards! Save time by prepping the fishcakes in advance (they're fridge and freezer friendly – whoop!). Whether cooked up on the hob, the grill or in the air fryer, serve them crispy on the outside. Their soft, lightly spiced centre is even better with the mint mayo drizzle...

Everyday Light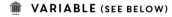

HOB-TOP METHOD
🗑 **20 MINS**

Add the diced potato to a pan of cold water (with a pinch of salt added if you want) and bring to the boil. Lower the heat and cook for 10 minutes until the potato is soft. Drain and mash well. Leave to one side to cool.

In a mixing bowl combine the tuna, spices and lime juice. Once the potato has cooled, add to the tuna and mix until well combined. We find it's best to use our hands to make sure the spices are fully incorporated. Taste the mix and add salt and pepper, if needed.

Add the egg and stir until the mixture comes together.

Divide the mixture into 12 small balls, place them on a plate and squash slightly to form small discs. Pop them in the fridge for 30 minutes to firm up.

Spray a frying pan with low-calorie cooking spray and place over a medium heat.

When the pan is hot, add the fishcakes and cook for 3 minutes on each side – you may find it easier to do this in batches.

While the fishcakes are cooking, put the tortillas in the microwave and heat for 60 seconds; this will make them a little more flexible.

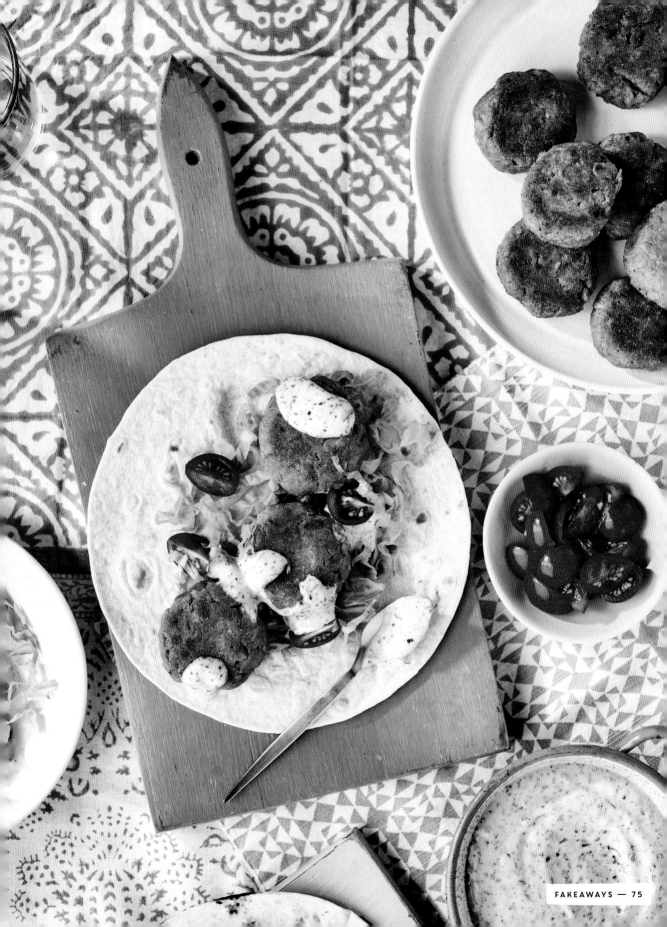

In a bowl, combine the mayo and mint sauce and mix well.

Once the fishcakes are cooked, you are ready to assemble the wraps. Add some thinly sliced lettuce and top with three of the fishcakes, drizzle with the mint mayo and add four tomato quarters.

Fold the sides of the wrap over the centre, or to seal in the filling, fold the bottom of the wrap towards the filling, then one side on top and then the final side on top. Add a small dab of water to the top edge of the wrap with your finger and press down firmly. Serve with a mixed salad if you like.

GRILL METHOD
20 MINS

Add the potato to a pan of cold water (with a pinch of salt added if you want) and bring to the boil. Lower the heat and cook for 10 minutes until the potato is soft. Drain and mash well. Leave to one side to cool.

In a mixing bowl combine the tuna, spices and lime juice. Once the mash has cooled, add to the tuna and mix until well combined. We find it's best to use our hands to make sure the spices are fully incorporated. Taste the mix and add salt and pepper, if needed.

Add the egg and stir until the mixture comes together.

Divide the mixture into 12 small balls, place them on a plate and squash slightly to form small discs. Pop them in the fridge for 30 minutes to firm up.

Preheat the grill to medium and spray a baking tray with low-calorie cooking spray.

When the grill is hot, add the fishcakes to the baking tray and spray the tops with low-calorie cooking spray. Cook for

10 minutes, turning over halfway through to get an even colour.

While the fishcakes are cooking, put the tortillas in the microwave and heat for 60 seconds; this will make them a little more flexible.

In a bowl, combine the mayo and mint sauce and mix well.

Once the fishcakes are cooked, you are ready to assemble the wraps. Add some thinly sliced lettuce and top with three of the fishcakes, drizzle with the mint mayo and add four tomato quarters.

Fold the sides of the wrap over the centre, or to seal in the filling, fold the bottom of the wrap towards the filling, then one side on top and then the final side on top. Add a small dab of water to the top edge of the wrap with your finger and press down firmly. Serve with a mixed salad if you like.

AIR-FRYER METHOD
10 MINS

SPECIAL EQUIPMENT
Air fryer

Add the potato to a pan of cold water (with a pinch of salt added if you want) and bring to the boil. Lower the heat and cook for 10 minutes until the potato is soft. Drain and mash well. Leave to one side to cool.

In a mixing bowl combine the tuna, herbs, spices and lime juice. Once the mash has cooled, add to the tuna and mix until well combined. We find it's best to use our hands to make sure the spices are fully incorporated. Taste the mix and add salt and pepper, if needed.

Add the egg and stir until the mixture comes together.

Divide the mixture into 12 small balls, place them on a plate and squash slightly to form small discs. Pop them in the fridge for 30 minutes to firm up.

Preheat the air fryer to 180°C and spray the air fryer basket with low-calorie cooking spray.

When the air fryer is hot, add the fishcakes and cook for 10 minutes, turning halfway through to get an even colouring. Depending on the size of your air fryer, you may need to do this in batches.

While the fishcakes are cooking, put the tortillas in the microwave and heat for 60 seconds; this will make them a little more flexible.

In a bowl, combine the mayo and mint sauce and mix well.

Once the fishcakes are cooked, you are ready to assemble the wraps. Add some thinly sliced lettuce and top with three of the fishcakes, drizzle with the mint mayo and add four tomato quarters.

Fold the sides of the wrap over the centre, or to seal in the filling, fold the bottom of the wrap towards the filling, then one side on top and then the final side on top. Add a small dab of water to the top edge of the wrap with your finger and press down firmly. Serve with a mixed salad if you like.

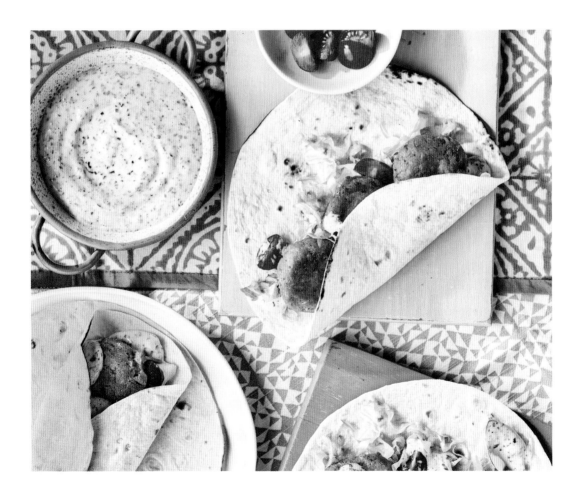

FREEZE ME

MEATBALLS ONLY

BATCH FRIENDLY

STUFFED MEATBALL TORTILLA SKEWERS

🕐 **15 MINS**   🗑 **20 MINS**   ✕ **SERVES 4**

PER SERVING:
315 KCAL / 20G CARBS
(4 per serving)

SPECIAL EQUIPMENT
16 bamboo toothpicks or
4 bamboo skewers, cut into
four lengths
Handheld stick blender
or food processor

FOR THE MEATBALLS
low-calorie cooking spray
500g 5%-fat minced pork
1 thin slice wholemeal bread,
    about 28g, made into
    breadcrumbs
2 tsp dried mixed herbs
1 tsp onion granules
1 tsp garlic granules
1 tsp paprika
½ tsp mild chilli powder
¼ tsp salt
¼ tsp ground black pepper
4 reduced-fat Babybel,
    quartered
2 low-calorie soft tortilla
    wraps

FOR THE SAUCE
low-calorie cooking spray
½ medium red onion, peeled
    and diced
1 garlic clove, peeled and
    crushed
200g tinned chopped
    tomatoes
1 tsp tomato puree
1 tsp white granulated
    sweetener
100ml boiling water
sea salt and freshly ground
    black pepper

These juicy pork meatballs come stuffed with a gooey, cheesy centre, alongside a rich marinara sauce. We're obsessed with the satisfying crunch from their crispy, tortilla-wrap coats! Rustle up a batch as a starter when you're feeling a bit fancy, or take them out and about as a light picnic bite.

Everyday Light ———————————————

Preheat the oven to 180°C (fan 160°C/gas mark 4), spray a baking tray with low-calorie cooking spray and set to one side. Soak the toothpicks or cut-up skewers in water.

In a mixing bowl, add all of the meatball ingredients apart from the Babybel and tortilla wraps. Mix well to combine. Take small amounts of the meatball mixture into your hands and press flat to cover the palm of your hand. Add a piece of cheese to the centre and roll the meat mixture firmly round the cheese. The mixture should make 16 meatballs.

Place the wraps flat on the work surface. Cut in half, then each half into half again horizontally. Finally cut each of these in half again vertically. You should now have 16 pieces of tortilla wrap.

Take a piece of tortilla wrap and wrap around one of the meatballs. Thread a toothpick or length of skewer through the centre to secure the wrap to the meatball and place it onto the lined tray. Repeat with the remaining meatballs.

Pop the tray into the oven for 15–20 minutes until the wraps are golden brown and the meatballs are cooked through.

While the meatballs are cooking, make the sauce. Spray a saucepan with low-calorie cooking spray, place over a medium heat, add the onion and garlic and fry for 5 minutes. Add the chopped tomatoes, tomato puree, sweetener and water. Turn down the heat and simmer, stirring, for 5 minutes until thickened. Blitz with a stick blender or food processor until smooth. Season with salt and pepper and set aside.

Once the meatballs are cooked, remove from the oven and serve with the tomato dipping sauce!

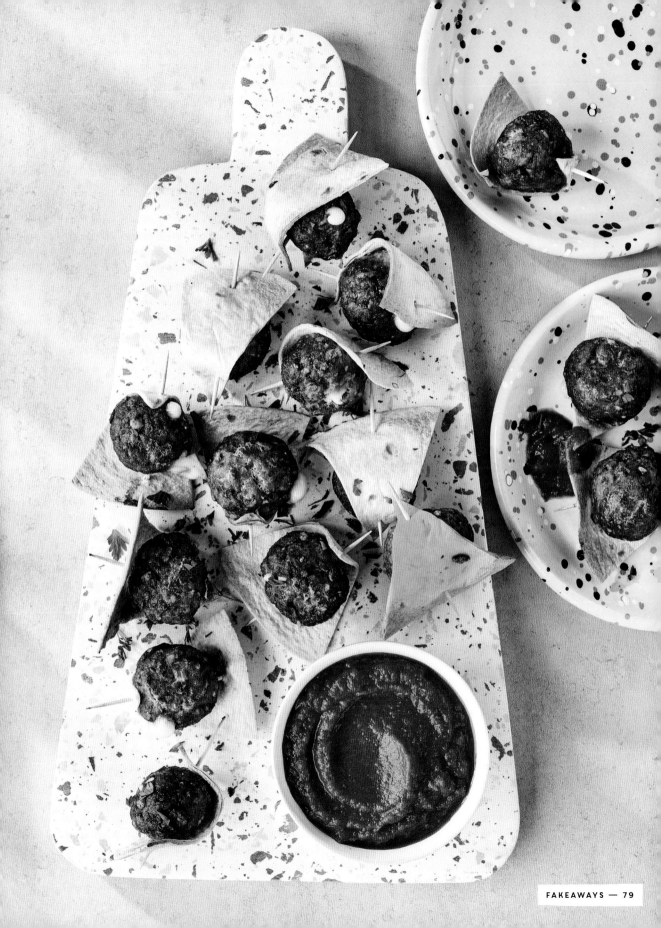

FREEZE ME

SAUCE ONLY

BATCH FRIENDLY

GLUTEN FREE

USE GF SPAGHETTI AND SOY SAUCE

SPICY SPAGHETTI BOLOGNESE

 10 MINS **1 HOUR** ✕ **SERVES 4**

PER SERVING:
557 KCAL / 70G CARBS

low-calorie cooking spray
500g 5%-fat minced beef
3cm (1¼in) piece root ginger,
   peeled and finely grated
3 garlic cloves, peeled and
   crushed
75ml dark soy sauce
2 tsp sriracha sauce
2 tbsp white granulated
   sweetener
6 spring onions, trimmed and
   sliced
1 carrot, peeled and coarsely
   grated
1 tbsp cornflour
300g dried spaghetti

FOR THE TOP
¼ medium red chilli,
   deseeded and thinly sliced
10g fresh coriander leaves,
   stalks removed and leaves
   roughly chopped

TO ACCOMPANY *(optional)*
80g green beans (+ 24 kcal
   per serving)

This pasta dish is a twist on a classic, adding some different flavours and spices to the mix. The beef is simmered in a rich, glossy, lightly spiced sauce and served with spaghetti. Sprinkle over fresh coriander leaves and red chilli to really make this simple dish something special.

Special Occasion ───────────────

Spray a medium saucepan with low-calorie cooking spray and place over a medium heat.

Add the minced beef, ginger and garlic and cook for 3–4 minutes, breaking up the mince with a wooden spoon, until the beef is sealed on all sides.

Add the soy sauce, sriracha sauce, sweetener, spring onions, carrot and 200ml water. Stir well. Cover and bring to the boil, then reduce the heat to low and simmer gently for 45 minutes, stirring occasionally.

In a small bowl, mix the cornflour with 1 tablespoon of water until smooth. Add to the beef mixture, stir and simmer, uncovered, for a further 3–4 minutes or until glossy and thickened slightly.

Meanwhile, bring a large saucepan of water to the boil and cook the spaghetti for about 8–10 minutes or according to the packet instructions. Drain well.

Serve the spicy Bolognese sauce on top of the spaghetti and sprinkle with chopped coriander leaves and slices of red chilli. Serve.

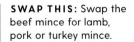 **SWAP THIS:** Swap the beef mince for lamb, pork or turkey mince.

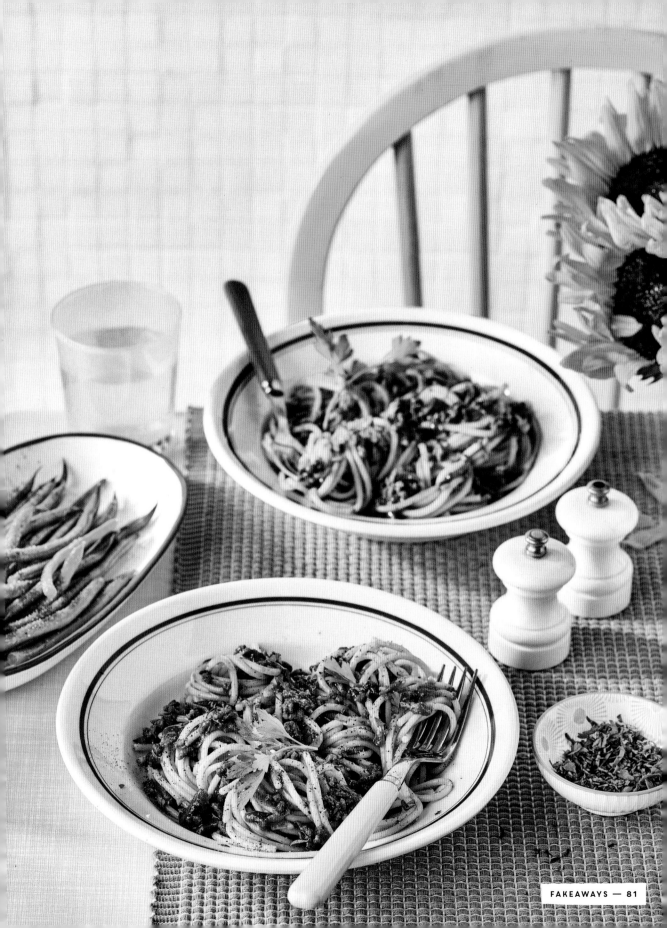

FREEZE ME

BATCH FRIENDLY

DAIRY FREE

GLUTEN FREE

USE GF STOCK
POT OR CUBE

GARLIC *and* GINGER CURRY

 10 MINS   🍲 **30 MINS**   ✗ **SERVES 4**

PER SERVING:
320 KCAL / 16G CARBS

low-calorie cooking spray
800g skinless, boneless
   chicken thighs (visible fat
   removed), cut into chunks
350ml chicken stock (1 stock
   pot or cube dissolved in
   350ml boiling water)
2 tsp fenugreek seeds
1 onion, peeled and diced
4 garlic cloves, peeled and
   crushed
3cm (1¼in) piece of root
   ginger, peeled and finely
   grated
1 green chilli, deseeded and
   finely chopped
1½ tsp garam masala
1½ tsp ground cumin
1 tsp ground turmeric
½ tsp chilli powder
½ tsp freshly ground black
   pepper
2 tbsp tomato puree
1 x 400g tin chopped tomatoes
1 tbsp mango chutney
a good handful of fresh
   coriander, roughly chopped
salt, to taste

TO ACCOMPANY
50g uncooked basmati
   rice per portion, cooked
   according to packet
   instructions (+ 173 kcal per
   125g cooked serving)
45g fat-free Greek yoghurt
   (+ 26 kcal per serving)

You're going to fall in love with this speedy curry! It builds so much flavour in so little time, and it's one of our favourites to batch cook because it keeps really well. Spicy, sweet and fragrant, serve it with a good dollop of fat-free Greek yoghurt and fluffy rice for the perfect fakeaway night.

Weekly Indulgence ——————————————————

Spray a wok with low-calorie cooking spray and place over a medium to high heat. When the pan is hot, add the chicken and fry for around 2 minutes until nicely browned. Do this in two batches to get even browning.

Remove the chicken from the pan and place to one side. If you have some brown crispy bits stuck to the bottom of the pan, add a splash of stock and scrape them up. These are full of flavour!

Spray the pan again with low-calorie cooking spray and add the fenugreek seeds. Toast for around a minute, until they begin to sizzle.

Add the onion and fry for 3 minutes over a medium heat, until starting to soften. Stir in the garlic, ginger and fresh chilli, and cook for another minute.

Add the garam masala, cumin, turmeric, chilli powder and black pepper and continue cooking for around a minute, until everything is well combined, and the spices are fragrant.

Add the tomato puree, chopped tomatoes and stock. Bring to the boil, then reduce the heat to a simmer and cook for 15–20 minutes, until the sauce has thickened and the chicken is cooked through.

Stir in the mango chutney, sprinkle over the coriander, season to taste with salt and serve with basmati rice and a dollop of Greek yoghurt if you like.

TIP: We'd call this a medium-spiced curry. If you prefer something milder, leave out the chilli.

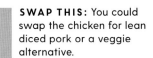

SWAP THIS: You could swap the chicken for lean diced pork or a veggie alternative.

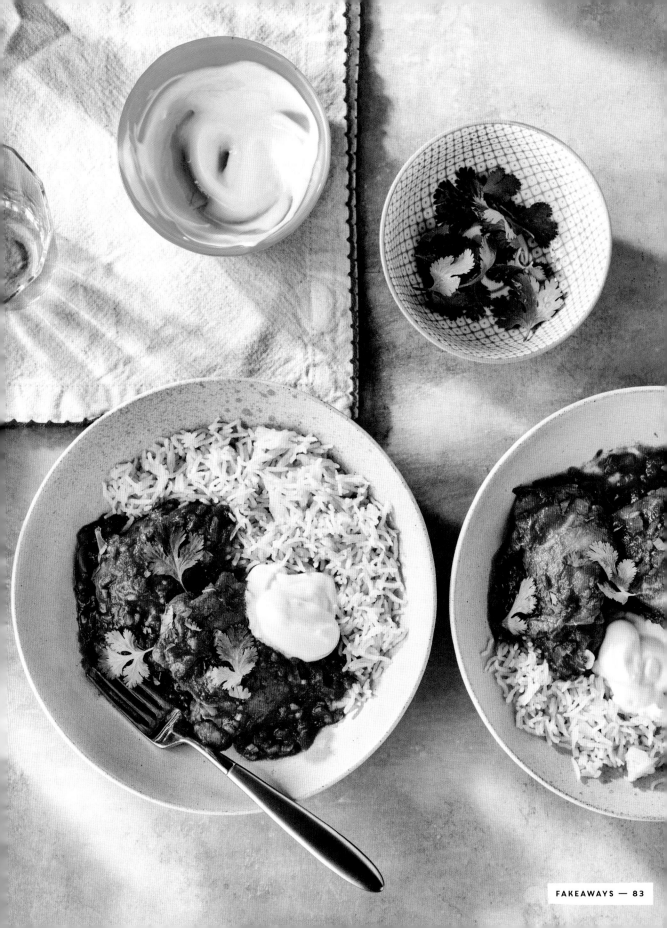

GLUTEN FREE

PIZZA NACHOS

🕐 **12 MINS**   🗑 **6 MINS**   ✕ **SERVES 4**

PER SERVING:
295 KCAL / 32G CARBS

170g lightly salted tortilla chips
½ red onion, peeled and finely sliced
½ green pepper, deseeded and finely sliced
6 cherry tomatoes, quartered
6 slices pepperoni, cut into strips
30g black olives, quartered
30g passata
1 tsp garlic granules
1 tsp dried mixed herbs
15g reduced-fat Cheddar cheese, grated
20g reduced-fat mozzarella cheese, grated

Ever thought of introducing your favourite pizza topping to a bowl of nachos? We tried it, and it turns out it's delicious! We've kept ours simple with onion, peppers, pepperoni and cheese, but everyone can get stuck in with their topping of choice. Why not try a bit of sweetcorn or ham and pineapple?

Everyday Light ——————————————

Preheat the grill to a high heat.

Spread the tortilla chips over a baking tray. Add the onion, pepper, cherry tomatoes, pepperoni and olives on top of the tortilla chips.

Add the passata, garlic granules and mixed herbs to a small dish and stir to combine. Drizzle the passata over the top of the tortilla chips.

Sprinkle over the Cheddar and mozzarella cheese and pop under the grill for 4–6 minutes until the cheese is melted and the tortilla chips are starting to brown.

SWAP THIS: You can swap the pepperoni for diced wafer-thin ham, or for a vegetarian meal, use meat-free cooked sausage.

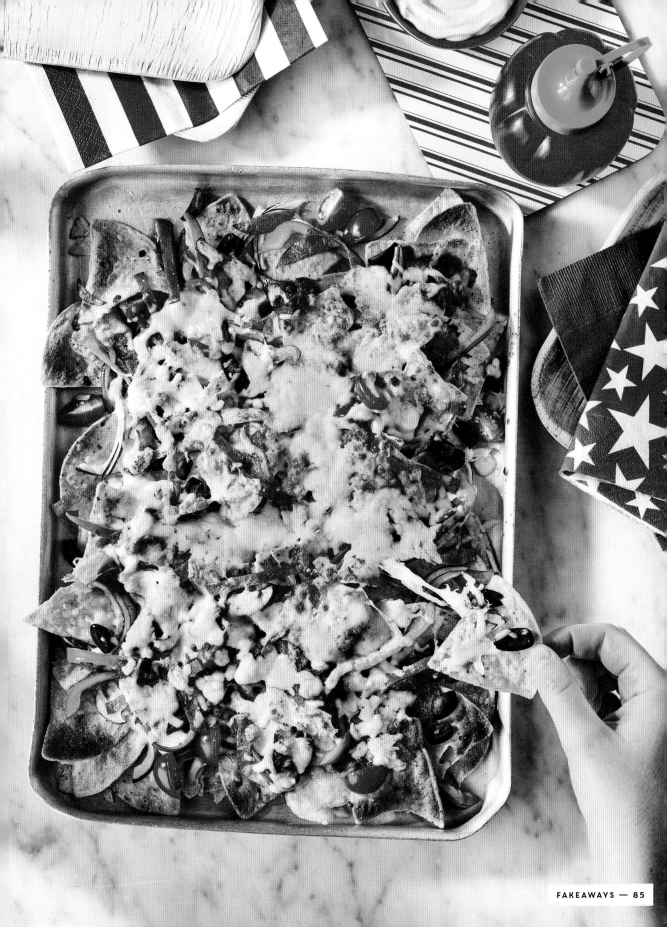

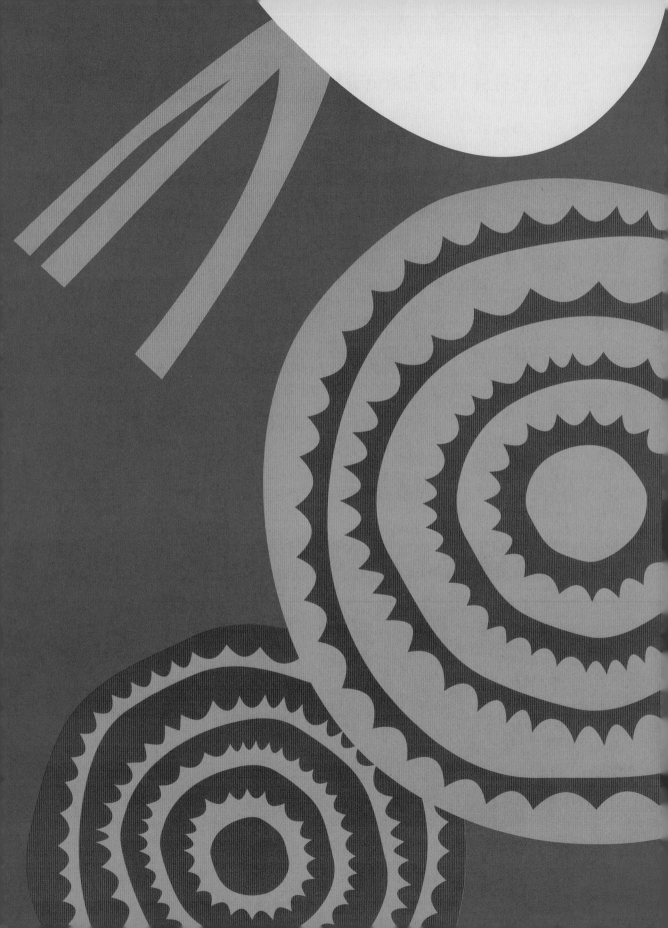

SOUPS
· and ·
STEWS

VEGGIE

FREEZE ME

BATCH FRIENDLY

GLUTEN FREE

USE GF STOCK CUBES

GARLIC MUSHROOM SOUP

 10 MINS   **40 MINS**   ✕ **SERVES 4**

PER SERVING:
125 KCAL / 18G CARBS

SPECIAL EQUIPMENT
Handheld stick blender or food processor

low-calorie cooking spray
1 onion, peeled and diced
500g mushrooms, sliced
6 garlic cloves, peeled and crushed
1.2 litres vegetable stock (2 vegetable stock cubes dissolved in 1.2 litres boiling water)
200g potato, peeled and diced
1 tbsp Henderson's relish
10g sprig of fresh thyme, leaves stripped from the woody stalks
75g low-fat cream cheese
sea salt and freshly ground black pepper

TO ACCOMPANY (optional)
60g wholemeal bread roll (+ 152 kcal per roll)

This garlicky soup will keep the vampires away! So luscious and creamy, you'd never think it could be low in calories. Mushrooms and garlic are always a match made in heaven, and we've simmered them together to make this simple yet delicious lunchtime recipe. Batch cook this soup and save a portion in the freezer for a rainy day.

Everyday Light

Spray a large saucepan with low-calorie cooking spray and place over a medium heat.

Add the onion to the pan and sauté for 5 minutes until softened.

Add the mushrooms and garlic and cook for another 5 minutes.

Pour in the stock, add the potato, Henderson's relish and most of the thyme leaves. Stir and bring to the boil.

Reduce the heat to a simmer and allow to cook for 30 minutes.

Stir in the cream cheese.

Remove half of the soup and, using a stick blender or food processor, blitz until smooth. Return to the other half in the pan and stir together. You can blitz the whole pan of soup if you prefer a smoother soup.

Garnish with the remaining thyme leaves, season with salt and pepper to taste and serve with a wholemeal bread roll if you wish.

SWAP THIS: We used chestnut mushrooms, but you can use any variety. The colour of your soup may differ depending on the mushrooms you use. You can replace the fresh thyme with a teaspoon of dried thyme. Add to the pan at the same time as the garlic. You could swap the low-fat cream cheese for half-fat crème fraîche.

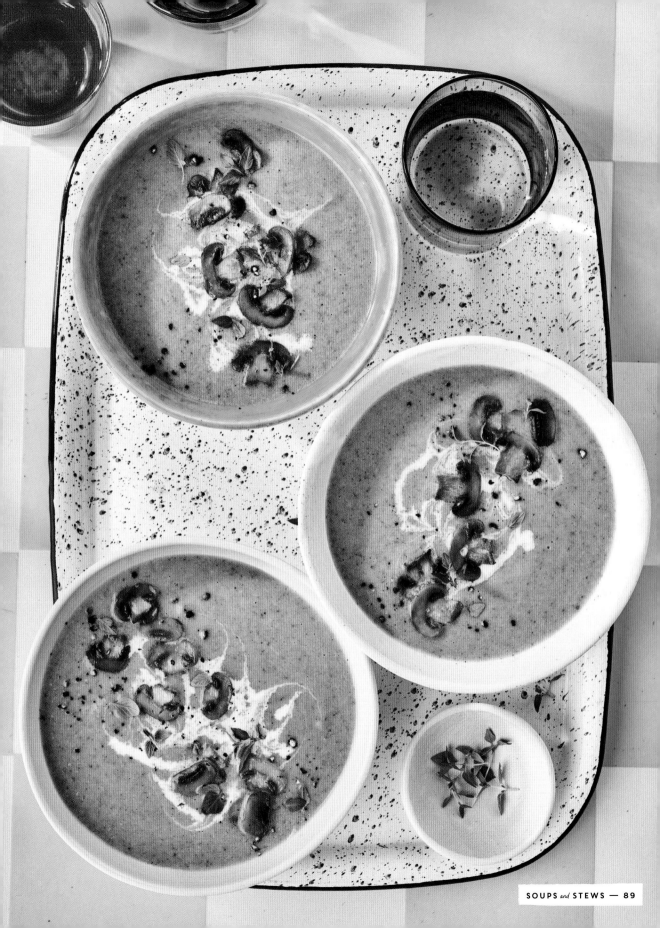

RAREBIT SOUP

🕐 **10 MINS** 🗑 **40 MINS** ✕ **SERVES 4**

PER SERVING:
241 KCAL / 25G CARBS

SPECIAL EQUIPMENT
Handheld stick blender or food processor

low-calorie cooking spray
2 leeks, trimmed of dark
  green leaves, rinsed and
  thinly sliced
350ml skimmed milk
1 litre vegetable stock
  (2 vegetable stock cubes
  dissolved in 1 litre boiling
  water)
400g potatoes, peeled and
  cut into 2cm (¾in) chunks
1 tsp mustard powder
2 bay leaves
3 tbsp Henderson's relish or
  Worcestershire sauce
120g reduced-fat mature
  Cheddar cheese, grated
freshly ground black pepper
1 tsp snipped chives for
  sprinkling (optional)

TO ACCOMPANY
60g wholemeal bread roll
  (+ 152 kcal per roll)

With tangy cheese and a spicy relish, this Rarebit Soup packs a punch! Named for the iconic flavours from the traditional Welsh dish, our low-calorie twist is simple and inexpensive to make. Combining potatoes and leeks with cheesy mustard, each bowlful is satisfying and delicious on its own (or even better with a crusty roll to mop up the leftovers!).

Everyday Light —————————————

Spray a large saucepan with low-calorie cooking spray and place over a medium to low heat. Add the leeks and gently fry for around 10 minutes, until they're soft but not browned.

Add the milk, stock, potatoes, mustard and bay leaves and bring to the boil. Turn the heat down to a simmer and allow to cook for 30 minutes, or until the potatoes are soft.

Remove the bay leaves and blitz the soup until smooth.

Return the soup to the pan and check on its consistency. If it's too thick, add a splash of water. If it's too thin, simmer for another few minutes until it reaches a consistency you like.

Add the Henderson's relish and the cheese. Stir until the cheese is melted. Don't allow the soup to boil after adding the cheese as it may become stringy and overcooked.

Season with some freshly ground black pepper and serve, sprinkled with some fresh chives (if using) and a crusty wholemeal roll.

SWAP THIS: You can swap the leeks for one large finely chopped onion.

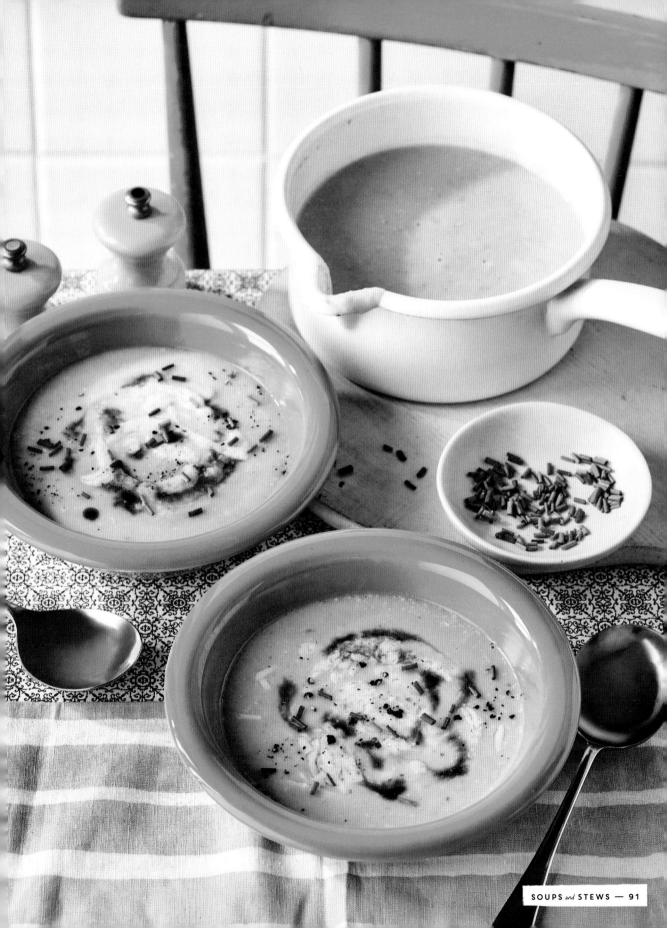

FREEZE ME

BATCH FRIENDLY

GLUTEN FREE

USE GF STOCK CUBES

BUTTERNUT, BACON *and* CHEDDAR SOUP

🕐 **15 MINS**   🗑 **45 MINS**   ✕ **SERVES 6**

PER SERVING:
177 KCAL /15G CARBS

SPECIAL EQUIPMENT
Food processor or stick blender

low-calorie cooking spray
1 large onion, peeled and
    chopped
2 garlic cloves, peeled and
    crushed
700g butternut squash,
    peeled, deseeded and cut
    into 2cm (¾in) chunks
150g white mushrooms,
    halved
4 smoked bacon medallions,
    cut into 2cm (¾in) pieces
1 litre chicken stock
    (2 chicken stock cubes
    dissolved in 1 litre boiling
    water)
1 tsp dried thyme
1 tsp dried oregano
¼ tsp mustard powder
120g reduced-fat mature
    Cheddar cheese, finely
    grated, plus extra to garnish
    (optional)
freshly ground black pepper
a few fresh thyme leaves, to
    garnish (optional)

TO ACCOMPANY *(optional)*
60g wholemeal bread roll
    (+ 152 kcal per roll)

You've just found your new favourite soup recipe! This big bowl of comfort is perfect to warm you up on a chilly day. Its perfect blend of veggies, salty bacon and smooth Cheddar make it rich and silky, even without cream. You'll want to serve this with a fresh wholemeal roll so you can soak up every last drop!

Everyday Light ————————————————————

Spray a large saucepan with low-calorie cooking spray and place over a medium heat. Add the onion and cook for 5 minutes until starting to soften and turning lightly golden.

Add the garlic, butternut squash, mushrooms and bacon and cook over a medium heat for 8–10 minutes until the onions are soft and the bacon is cooked.

Add the chicken stock, thyme, oregano and mustard powder and stir well. Reduce the heat to low, cover with a lid and simmer for 20–25 minutes until the butternut squash is soft when tested with a sharp knife.

Blitz the soup until smooth, using a food processor or stick blender, taking care not to splash yourself with hot soup. You may need to do this in several batches.

Return the blitzed soup to the saucepan and place over a low heat. Add the cheese and stir for a few minutes until completely melted. Season to taste with black pepper.

Garnish with a little extra cheese (5g each is an additional 15 kcal per serving) and a few fresh thyme leaves, if you wish. Serve with a wholemeal bread roll or other accompaniment of your choice.

TIP: Take care when peeling and cutting the butternut squash as they are very hard, heavy and can roll around. Cut off each end first with a large sharp knife, then cut in half across the width. Then you can use a peeler or a sharp knife to remove the skin. Cut the round bottom section in half and scoop out the seeds and discard. Next, square off any round edges to stop the squash from rolling around and carefully cut the butternut squash into chunks.

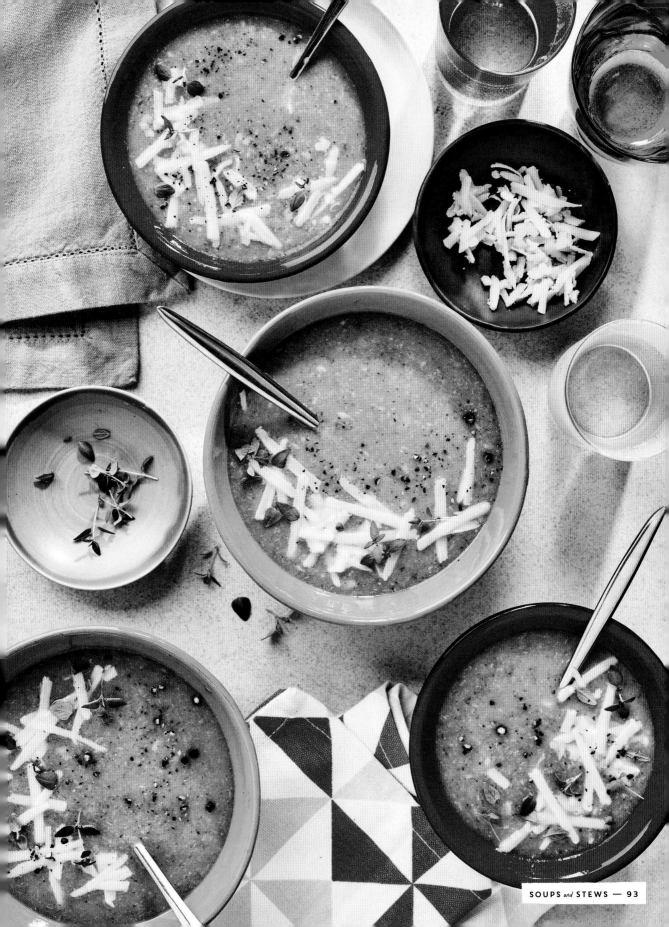

ROOT VEGETABLE CASSOULET

🕐 **15 MINS**   🗑 **VARIABLE** (SEE BELOW)   ✕ **SERVES 4**

PER SERVING:

242 KCAL / 39G CARBS

low-calorie cooking spray
2 shallots, peeled and finely sliced
1 leek, trimmed and finely sliced
1 tsp dried herbes de Provence
1½ tsp garlic granules
1 tsp mustard powder
250g carrots, peeled and cut into 1.5cm (½in) dice
250g swede, peeled and cut into 1.5cm (½in) dice
250g potatoes, peeled and cut into 1.5cm (½in) dice
1 litre vegetable stock (1 vegetable stock cube dissolved in 1 litre boiling water)
1 tsp white wine vinegar
1 white wine stock pot
1 tsp tomato puree
2 x 400g tins cannellini beans, rinsed and drained
sea salt and freshly ground black pepper
handful of chopped parsley, to serve

TO ACCOMPANY

60g wholemeal bread roll (+ 152 kcal per roll)

> **TIP:** If you can't get white wine stock pots, use an extra vegetable stock cube and replace 100ml of the water with 100ml of dry white wine. Adjust the calories accordingly.

> **SWAP THIS:** You can swap the cannellini beans with butter beans.

This hearty vegetarian dish is inspired by the flavours of a rich French cassoulet. Our veggie take on the traditional recipe which usually uses pork or sausage, is packed with root vegetables and beans. Whether you use your slow cooker, pop it in the oven, or let it simmer away on the hob – you'll be rewarded with a big bowl of wholesome comfort food.

Everyday Light ————————————————

OVEN METHOD
🍲 **1 HOUR 25 MINS**

SPECIAL EQUIPMENT

30cm (12in) casserole dish with a tight-fitting lid

Preheat the oven to 160°C (fan 140°C/gas mark 3).

Spray the casserole dish with low-calorie cooking spray and place over a medium heat. Add the shallots and leek and sauté for 8–10 minutes until they are soft and golden in colour.

Add the herbs, garlic granules and mustard powder and stir well. Add the carrots, swede and potatoes.

Pour in the stock and add the white wine vinegar, white wine stock pot and tomato puree. Stir well to dissolve the stock pot and bring to the boil. Cover with a tight-fitting lid and place in the oven to cook for 1 hour. Give the cassoulet a stir halfway through, and check that it is not drying out.

After 1 hour, stir in the beans, replace the lid and return to the oven for 15 minutes until the vegetables are tender. You can add a little extra water at this point if it seems too dry.

Season with a little salt and freshly ground pepper if you wish, and sprinkle with the parsley. Serve in warm bowls. We love to have a wholemeal crusty roll to mop up the delicious sauce!

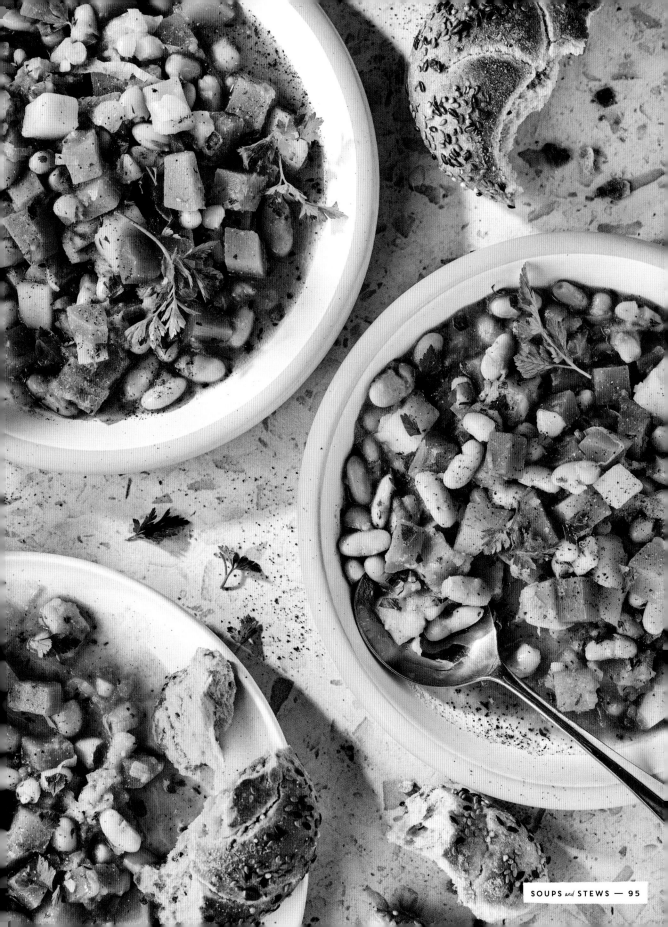

HOB-TOP METHOD
🍲 1 HOUR 10 MINS

SPECIAL EQUIPMENT
**30cm (12in) casserole dish
with a tight-fitting lid**

Spray the casserole dish with low-calorie cooking spray and place over a medium heat.

Add the shallots and leek and sauté for 8–10 minutes until they are soft and golden in colour.

Add the herbs, garlic granules and mustard powder and stir well. Add the carrots and swede.

Pour in the stock and add the white wine vinegar, white wine stock pot and tomato purée. Stir well to dissolve the stock pot and bring to the boil. Turn the heat down to low, cover with a tight-fitting lid and simmer for 40 minutes.

After 40 minutes, add the beans and potatoes, replace the lid and continue cooking for 20 minutes until the vegetables are tender.

Season with a little salt and freshly ground pepper if you wish. Serve in warm bowls. We love to have a wholemeal crusty roll to mop up the delicious sauce.

SLOW-COOKER METHOD
🍲 LOW: 5 HOURS 40 MINS

SPECIAL EQUIPMENT
Slow cooker

Turn on your slow cooker to the low setting.

Spray a frying pan with low-calorie cooking spray and place over a medium heat.

Add the shallots and leek and sauté for 8–10 minutes until they are soft and golden in colour.

Transfer into the slow cooker and add all the remaining ingredients, except for the beans and salt and pepper. Stir well and cover with the lid.

Cook for 5 hours on low. Try not to lift the lid as the slow cooker will lose heat and your cooking time will increase.

After 5 hours, the veggies should be cooked through. Stir in the beans and replace the lid. Cook for a further 30 minutes until the beans are thoroughly heated through.

Season with a little salt and freshly ground pepper if you wish. Serve in warm bowls. We love to have a wholemeal crusty roll to mop up the delicious sauce.

"
You're making my slimming journey a thoroughly tasty one!

—— CHLOE

DIJON CHICKEN *and* DUMPLINGS

🕐 **15 MINS**   🗑 **VARIABLE** (SEE BELOW)   ✕ **SERVES 4**

PER SERVING:
340 KCAL / 33G CARBS

low-calorie cooking spray
2 onions, peeled and
   chopped
3 garlic cloves, peeled and
   crushed
600g diced chicken breast
200g button mushrooms,
   halved
700ml chicken stock
   (1 chicken stock cube,
   dissolved in 700ml boiling
   water)
1 white wine stock pot
3 tbsp Dijon mustard
½ tsp mustard powder
1 tsp dried mixed herbs
1 tbsp cornflour
40g baby spinach leaves

FOR THE DUMPLINGS
100g self-raising flour
¼ tsp baking powder
sea salt and freshly ground
   black pepper
2 medium egg yolks

TO ACCOMPANY *(optional)*
80g steamed vegetables
   (+ 38 kcal per serving)

> **SWAP THIS:** You can
> use diced chicken thighs
> instead of chicken breasts.
> You can swap spinach for
> frozen peas. You could use
> wholegrain Dijon mustard
> in this recipe instead of
> smooth Dijon mustard but
> we wouldn't recommend
> swapping for English
> mustard as it's much hotter!

You can't beat the warming comfort of a stew topped with dumplings! We've used tender chicken pieces, mushrooms, spinach and a helping of Dijon mustard to make this hugely satisfying midweek meal. Our dumplings are made without a gram of suet in sight, and we're so happy with the deliciously light results!

Everyday Light ———————————————

HOB-TOP METHOD
🗑 **1 HOUR 30 MINS**

SPECIAL EQUIPMENT
26cm (10in) lidded casserole dish

Preheat the oven to 160°C (fan 140°C/gas mark 3). Spray the casserole dish with low-calorie cooking spray and place over a medium heat. Add the onions and cook for 5 minutes until starting to soften.

Add the garlic and chicken and cook for a further 5 minutes, until the chicken is sealed and lightly browned.

Add the mushrooms, chicken stock, white wine stock pot, Dijon mustard, mustard powder and mixed herbs. Stir well until the stock pot has dissolved.

Cover with a tight-fitting lid and place in the preheated oven for 1 hour, stirring halfway through.

Meanwhile, make the dumplings. Sift the flour and baking powder into a small bowl. Season with a little salt and black pepper, then add the egg yolks and mix slightly with a fork. Using your fingertips, rub in the egg yolk until the mixture resembles breadcrumbs.

Add 3–4 tablespoons of cold water, a little at a time, and stir with a round-bladed knife until it comes together to form a dough.

You will need a firm dough that's not too wet, so the amount of water you need will depend on the size of your egg yolks. Shape the dough into four equal-sized dumplings and set aside in the fridge for later.

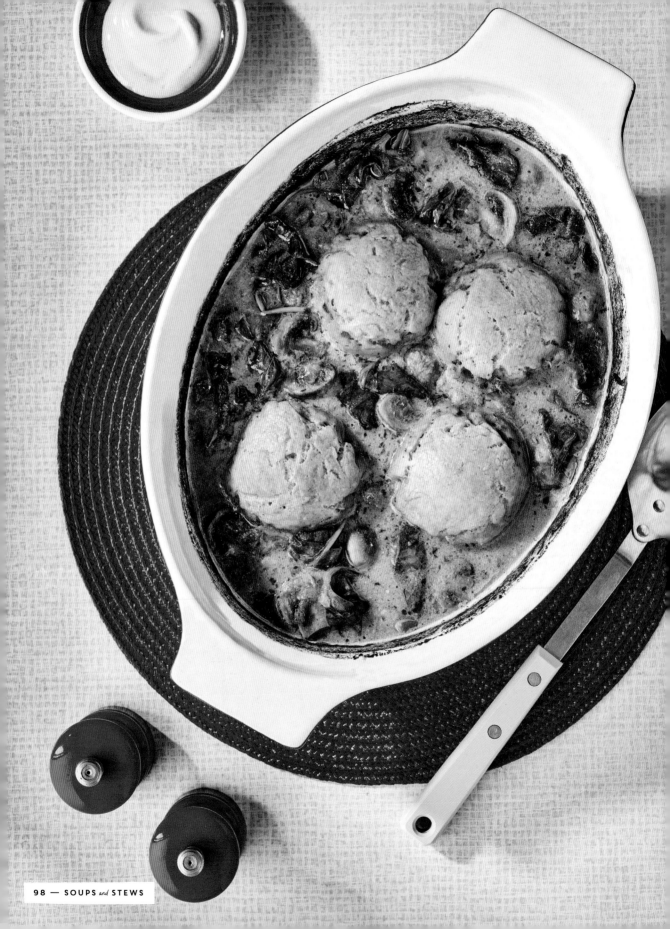

After the stew has been cooking for 1 hour, mix the cornflour with 1 tablespoon of cold water until smooth. Remove the stew from the oven and stir in the cornflour mixture.

Stir in the spinach leaves for a minute or two, until wilted, then place the dumplings on top of the stew. Replace the lid and return to the oven for another 20–25 minutes, until the stew has thickened slightly and the dumplings have puffed up. Remove the lid for the last 10 minutes if you want the dumplings to be golden.

Remove from the oven and serve with steamed vegetables or an accompaniment of choice.

SLOW-COOKER METHOD
🍲 **HIGH: 3 HOURS 50 MINS**

SPECIAL EQUIPMENT
Slow cooker

Spray a large frying pan with low-calorie cooking spray and place over a medium heat. Add the onions and cook for 5 minutes until starting to soften.

Add the garlic and chicken and cook for a further 5 minutes, until the chicken is sealed and lightly browned. Place the mixture in the slow cooker.

Add the mushrooms, chicken stock, white wine stock pot, Dijon mustard, mustard powder and mixed herbs to the slow cooker.

Stir well until the stock pot has dissolved. Cover with the lid and cook on high for 3 hours.

Meanwhile, make the dumplings: sift the flour and baking powder into a small bowl. Season with a little salt and black pepper, then add the egg yolks and mix slightly with a fork. Using your fingertips, rub in the egg yolk until the mixture resembles breadcrumbs.

Add 3–4 tablespoons of cold water, a little at a time, and stir with a round-bladed knife until it comes together to form a dough.

You will need a firm dough that's not too wet, so the amount of water you need will depend on the size of your egg yolks. Shape the dough into four equal-sized dumplings and set aside in the fridge for later.

After 3 hours cooking, mix the cornflour with 1 tablespoon of cold water until smooth. Stir the cornflour mixture into the stew.

Stir in the spinach leaves for a minute or two, until wilted, then place the dumplings on top of the stew. Replace the lid and cook on high for a further 40 minutes, until the stew has thickened slightly, and the dumplings have puffed up.

Serve with steamed vegetables or an accompaniment of choice.

FREEZE ME

DAIRY FREE

GLUTEN FREE

USE GF STOCK CUBE AND HENDERSON'S RELISH

CHICKEN GUMBO

🕐 **10 MINS**   🍲 **30 MINS**   ✗ **SERVES 4**

PER SERVING:
195 KCAL / 13G CARBS

low-calorie cooking spray
500g diced chicken breast
2 green peppers, deseeded
    and diced
1 onion, peeled and diced
2 celery sticks, sliced
1 courgette, sliced
4 garlic cloves, peeled and
    crushed
1 red chilli, deseeded and
    finely chopped
1 tsp dried oregano
1 tsp ground cumin
1 tsp ground coriander
1 tsp smoked paprika
½ tsp cayenne pepper
1 x 400g tin chopped
    tomatoes
400ml chicken stock
    (1 chicken stock cube
    dissolved in 400ml boiling
    water)
1 tbsp Henderson's relish or
    Worcestershire sauce
handful of coriander leaves,
    to garnish

TO ACCOMPANY (optional)
50g uncooked basmati
    rice per portion, cooked
    according to packet
    instructions (+ 173 kcal per
    125g cooked serving)

Inspired by the popular spicy stew from Southern USA, our Chicken Gumbo is a healthy, hearty meal the whole family will love. To keep it slimming friendly, we've used a tomato-based sauce, enriched with the gumbo 'holy trinity' of green peppers, onion and celery. This perfect weeknight dinner, served with a side of fluffy boiled rice, can be on the table in under an hour.

Everyday Light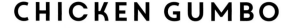

Spray a large saucepan with low-calorie cooking spray and place over a medium heat. Add the chicken and cook for 3–4 minutes until sealed. Remove from the pan and put to one side.

Give the pan another spray and add the peppers, onion and celery. Cook for 5 minutes until softened. Return the chicken to the pan and add the courgette, garlic, red chilli, herbs and spices and cook for a minute to release the flavours.

Stir in the chopped tomatoes, stock and Henderson's relish. Bring to the boil, then reduce the heat and simmer for 20 minutes.

Serve sprinkled with coriander and with rice or an accompaniment of your choice.

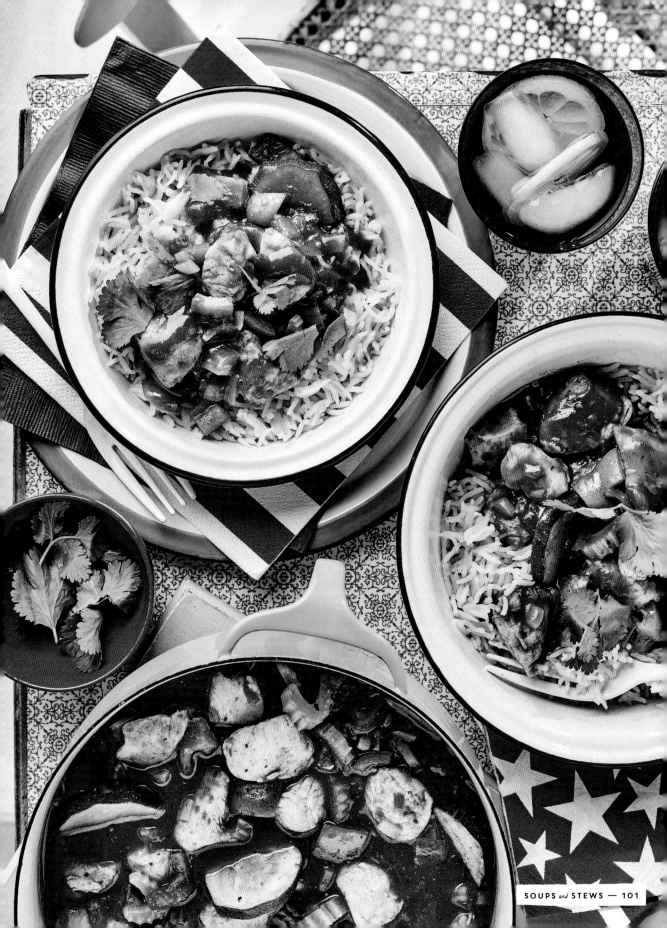

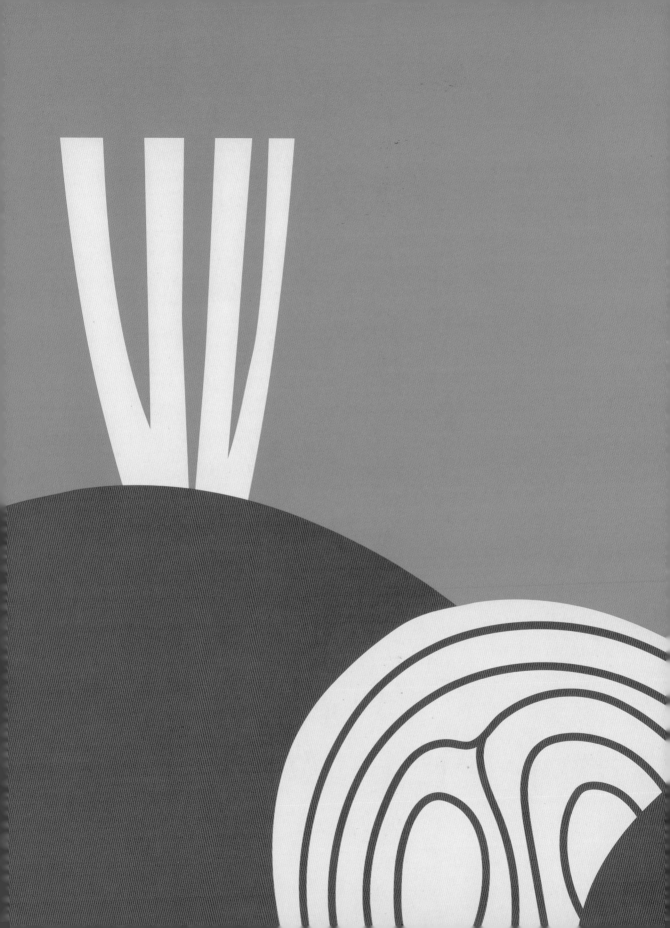

BAKES, ROASTS AND ONE POTS

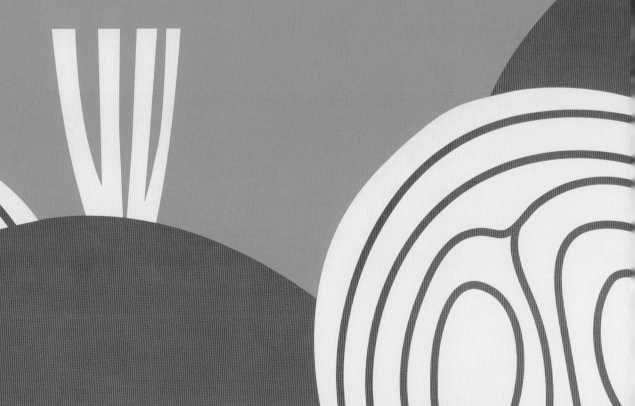

BEEF OLIVES

 40 MINS* 🗑 **VARIABLE** (SEE BELOW) ✕ **SERVES 6**

***PLUS 30 MINS CHILLING**

PER SERVING:
348 KCAL / 16G CARBS

SPECIAL EQUIPMENT
Cooking string

FOR THE STUFFING
2 slices wholemeal bread
low-calorie cooking spray
1 large onion, peeled and
  very finely chopped
1 large leek, trimmed and
  very finely chopped
1 garlic clove, peeled and
  crushed
200g button mushrooms,
  very finely chopped
6 unsmoked bacon
  medallions, minced
1 tbsp finely chopped fresh sage
sea salt and freshly ground
  black pepper

FOR THE STEAKS
6 thin beef frying steaks,
  about 130g each
25g plain flour
3 tsp Dijon mustard
low-calorie cooking spray

FOR THE GRAVY
800ml beef stock (1 stock
  cube dissolved in 800ml
  boiling water)
1 red wine stock pot
200g passata
1 tbsp Worcestershire sauce
  or Henderson's relish
1 tsp Dijon mustard
1 tsp garlic granules
sea salt and black pepper
low-calorie cooking spray

TO ACCOMPANY *(optional)*
80g steamed vegetables
  (+ 38 kcal per serving)
Honey Garlic Potatoes (see
  page 202; + 130 kcal per
  serving)

Despite the name, there are no olives in this recipe!
Our Beef Olives dish is inspired by the traditional Scottish
recipe, which dates back to the 1600s, and they're parcels
of beef steak, stuffed with bacon and mushrooms,
simmered in a rich, meaty gravy. When it comes to
comfort food, it doesn't get better than this!

Special Occasion ─────────────────────

OVEN METHOD
🗑 **3 HOURS 20 MINS**

SPECIAL EQUIPMENT 30cm (12in) lidded casserole dish

For the stuffing: place the bread in a food processor and
blitz until it becomes fine breadcrumbs.

Spray a large frying pan with low-calorie cooking spray and
place over a medium heat. Add the onion and leek and fry
for 10 minutes, stirring occasionally, until slightly softened and
golden brown. Add the garlic, mushrooms and bacon and cook
for a further 5–7 minutes, or until the bacon is just cooked.
Tip the mixture into a bowl. Add the breadcrumbs, sage and
season with salt and black pepper. Mix well and set aside
to cool. Preheat the oven to 170°C (fan 150°C/gas mark 3).

Place a sheet of cling film on a large chopping board. Place one
of the steaks on top and cover with another sheet of cling film.
Using a rolling pin, beat the steak flat until it is very thin. Repeat
with the five remaining steaks. Place the flour on a large plate.
Dip both sides of each steak in the flour to lightly coat. Lay the
floured steaks out on a large chopping board. Spread one side
of each one with ½ teaspoon Dijon mustard.

When the stuffing is cold, divide into six and shape into short
sausage shapes. Lay one sausage on the short end of the first
steak and roll up around the stuffing. Secure with a cocktail
stick, then tie cooking string securely around all sides. Repeat
with the remaining stuffing and steaks. Place the beef parcels
in the fridge to chill and firm up for about 30 minutes.

Spray low-calorie cooking spray into the frying pan and place
over a high heat. When the pan is hot, add the parcels and brown

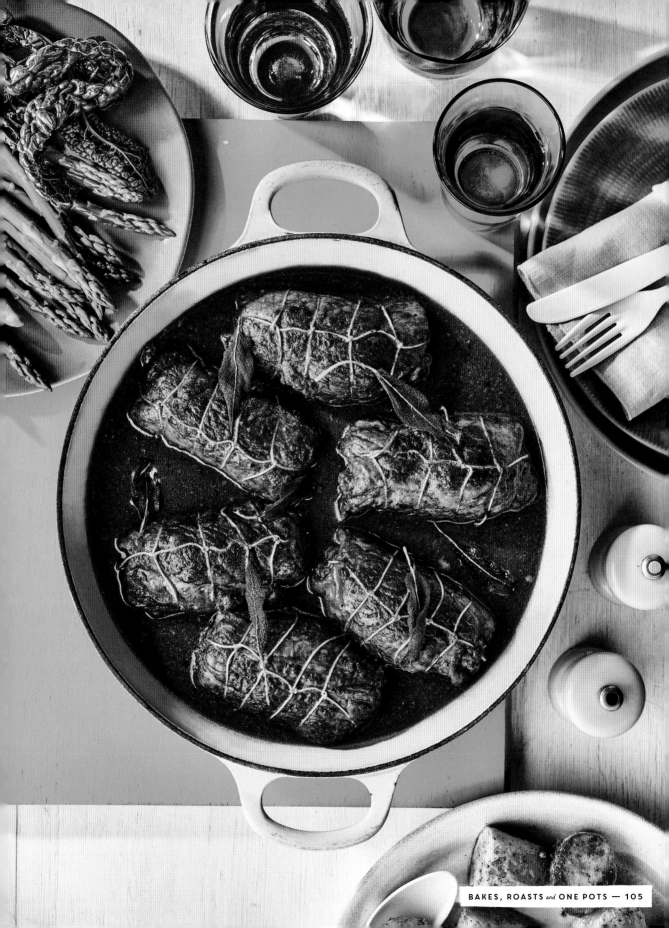

for 1–2 minutes on all sides, including the ends. Set aside on a plate.

To make the gravy, mix together the beef stock, stock pot, passata, Worcestershire sauce, Dijon mustard and garlic granules. Pour into the casserole dish. Remove the cocktail sticks from the beef parcels. Carefully place the beef parcels, seam side down, in a single layer in the casserole dish.

Put the lid on the casserole dish and place in the oven for 2½–3 hours. Turn the beef parcels over once during cooking. Towards the end of cooking, check the consistency of the gravy. It should be only slightly thickened so add a little more boiling water if needed.

When cooked, carefully snip off the cooking string and discard. Serve with steamed vegetables or your choice of accompaniment.

SLOW-COOKER METHOD
🥘 6 HOURS

SPECIAL EQUIPMENT
Slow cooker

Place the bread in a food processor and blitz until it becomes fine breadcrumbs.

Spray a large frying pan with low-calorie cooking spray and place over a medium heat. Add the onion and leek and fry for 10 minutes, stirring occasionally, until slightly softened and golden brown. Add the garlic, mushrooms and bacon and cook for a further 5–7 minutes, or until the bacon is just cooked. Tip the mixture into a bowl. Add the breadcrumbs, sage and season with salt and black pepper. Mix well and set aside to cool.

Place a sheet of cling film on a large chopping board. Place one of the steaks on top and cover with another sheet of cling film. Using a rolling pin, beat the steak flat until it is very thin. Repeat with the five remaining steaks. Place the flour on a large plate. Dip both sides of each steak in the flour to lightly coat. Lay the floured steaks out on

a large chopping board. Spread one side of each one with ½ teaspoon Dijon mustard.

When the stuffing is cold, divide into six and shape into short sausage shapes. Lay one sausage on the short end of the first steak and roll up around the stuffing. Secure with a cocktail stick, then tie cooking string securely around all sides. Repeat with the remaining stuffing and steaks. Place the beef parcels in the fridge to chill and firm up for about 30 minutes.

Spray low-calorie cooking spray into the frying pan and place over a high heat. When the pan is hot, add the beef parcels and brown for 1–2 minutes on all sides, including the ends. Set aside on a plate.

To make the gravy, mix together the beef stock, stock pot, passata, Worcestershire sauce, Dijon mustard and garlic granules. Pour into the slow cooker. Remove the cocktail sticks from the beef parcels. Carefully place the beef parcels, seam side down, in a single layer in the slow cooker.

Put the lid on and turn on to the low setting. Leave to cook for 5½ hours, turning the beef parcels over once during cooking if you can. After 5½ hours, remove the lid, turn up to high and continue to cook for another 30 minutes. This will reduce the gravy down and thicken it slightly.

When cooked, carefully snip off the cooking string and discard. Serve with steamed vegetables or your choice of accompaniment.

HOB-TOP METHOD
🥘 1 HOUR 50 MINS

Place the bread in a food processor and blitz until it becomes fine breadcrumbs.

Spray a large, deep frying pan with low-calorie cooking spray and place over a medium heat. Add the onion and leek and fry for 10 minutes, stirring occasionally, until slightly softened and golden brown. Add the garlic, mushrooms and bacon and cook for a further 5–7 minutes, or until the bacon is just cooked. Tip the mixture into a bowl. Add the breadcrumbs, sage and season with salt and black pepper. Mix well and set aside to cool.

Place a sheet of cling film on a large chopping board. Place one of the steaks on top and cover with another sheet of cling film. Using a rolling pin, beat the steak flat until it is very thin. Repeat with the five remaining steaks. Place the flour on a large plate. Dip both sides of each steak in the flour to lightly coat. Lay the floured steaks out on a large chopping board. Spread one side of each one with ½ teaspoon Dijon mustard.

When the stuffing is cold, divide into six and shape into short sausage shapes. Lay one sausage on the short end of the first steak and roll up around the stuffing. Secure with a cocktail stick, then tie cooking string securely around all sides. Repeat with the remaining stuffing and steaks. Place the beef parcels in the fridge to chill and firm up for about 30 minutes.

Spray low-calorie cooking spray into the frying pan and place over a high heat. When the pan is hot, add the beef parcels and brown for 1–2 minutes on all sides, including the ends. Set aside on a plate.

To make the gravy, mix together the beef stock, stock pot, passata, Worcestershire sauce, Dijon mustard and garlic granules. Pour into the frying pan. Remove the cocktail sticks from the beef parcels. Carefully place the beef parcels, seam side down, in a single layer in the frying pan.

Put the lid on the frying pan or cover tightly with kitchen foil. Place over a low heat and simmer gently for 1 hour until tender. Turn the beef parcels over once during cooking.

After 1 hour, remove the lid or kitchen foil and simmer for a further 30 minutes until the gravy has reduced and thickened slightly.

When cooked carefully snip off the cooking string and discard. Serve with steamed vegetables or your choice of accompaniment.

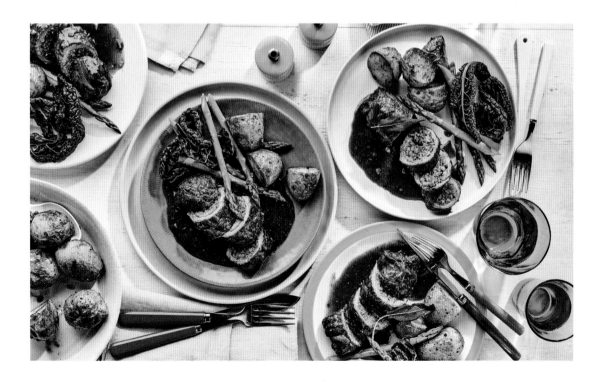

FREEZE ME

DAIRY FREE

USE DF CHEESE AND MILK

GLUTEN FREE

USE HENDERSON'S RELISH AND GF STOCK CUBES

COTTAGE PIE *with* A CHEESY CAULIFLOWER TOP

🕐 **20 MINS**   🍲 **50 MINS**   ✗ **SERVES 4**

PER SERVING:
427 KCAL / 21G CARBS

SPECIAL EQUIPMENT
18 x 27cm (7 x 10½in)
ovenproof dish

FOR THE FILLING
low-calorie cooking spray
2 onions, peeled and chopped
500g 5%-fat minced beef
2 medium carrots, peeled
  and cut into 1cm (½in) dice
2 celery sticks, thinly sliced
1 beef stock cube, dissolved
  in 500ml boiling water
1 tbsp Worcestershire sauce
  or Henderson's relish
1 tsp dried thyme
sea salt and freshly ground
  black pepper

**FOR THE CHEESY
CAULIFLOWER MASH**
500g cauliflower, cut into
  florets
60ml semi-skimmed milk
100g reduced-fat mature
  Cheddar cheese, finely grated
sea salt and freshly ground
  black pepper

TO SPRINKLE ON TOP
20g reduced-fat mature
  Cheddar cheese, finely grated

TO ACCOMPANY *(optional)*
80g steamed vegetables
  (+ 38 kcal per serving)

SWAP THIS: Swap the
beef mince for lamb, pork
or turkey mince.

How does cottage pie-meets-cauliflower cheese sound? We've given our timeless Cottage Pie a seriously cheesy twist by swapping out the mashed potato for a much lighter cauliflower topping. There's cheese mixed into the cauli mash and sprinkled over the top too, so just wait until this starts bubbling in the oven – it smells incredible!

Weekly Indulgence

Preheat the oven to 200°C (fan 180°C/gas mark 6).

To make the filling, spray a large frying pan (for which you have a lid) with low-calorie cooking spray and place over a medium heat. Add the onions and fry for about 5 minutes until starting to soften. Add the minced beef and fry, breaking it up with a wooden spoon, for 5 minutes, until lightly browned on all sides, then add the carrots, celery, beef stock, Worcestershire sauce or Henderson's relish and thyme. Season with salt and black pepper.

Cover and simmer over a medium heat for 20 minutes, taking the lid off for the last 5 minutes to reduce the gravy a little.

While the filling is cooking, make the cheesy cauliflower mash. Place the cauliflower florets in a large saucepan of boiling water, cover and simmer over a medium heat for about 15 minutes until soft.

Drain the cauliflower well and return it to the saucepan. Mash with the milk and cheese until smooth. Season well with salt and black pepper, to taste.

Place the beef filling in the ovenproof dish and spread it out evenly. Spoon the cheesy cauliflower mash on top and spread it out to cover the filling. Texture the top with a fork. Sprinkle the remaining cheese on the top and place on a baking tray. Place in the preheated oven for 20 minutes, until golden brown and piping hot throughout.

Serve at once with steamed vegetables or an accompaniment of your choice.

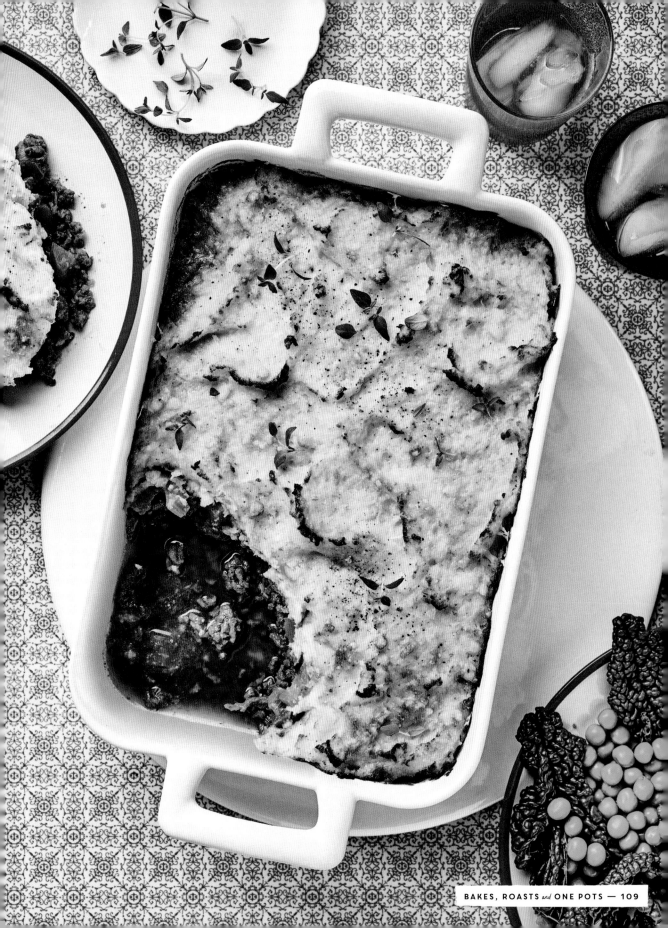

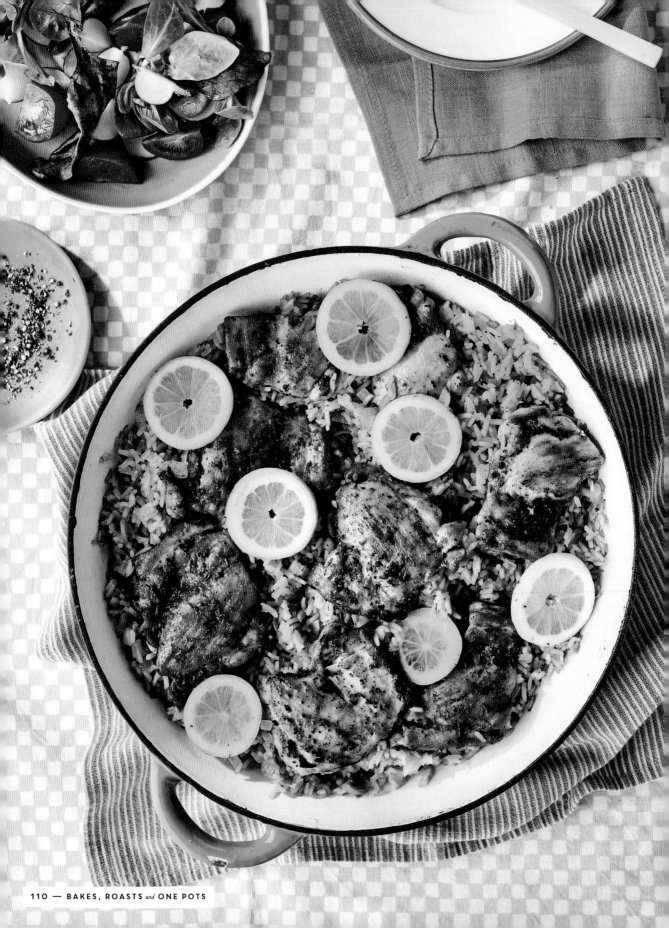

OVEN-BAKED GARLIC CHICKEN *and* RICE

🕐 **10 MINS** 🍲 **40 MINS** ✗ **SERVES 4**

FREEZE ME

DAIRY FREE

GLUTEN FREE

USE GF
STOCK CUBE

PER SERVING:
459 KCAL / 61G CARBS

SPECIAL EQUIPMENT
30cm (12in) lidded ovenproof and hob-proof casserole dish

low-calorie cooking spray
600g skinless, boneless chicken thighs (visible fat removed)
2 onions, peeled and finely diced
3 garlic cloves, peeled and crushed
275g long-grain rice
650ml chicken stock (1 chicken stock cube dissolved in 650ml boiling water)
1 lemon, sliced

FOR THE SEASONING MIX
1 tsp Italian mixed herbs
1 tsp garlic granules
½ tsp paprika
good pinch of salt and pepper

TO ACCOMPANY *(optional)*
75g mixed salad (+ 15 kcal per serving)

Big flavours, minimal effort and on the table in just 50 minutes – what more could you want from a one-pot dish? This is an easy crowd-pleaser to build a light family dinner around. We like this garlicky rice dish with salad. All the better with a squeeze of lemon!

Weekly Indulgence ───────────────

Preheat the oven to 180°C (fan 160°C/gas mark 4).

Combine the spices for the seasoning mix in a small bowl. Spray the chicken with low-calorie cooking spray and rub in the seasoning mix.

Spray the casserole dish with low-calorie cooking spray and place over a medium to high heat. Add the chicken thighs and seal on each side for 1 minute. Remove from the pan and set aside.

Add the onions to the pan and sauté for 5 minutes, until beginning to soften. Add the garlic and continue to cook for 1 minute.

Add the rice and stir around until well mixed with the garlic and onions. Pour in the stock and bring to the boil. Turn off the heat.

Lay the chicken thighs on top, and scatter over the lemon slices. Cover with a tight-fitting lid and place in the oven for 25 minutes.

When cooked, fluff up the rice with a fork and serve, with a mixed salad if you like.

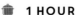

PESHAWARI-STYLE BAKED CHICKEN THIGHS

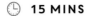 **15 MINS** 🍲 **1 HOUR** ✕ **SERVES 4**

PER SERVING:
349 KCAL / 19G CARBS

SPECIAL EQUIPMENT
Large, shallow ovenproof and hob-proof casserole dish or sauté pan
Blender or food processor

1 onion, peeled and roughly chopped
1 red chilli, deseeded
4 garlic cloves, peeled
5cm (2in) piece of ginger, peeled
low-calorie cooking spray
600g skinless, boneless chicken thighs (visible fat removed)
juice of ½ lemon
1 tbsp tomato puree
2 tsp garam masala
1 yellow or red pepper, deseeded and sliced
400ml coconut dairy-free milk alternative
250ml chicken stock (1 chicken stock cube dissolved in 250ml boiling water)
50g ground almonds
50g sultanas
handful of coriander leaves

TO ACCOMPANY *(optional)*
50g basmati rice per portion, cooked according to packet instructions (+ 173 kcal per 125g cooked serving)

TIP: If you like plenty of spice, leave the seeds in the chilli.

We've used low-calorie swaps to borrow the flavours from our favourite Peshawari naan bread for this recipe. It's so easy to make: leave everything to simmer in the pan and let the heat do all the work for you! The sweet and nutty mix of sultanas and almonds, combined with creamy coconut, make this chicken dinner a surefire favourite.

Special Occasion

Preheat the oven to 160°C (fan 140°C/gas mark 3).

Place the onion, chilli, garlic and ginger in a blender or food processor and blitz to a paste.

Spray the casserole dish with low-calorie cooking spray and place over a medium heat. When hot, add the chicken thighs and brown for 2 minutes on each side. Remove to a plate and place to one side.

Add the lemon juice to deglaze the dish, scraping up any crispy brown bits stuck to the bottom.

Give the dish another spritz with low-calorie cooking spray and then add the onion paste. Cook for 6 minutes, stirring well. Add the tomato puree and garam masala and stir well. Add the pepper.

Pour in the coconut milk and stock, then add the almonds and sultanas. Stir well and bring to a simmer. Return the thighs to the dish, then cover with a tight-fitting lid and place in the preheated oven for 30 minutes.

After 30 minutes, remove the lid and stir well. Return to the oven, uncovered for 15 minutes.

Sprinkle over the coriander leaves and serve with rice, or an accompaniment of your choice.

SWAP THIS: We used a plant-based dairy alternative coconut milk to save on fat and calories, but you can use tinned coconut milk if you prefer, but adjust the nutritional values accordingly!

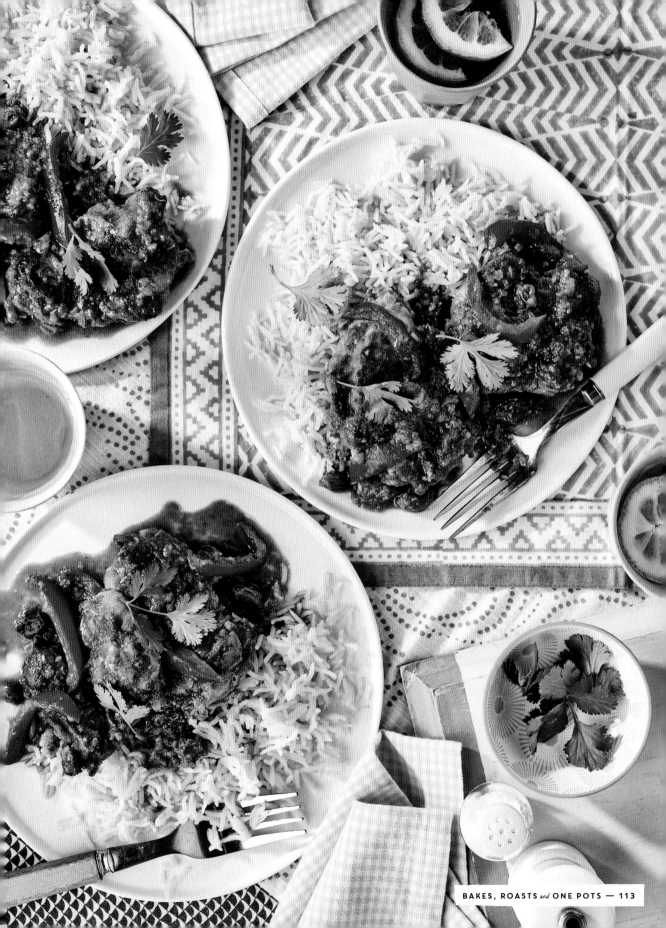

VEGGIE

USE VEGETARIAN
HARD CHEESE

FREEZE
ME

MINESTRONE PASTA BAKE

🕐 **10 MINS**　🗑 **15 MINS**　✕ **SERVES 4**

PER SERVING:
212 KCAL / 30G CARBS

SPECIAL EQUIPMENT
24cm (9½in) ovenproof dish

100g dried pasta
low-calorie cooking spray
1 onion, peeled and diced
1 red pepper, deseeded and
　diced
3 garlic cloves, peeled and
　crushed
1 courgette, diced
1 tbsp tomato puree
1 tsp balsamic vinegar
1 tsp dried mixed herbs
100ml boiling water
1 vegetable stock cube
200g tinned baked beans in
　tomato sauce
5 fresh basil leaves, thinly
　sliced
sea salt and freshly ground
　black pepper
10g vegetarian hard cheese
　or Parmesan, finely grated
30g reduced-fat Cheddar
　cheese, finely grated

This Minestrone Pasta Bake is a super-easy midweek meal that'll make the best of your veggies in a flash. We've stuck to traditional minestrone flavours in this homely dish with onions, beans and peppers stirred through. There's also a golden, bubbling layer of cheese on top because, well, why not?

Everyday Light ────────────────────

Add the pasta to a saucepan of boiling water and cook according to the packet instructions. This should usually take about 10 minutes.

While the pasta is cooking, spray a frying pan with low-calorie cooking spray and place over a medium heat. Add the onion and fry for 5 minutes, until just softening. Add the pepper, garlic and courgette and continue to fry for 2 minutes.

Add the tomato puree, balsamic vinegar, mixed herbs and boiling water in a jug. Crumble in the stock cube and stir. Add to the pan with the onion and peppers.

Add the baked beans to the pan, add the sliced basil and season with salt and pepper to taste. Allow the pan to simmer to heat the beans through.

When the pasta is cooked, drain well and add to the frying pan. Give the pan a good stir to coat the pasta. Preheat your grill.

Pour into the ovenproof dish and sprinkle over the Parmesan and Cheddar cheese. Pop under the grill for 5 minutes until the cheese is melted and golden. Enjoy!

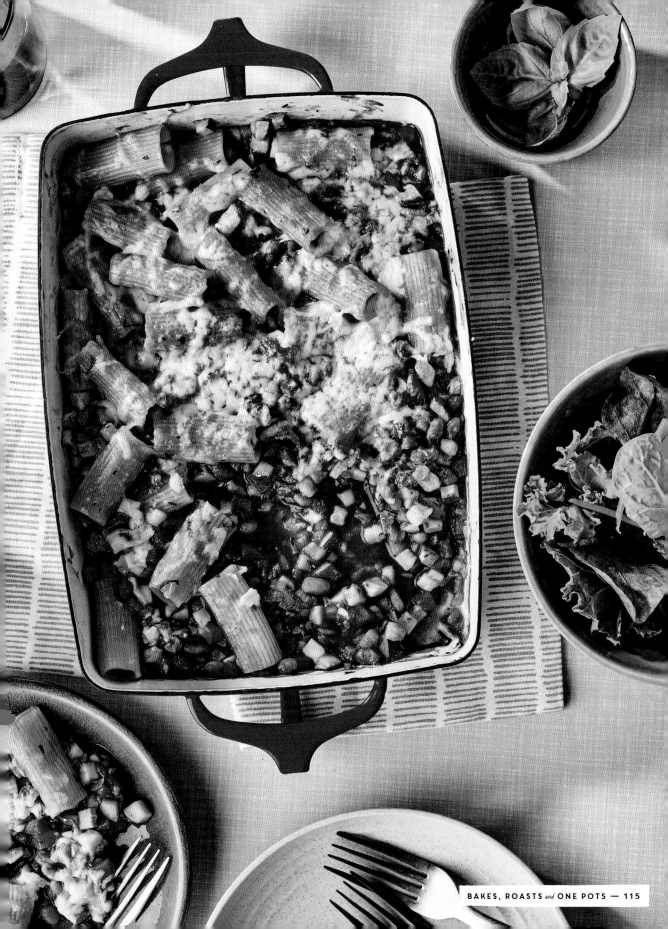

MINI CHICKEN KYIV BALLS

🕐 **20 MINS***   🗑 **VARIABLE** (SEE BELOW)   ✕ **SERVES 4**

*PLUS 35 MINS FREEZING

PER SERVING:
333 KCAL / 17G CARBS
(3 per serving)

SPECIAL EQUIPMENT
**Food processor or
mini chopper**

FOR THE FILLING
2 garlic cloves, peeled and
   crushed
4g fresh flat-leafed parsley,
   finely chopped
1 vegetable stock pot
¼ tsp onion granules
90g reduced-fat spread

FOR THE KYIVS
400g minced chicken breast
¼ tsp onion granules
2g fresh flat-leafed parsley,
   finely chopped
sea salt and freshly ground
   black pepper

FOR THE COATING
60g wholemeal bread
2 tbsp cornflour
1 egg, beaten

TO ACCOMPANY *(optional)*
75g mixed salad (+ 15 kcal
   per serving)

> **SWAP THIS:** You can
> replace the minced
> chicken breast with
> minced turkey breast.

These nifty baked bites are bursting with big Kyiv flavour! Stuffed with tasty garlic and parsley 'butter', we've even covered them in a crispy, golden breadcrumb shell.

Everyday Light ——————————————

OVEN METHOD
🕐 **20 MINS**

First make the filling. Add the garlic, parsley, vegetable stock pot, onion granules and reduced-fat spread to a mini chopper or food processor. Whizz until the garlic and parsley are fully combined.

Line a baking tray with greaseproof paper. Using a teaspoon, scoop out 12 mounds of the filling mixture and set on the baking tray. They don't have to be neat, but don't spread them out too much. Place the baking tray into the freezer for 35 minutes, until firm.

Meanwhile add the chicken mince, onion granules, parsley and a pinch of salt and pepper to a mixing bowl. Mix together using your hands, then cover and pop into the fridge.

Using an electric chopper or food processor, whizz the bread into fine breadcrumbs. Prepare three bowls with the breadcrumbs, cornflour and egg, ready for dipping the mini Kyivs. Preheat the oven to 200°C (fan 180°C/gas mark 6).

Take a walnut-sized amount of the chicken mixture and flatten it in your hand. Add a piece of the frozen spread mixture to the centre and encase it with the chicken mixture. Roll it a little between your hands to make a small ball. Repeat with the rest of the mixture to make 12 mini Kyivs. Roll a ball in the cornflour, then the beaten egg and, finally, into the breadcrumbs. Roll to coat on all sides and repeat with the rest of the Kyiv balls.

Line a baking tray with greaseproof paper and add the balls to the tray. Bake in the oven for 20 minutes, turning halfway through.

Serve with salad or your choice of accompaniment.

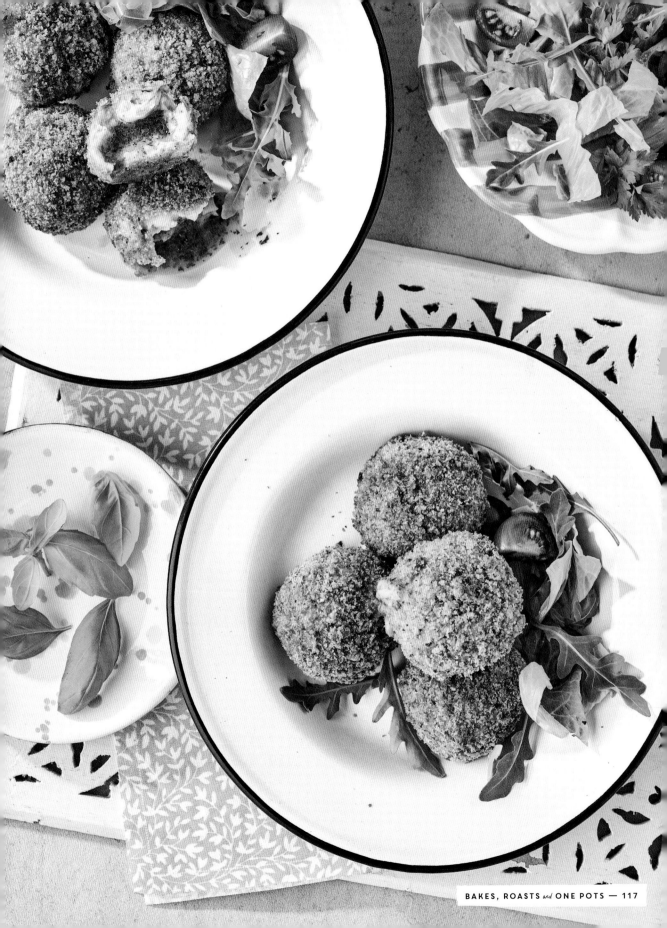

AIR-FRYER METHOD
🍳 15 MINS

SPECIAL EQUIPMENT
Air fryer

First make the filling. Add the garlic, parsley, vegetable stock pot, onion granules and reduced-fat spread to a mini chopper or food processor. Whizz until the garlic and parsley are fully combined.

Line a baking tray with greaseproof paper. Using a teaspoon, scoop out 12 mounds of the mixture and set on the baking tray. They don't have to be neat, but don't spread them out too much. Place the baking tray into the freezer for 35 minutes, until firm.

While the filling is in the freezer, prepare the chicken mixture. Add the chicken mince, onion granules, parsley and a pinch of salt and pepper to a mixing bowl. Mix together using your hands, then cover and pop into the fridge.

Using an electric chopper or food processor, whizz the bread into fine breadcrumbs. Prepare three bowls with the breadcrumbs, cornflour and egg, ready for dipping the mini Kyivs.

Preheat the air fryer to 180°C.

Take a walnut-sized amount of the chicken mixture and flatten it in your hand. Add a piece of the frozen spread mixture to the centre and encase it with the chicken mixture. Roll it a little between your hands to make a small ball. Repeat with the rest of the mixture to make 12 mini Kyivs.

Roll a ball in the cornflour, then the beaten egg and, finally, into the breadcrumbs. Roll to coat on all sides and repeat with the rest of the Kyiv balls.

Add the balls to the air fryer basket and cook for 15 minutes, turning halfway through to get an even golden colour. You may need to do this in batches, depending on the size of your air fryer.

Serve with a mixed salad or your choice of accompaniment.

> **TIPS:** If you don't have a mini chopper or food processor, chop the parsley and garlic really finely and mix together with the reduced-fat spread. If your air fryer doesn't have a preheat function, we suggest heating at cooking temperature for a few minutes before cooking your food.

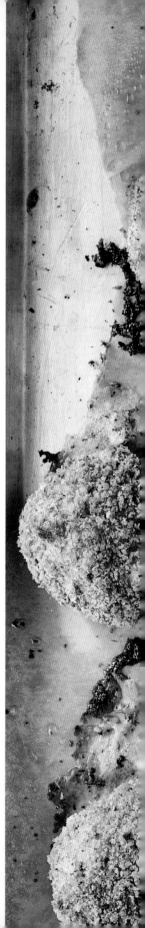

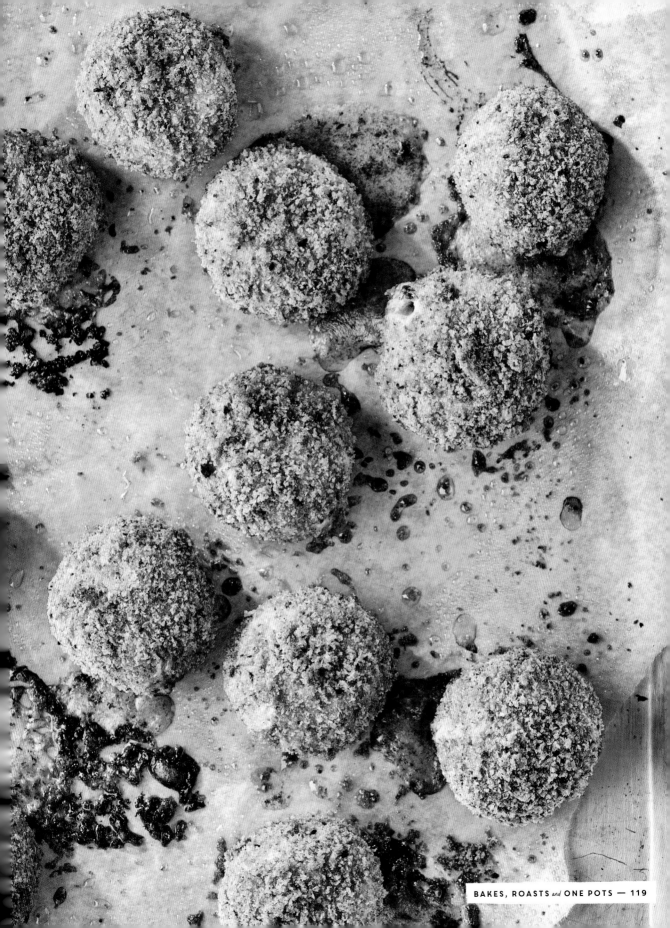

STEAK *and* KIDNEY PIE

 25 MINS   **2 HOURS 40 MINS**   ✕ **SERVES 4**

PER SERVING:
423 KCAL / 36G CARBS

SPECIAL EQUIPMENT
27 x 16cm (10½ x 6in) ovenproof dish

250g lamb kidneys
low-calorie cooking spray
1 onion, peeled and chopped
500g diced beef (visible fat removed)
2 tbsp cornflour
300ml beef stock (1 beef stock cube dissolved in 300ml boiling water)
1 tbsp Worcestershire sauce or Henderson's relish
2 dried bay leaves
½ tsp dried thyme
½ tsp dried parsley
200g button mushrooms, halved
sea salt and freshly ground black pepper

FOR THE TOP
4 sheets of filo pastry, about 180g
1 medium egg, beaten
fresh thyme leaves (optional)

TO ACCOMPANY *(optional)*
Roasted Garlic Mashed Potato (+ 250 kcal per portion)

SWAP THIS: You can swap the kidneys for an additional 250g diced beef.

We adore creating slimming-friendly versions of classic British dishes, and you can't get much more classic than a Steak and Kidney Pie. Say goodbye to the usual calorie-laden pastry topping – our light filo pastry is just as crisp and satisfying. Delicious gravied beef, kidneys, mushrooms and onions will feed the whole family – just serve creamy mash on the side.

Weekly Indulgence

Rinse the kidneys under cold running water and pat dry with kitchen paper. Place on a board. Cut the kidneys in half lengthways with a sharp knife. Use small sharp kitchen scissors to snip out the white core from the centre of each kidney half. Pull out all white parts and discard. Cut the kidneys into 2cm (¾in) pieces and set aside.

Spray a medium saucepan with low-calorie cooking spray and place over a medium heat. Add the onion and cook, stirring, for 5 minutes until lightly golden.

Add the beef and kidneys and cook for 4–5 minutes, until browned on all sides. Add the cornflour, stir in and cook for about 1 minute. Add the stock, Worcestershire sauce or Henderson's relish, bay leaves, thyme and parsley and stir well. Bring to the boil, then reduce the heat to low. Cover completely with a lid and simmer gently for 1½ hours, stirring frequently.

Add the mushrooms and stir in. Cover completely with a lid and simmer gently for 15 minutes. Preheat the oven to 180°C (fan 160°C/gas mark 4).

Remove the lid and continue to simmer for a further 15 minutes until the mushrooms are tender and the gravy has thickened.

Remove the bay leaves and season to taste with salt and black pepper. Transfer the filling into the ovenproof dish and spread it out evenly.

For the pastry top, cut the filo sheets into single-layer strips about 5cm (2in) wide.

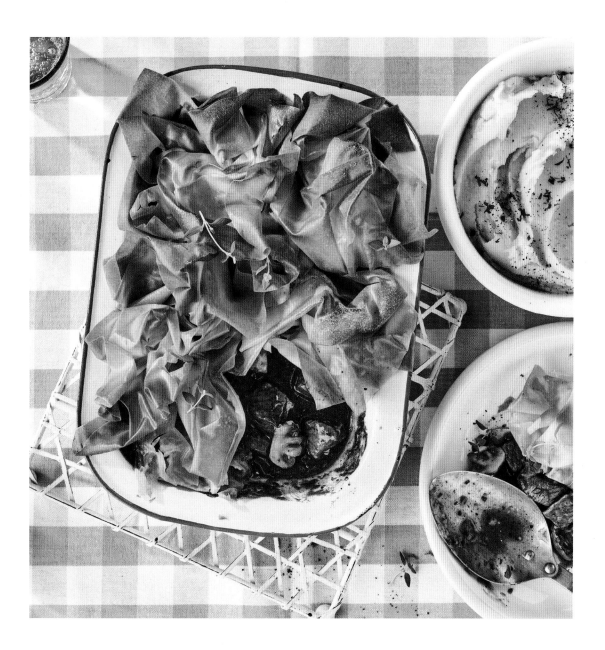

TIP: We used lamb kidneys, but any type will be fine. If they are covered with a membrane, make a cut with a small sharp knife, peel the membrane away and discard (most kidneys from supermarkets will already have the membrane removed).

Lay single-layer pastry strips over the filling, folding and curling them like ribbons. Don't worry if some strips break, it doesn't need to be perfect! Alternatively, scrunch up the single sheets and use them to cover the filling.

Carefully brush the pastry top with beaten egg and place on a baking tray. Place in the preheated oven and bake for 25–30 minutes until golden brown and piping hot throughout.

Serve sprinkled with thyme (if liked) and with Roasted Garlic Mashed Potato or another accompaniment of your choice.

BAKED COD BALLS

🕐 **10 MINS**   🗑 **VARIABLE** (SEE BELOW)   🍴 **SERVES 4**

PER SERVING:
287 KCAL /25G CARBS
(4 per serving)

1 medium potato, peeled and
   chopped into chunks
400g cod fillets, skinless and
   boneless
150ml skimmed milk
sea salt and freshly ground
   black pepper
1 leek, trimmed and
   finely diced
1 tsp garlic granules
grated zest of 1 lemon
2g fresh flat-leafed parsley
   leaves, finely chopped
2 eggs, beaten
80g panko breadcrumbs
low-calorie cooking spray

FOR THE SAUCE
2 tbsp tartare sauce
2 tbsp fat-free Greek-style
   yoghurt
1 tbsp lemon juice

These bite-size Baked Cod Balls are so much quicker to make than you might expect. In around half an hour, you'll be plating them up with some chips, or serving them as a tasty snack. Don't forget to dip them into the zingy tartare, lemon and yoghurt sauce!

Everyday Light ─────────────────────

OVEN METHOD
🗑 **22 MINS**

Preheat the oven to 180°C (fan 160°C/gas mark 4) and line a baking tray with non-stick baking paper.

Add the potato to a pan of cold water and bring to the boil. Cover with a lid, lower the heat to a simmer and cook for 7 minutes until the potatoes are soft. Drain well and mash. Leave to one side to cool.

While the potato is cooking, add the cod fillets to a small saucepan, pour over the skimmed milk and season with salt and pepper. Place over a low heat and cook for 7 minutes until the fish is flaky. Drain and discard the milk. Break the fish up with a fork and leave to cool.

Add the leek, garlic granules, lemon zest, parsley and a little salt and pepper to a large bowl. Add the fish and mashed potato and mix together until smooth and combined. Divide the mixture into 16 balls.

Add the beaten eggs to a bowl and the panko breadcrumbs to a plate. Dip a cod ball in the egg, being careful not to submerge it for too long as it may break up. Then roll the cod ball in the breadcrumbs.

Add the cod ball to the lined baking tray and repeat with the remaining balls. Spray with low-calorie cooking spray and place the tray into the oven for 15 minutes, until the breadcrumbs are lightly golden.

While the cod balls are cooking, add the tartare sauce, yoghurt and lemon juice to a small bowl and mix until smooth. Serve the cod balls alongside the sauce.

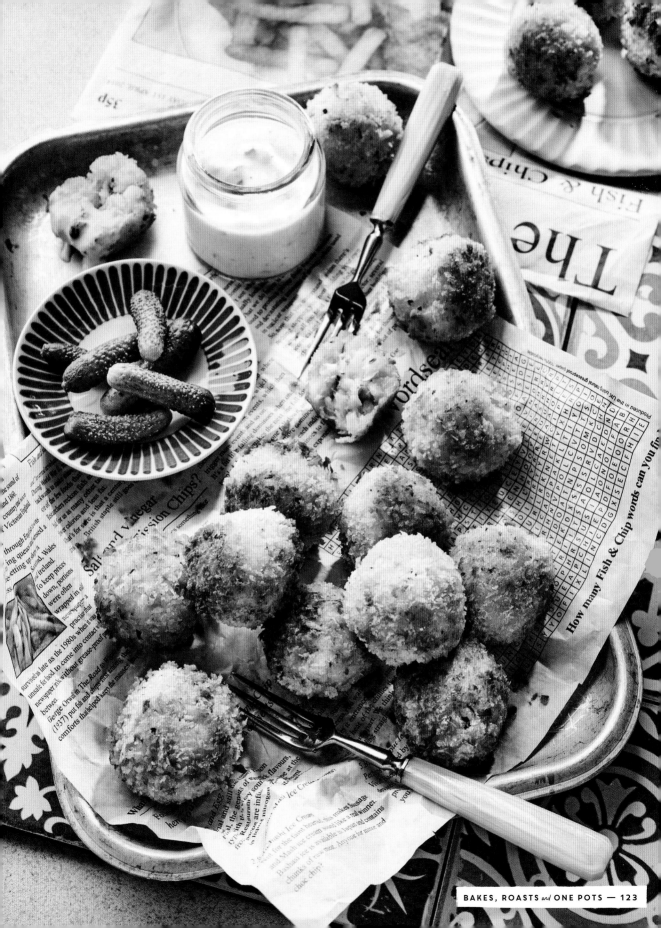

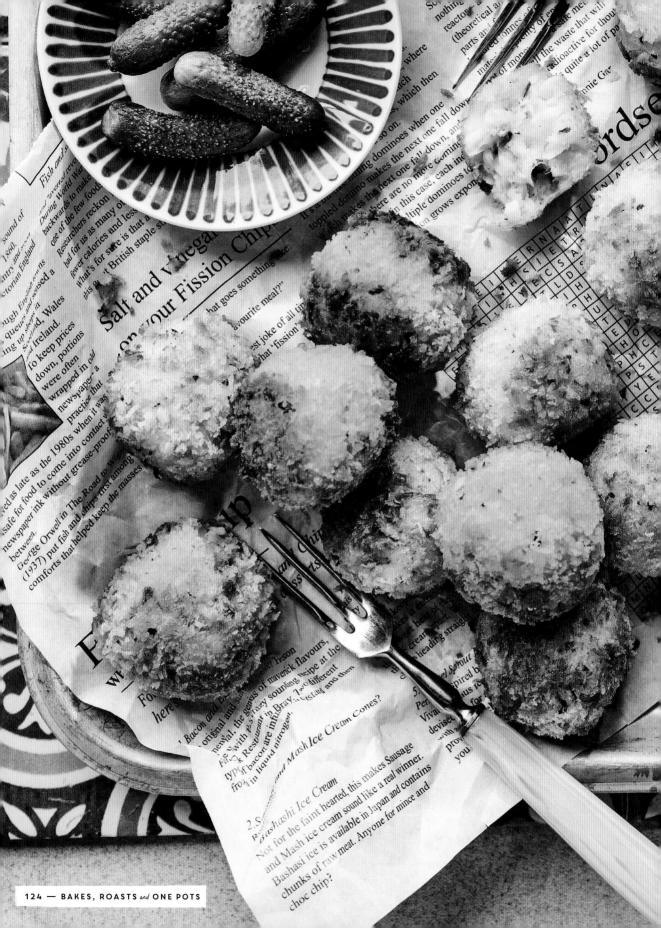

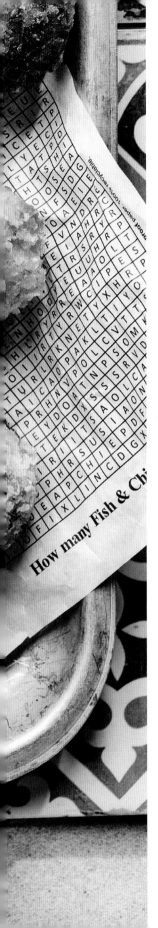

AIR-FRYER METHOD
🫓 12 MINS

SPECIAL EQUIPMENT
Air fryer

Preheat the air fryer to 170°C.

Add the potato to a pan of cold water and bring to the boil. Cover with a lid, lower the heat to a simmer and cook for 7 minutes until the potatoes are soft. Drain well and mash. Leave to one side to cool.

While the potatoes are cooking, add the cod fillets to a small saucepan, pour over the skimmed milk and season with salt and pepper. Place over a low heat and cook for 7 minutes until the fish is flaky. Drain and discard the milk. Break the fish up with a fork and leave to cool.

Add the leek, garlic granules, lemon zest, parsley and a little salt and pepper to a large bowl. Add the fish and mashed potato and mix until smooth and combined. Divide the mixture into 16 balls.

Add the beaten eggs to a bowl and the panko breadcrumbs to a plate. Dip a cod ball in the egg, being careful not to submerge it for too long as it may break up. Then roll the cod ball in the breadcrumbs. Repeat with the remaining cod balls.

Add the cod balls to the air fryer basket and spray with low-calorie cooking spray. Cook for 12 minutes until lightly golden. You may need to cook in batches, depending on the size of your air fryer.

While the cod balls are cooking, add the tartare sauce, yoghurt and lemon juice to a small bowl and mix until smooth. Serve the cod balls alongside the sauce.

"

Who'd have thought that with Pinch of Nom, weight loss could be so tasty?

— **PHILIPPA**

RAS EL HANOUT CHICKEN
and ORZO BAKE

🕐 **15 MINS** 🍲 **55 MINS** ✕ **SERVES 4**

PER SERVING:
523 KCAL / 66G CARBS

SPECIAL EQUIPMENT
Large lidded hob-proof and ovenproof casserole dish

600g skinless, boneless chicken thighs (visible fat removed)
low-calorie cooking spray
4 tsp ras el hanout
1 onion, peeled and finely chopped
2 mixed peppers, deseeded and diced
100g butternut squash, peeled and cut into 1cm (½in) dice
6 garlic cloves, peeled and crushed
1 x 400g tin chopped tomatoes
500ml chicken stock (2 chicken stock cubes dissolved in 500ml boiling water)
juice of 1 lemon
30g sultanas
250g orzo
handful of fresh coriander, roughly chopped

TO ACCOMPANY *(optional)*
75g mixed salad (+ 15 kcal per serving)

SWAP THIS: You could swap the sultanas for diced dried apricots.

This recipe is derived from one of our most popular recipes, One Pot Mediterranean-style Chicken and Orzo Bake. We've made it sweet and spicy (but not too spicy) to give it a Moroccan-style twist with the ras el hanout, tomatoes and a few sweet sultanas. Cooked all in one pot, because who wants to wash lots of pans, and only 523 calories, this is great for calorie counters or those following popular weight-loss plans.

Special Occasion ────────────

Preheat the oven to 180°C (fan 160°C/gas mark 4).

Cut the chicken thighs in half, place in a bowl and spray lightly with low-calorie cooking spray. Sprinkle over 2 teaspoons of ras el hanout and rub into the thighs until they are well covered.

Spray the casserole dish with low-calorie cooking spray and place over a medium heat. When hot, add the chicken thighs and seal for about 2 minutes on each side. Remove from the dish and set to one side.

Spray the same dish with low-calorie cooking spray and add the onion, peppers and butternut squash. Cook over a medium heat for around 5 minutes, until the vegetables are beginning to soften.

Add the garlic and remaining 2 teaspoons of ras el hanout. Stir in and cook for a minute to release the spice flavours. Add the tomatoes and 250ml of the stock. Return the chicken thighs back to the dish, cover and place in the oven for 15 minutes.

After 15 minutes, carefully remove the dish from the oven. Stir in the remaining stock and the lemon juice, the sultanas and the orzo and return, uncovered, to the oven. Cook for a further 20–25 minutes, stirring halfway through to ensure even cooking. The orzo should absorb most of the liquid, but still be moist. Add a little water when you stir it if it looks like it is drying out too much.

Sprinkle with the chopped coriander and serve with mixed salad or an accompaniment of your choice.

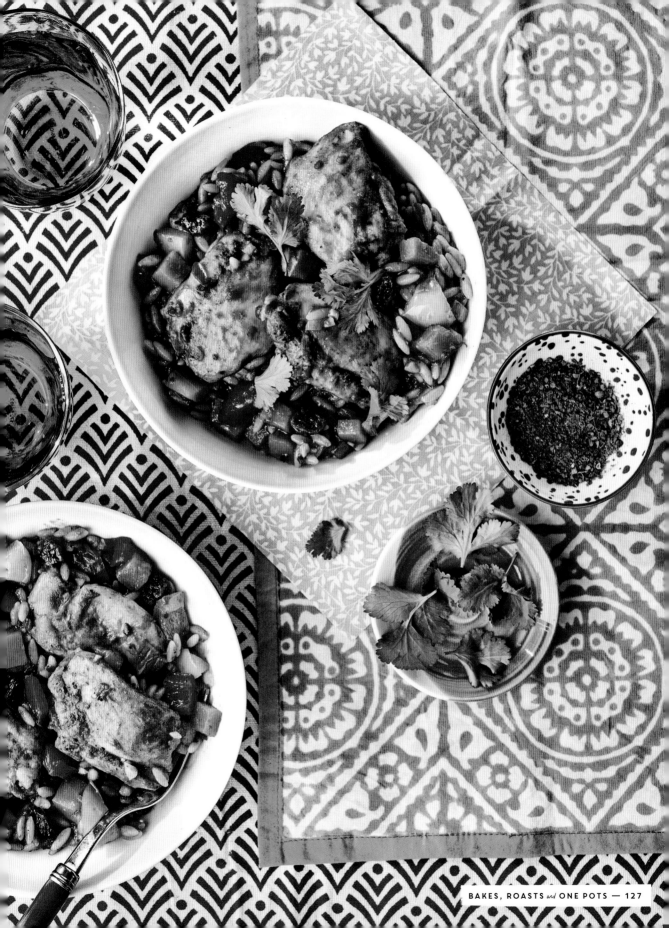

VEGAN BAKES

🕐 **15 MINS**   🗑 **20 MINS**   ✕ **SERVES 6**

PER BAKE:
177 KCAL / 27G CARBS

100g potato, peeled and cut
   into 1cm (½in) dice
40g carrot, peeled and cut
   into 1cm (½in) dice
25g parsnip, peeled and cut
   into 1cm (½in) dice
low-calorie cooking spray
200g meat-free mince
½ small onion, peeled and
   diced
100ml boiling water
½ vegetable stock cube
1 tbsp Henderson's relish
2 tsp Marmite
½ tsp onion granules
¼ tsp Dijon mustard
freshly ground black pepper
6 white or wholemeal
   sandwich thins
2 tbsp almond milk

TO ACCOMPANY (optional)
2 tbsp tomato ketchup (+ 15
   kcal per tbsp)

Trying to eat less meat? A vegan-friendly twist on a traditional Cornish pasty, these Vegan Bakes deliver all the flavours you're craving, so you'll never feel you're missing out. We've dropped calories by using sandwich thins instead of pastry. This is a yummy meat-free bite you can take on the go.

Everyday Light

Line a large baking tray with a sheet of non-stick baking paper.

Add the vegetables to a saucepan and cover with cold water. Place over a medium heat and bring to the boil. Cook for 6 minutes until softened, but holding shape. Drain and set aside.

While the vegetables are cooking, spray a frying pan with low-calorie cooking spray and place over a medium heat. Flake the meat-free mince into the pan and fry for 1–2 minutes, leaving it untouched. Add the onion and cook for 4 minutes, stirring.

Add the boiling water, crumbled stock cube, Henderson's relish, Marmite, onion granules and Dijon mustard to a measuring jug and stir to mix.

Add the softened vegetables to the pan. Pour in the stock and simmer, uncovered, for 4–5 minutes until thickened. Taste and season with black pepper. Allow to cool slightly.

Preheat the oven to 180°C (fan 160°C/gas mark 4). Split the sandwich thins in half and lay out on a chopping board.

Divide the mixture into six portions in the pan. Place a portion of the slightly cooled mixture onto six sandwich thin halves, leaving a 1cm (½in) gap around the edges. Brush the milk around the edges and place a sandwich thin half on top of the filling. Press the centre of the lid down gently with a flat hand, then press around the edges to seal. Use a fork to crimp the edges and seal well. Repeat until you've made six bakes. Place the bakes on the lined baking tray and brush all over with the remaining milk. Place in the oven and bake for about 10 minutes or until golden brown.

Transfer the bakes to a wire rack to cool before serving with tomato ketchup, if liked.

TIPS: Try not to stir the meat-free mince too much, as it may turn mushy and clump together in the pan. Cool the bakes on a rack rather than on the baking tray, otherwise the bases may become soggy.

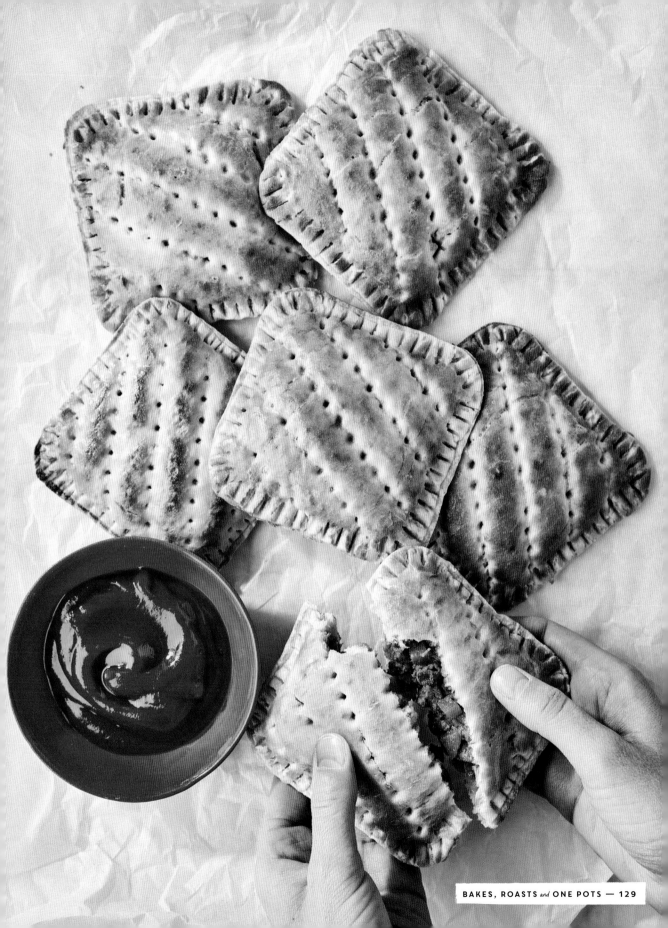

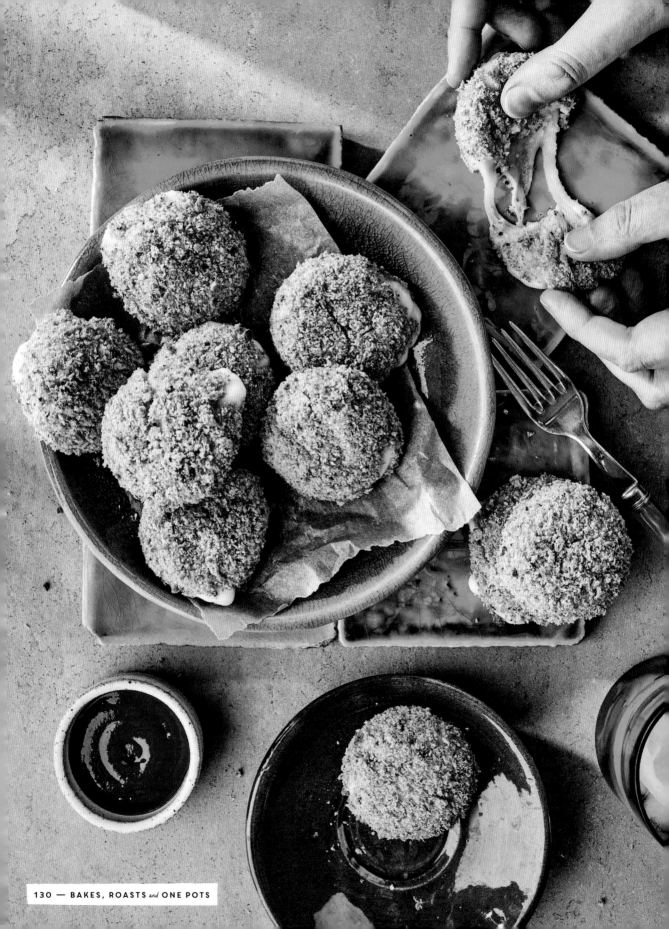

CRISPY HAM *and* CHEESE NUGGETS

🕐 **25 MINS***   🗑 **VARIABLE** (SEE BELOW)   ✗ **SERVES 4**

***PLUS 30 MINS CHILLING**

PER NUGGET:
219 KCAL / 26.8G CARBS
(3 nuggets per serving)

SPECIAL EQUIPMENT
**Food processor or
mini chopper**

300g potatoes, peeled and
  cut into chunks
sea salt and freshly ground
  pepper
150g wafer-thin ham
1 tsp wholegrain mustard
1 tbsp chopped chives
1 egg yolk
6 light Babybel, sliced in half
  widthways to form 12 discs
1 medium slice of wholemeal
  bread, about 60g
low-calorie cooking spray

TO ACCOMPANY *(optional)*
¼ tin baked beans (+ 95 kcal
  per portion)
70g corn on the cob (+ 32 kcal
  per portion)
2 tbsp tomato ketchup
  (+ 15 kcal per tbsp)

TIPS: These can be served straight from the oven as a main meal (3 nuggets per portion) for 219 kcal per serving. Alternatively, cool and serve chilled for a picnic or buffet. Toasting the breadcrumbs gives the nuggets an extra-crispy coating, which we love. Your nuggets will still be delicious even if you skip this step!

We've got three words for you: gooey cheese centre. Bite into these crispy nuggets when they're freshly cooked and you'll be rewarded with a mouthful of melty, cheesy deliciousness. Don't get us wrong, these are just as good cold too, so they'll be your new favourite thing to pack in a picnic or lunchbox.

Everyday Light ─────────────

OVEN METHOD
🗑 **40 MINS**

Cook the potatoes in a pan of salted boiling water for around 15 minutes, until soft. Drain well and mash. Leave aside to cool.

Using a food processor or mini chopper, blitz the ham to a fine crumb. Place in a bowl and add the cooled potatoes, mustard and chives. Mix together, taste and season with some salt and pepper if you wish.

Add the egg yolk and mix well. This will help the mixture stick together.

Divide the mixture into 12 portions and wrap each one around a Babybel disc. Form into mini burger shapes, ensuring the cheese is fully enclosed. Cover and place in the fridge to chill for 30 minutes.

Preheat the oven to 180°C (fan 160°C/gas mark 4). While the nuggets chill, blitz the bread to crumbs in a food processor. Spread evenly on a baking tray and place in the oven to toast for around 10 minutes. Remove and place on a plate to cool.

Increase the oven temperature to 200°C (fan 180°C/gas mark 6) and spray a baking tray with low-calorie cooking spray. Carefully dip each nugget into the breadcrumbs to lightly coat, and place on the baking tray, reshaping if needed.

Spray well with low-calorie cooking spray and bake in the oven for 12–15 minutes until crispy and golden. Serve with beans, corn on the cob and ketchup if liked.

AIR-FRYER METHOD
🍲 35 MINS

SPECIAL EQUIPMENT
Air fryer

Cook the potatoes in a pan of salted boiling water for around 15 minutes, until soft. Drain well and mash. Leave aside
to cool.

Using a food processor or mini chopper, blitz the ham to a fine crumb. Place in a bowl and add the cooled potatoes, mustard and chives. Mix together, taste and season with some salt and pepper if you wish.

Add the egg yolk and mix well. This will help the mixture stick together.

Divide the mixture into 12 portions and wrap each one around a Babybel disc. Form into mini burger shapes, ensuring the cheese is fully enclosed. Cover and place in the fridge to chill for 30 minutes.

Preheat the air fryer to 200°C.

While the nuggets chill, blitz the bread to crumbs in a food processor. Spread evenly on a baking tray and place in the oven to toast for around 10 minutes. Remove and place on a plate to cool.

Carefully dip each nugget into the breadcrumbs to lightly coat and place on the baking tray, reshaping if needed.

Spray well with low-calorie cooking spray and cook in the air fryer for 8–10 minutes, until crispy and golden. Try not to overload the air fryer to ensure even cooking. You may need to do this in two batches, depending on the size of your air fryer. Serve with beans, corn on the cob and ketchup if liked.

"

Loving cooking all of these recipes, not had a bad one yet!

—— AMY

CRISPY TOFU NUGGETS

🕐 **15 MINS** 🗑️ **VARIABLE** (SEE BELOW) 🍴 **SERVES 4**

PER SERVING:
149 KCAL /22G CARBS
(8 nuggets per serving)

FOR THE NUGGETS
low-calorie cooking spray
280g extra-firm tofu, thickly
  sliced
40g cornflour
1¼ tsp garlic granules
1¼ tsp onion granules
1¼ tsp smoked paprika
50g panko breadcrumbs
¼ tsp salt
¼ tsp ground black pepper
100ml unsweetened almond
  milk

FOR THE SPICY KETCHUP
3 tbsp reduced sugar and salt
  tomato ketchup
2 tsp maple syrup
1 tsp chipotle paste

TO ACCOMPANY (optional)
Homemade Oven Chips (from
  Pinch of Nom website) (+ 96
  kcal per portion)
¼ tin baked beans (+ 95 kcal
  per portion)

TIP: Make sure you really squeeze the moisture from the tofu, or the nuggets will be too wet!

SWAP THIS: You can swap the maple syrup for honey and the almond milk for coconut milk.

Who doesn't love nuggets? These vegan-friendly ones will put a smile on everyone's face! If you're not sure about tofu, we promise this recipe turns it into something special. These crispy nuggets make great finger food for snacking, as well as a cheeky midweek meal if you add some of our Homemade Oven Chips and beans. Don't worry, we didn't forget you need something to dip them in – this spicy ketchup is perfection!

Everyday Light ─────────────────

OVEN METHOD
🗑️ **30 MINS**

Preheat the oven to 200°C (fan 180°C/gas mark 6) and spray a baking tray with low-calorie cooking spray.

Place the tofu pieces between a clean folded tea towel. Gently press down on the tofu to remove the moisture. You may need to do this a few times to ensure the tofu is dry.

Add the cornflour to a plate and add ¼ teaspoon of the garlic granules, ¼ teaspoon of the onion granules and ¼ teaspoon of the smoked paprika. Mix until combined. Add the breadcrumbs to another plate and add the rest of the garlic and onion granules, paprika, salt and black pepper. Mix until combined.

Cut the tofu lengthways into four slices and then cut each slice into eight bite-sized pieces. Pour the almond milk into a shallow bowl and dip a piece of your tofu into the cornflour mixture first to lightly coat it, then dip it into the milk. Dip again into the cornflour and then into the milk, before adding to the breadcrumb mixture. Roll the tofu until coated on all sides. Add to the baking tray and repeat with all the nuggets.

Spray the tops of the nuggets with low-calorie cooking spray and place in the oven for 30 minutes, until crisp and golden, turning halfway through.

While the nuggets are cooking, add the tomato ketchup, maple syrup and chipotle paste to a small bowl and mix until combined. Serve the nuggets with the spicy ketchup dip, Homemade Oven Chips and baked beans if liked.

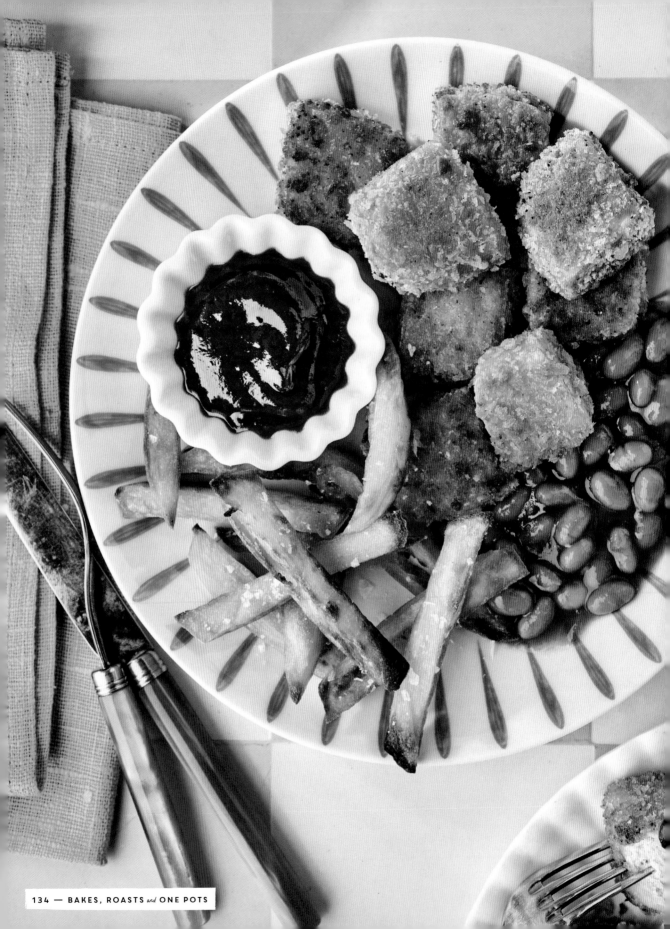

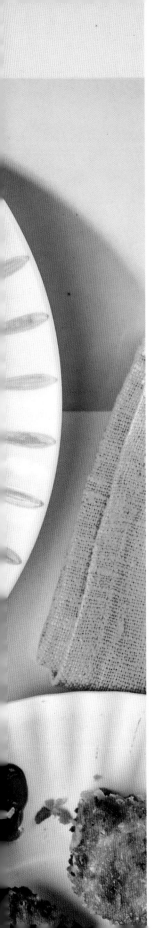

AIR-FRYER METHOD
🕐 15 MINS

SPECIAL EQUIPMENT
Air fryer

Preheat the air fryer to 180°C.

Place the tofu pieces between a clean folded tea towel. Gently press down on the tofu to remove the moisture. You may need to do this a few times to ensure the tofu is dry.

Add the cornflour to a plate and add ¼ teaspoon of the garlic granules, ¼ teaspoon of the onion granules and ¼ teaspoon of the smoked paprika. Mix until combined.

Add the breadcrumbs to another plate and add the rest of the garlic and onion granules, paprika, salt and black pepper. Mix until combined.

Cut the tofu lengthways into four slices and then cut each slice into eight bite-sized pieces. Pour the almond milk into a shallow bowl and dip a piece of your tofu into the cornflour mixture first to lightly coat it, then dip it into the milk. Dip again into the cornflour and then into the milk, before adding to the breadcrumb mixture. Roll the tofu until completely coated on all sides. Add to the baking tray and repeat with all the nuggets.

Place the nuggets into the air fryer basket. Spray the top of the nuggets with low-calorie cooking spray and cook for 15 minutes until crisp and golden, turning halfway through. You may need to do this in two batches, depending on the size of your air fryer.

While the nuggets are cooking, add the tomato ketchup, maple syrup and chipotle paste to a small bowl and mix until combined.

Serve the nuggets with the spicy ketchup dip, Homemade Oven Chips and baked beans if liked.

VEGGIE

USE VEGETARIAN
ITALIAN HARD
CHEESE

FREEZE
ME

GLUTEN
FREE

HERBY QUICHE *with a* POTATO CRUST

🕐 **20 MINS**　　🗑 **1 HOUR**　　✗ **SERVES 6**

PER SERVING:
211 KCAL /15G CARBS

SPECIAL EQUIPMENT
23cm (9in) round flan dish
Mandoline (useful but
not essential)

FOR THE POTATO CRUST
low-calorie cooking spray
350g medium potatoes,
　peeled and cut into very
　thin slices (around 2.5mm
　thick)
½ tsp garlic granules
sea salt and freshly ground
　black pepper
30g reduced-fat Cheddar
　cheese, finely grated

FOR THE FILLING
low-calorie cooking spray
1 small red onion, peeled and
　finely chopped
2 garlic cloves, peeled and
　crushed
6 spring onions, sliced
5 medium eggs
200ml skimmed milk
60g reduced-fat Cheddar
　cheese, finely grated
30g Parmesan cheese, finely
　grated
5g fresh dill, stalks removed
　and fronds roughly chopped
5g flat-leafed parsley, stalks
　removed and roughly chopped

TO ACCOMPANY *(optional)*
75g mixed salad (+ 15 kcal
　per serving)

Rather than calorific pastry, this light quiche has a crust made from potatoes! It's amazing what the humble spud can do: here it adds the perfect crunch to the filling. Try to slice your potatoes as thinly as possible (using a mandoline, if you have one) so they'll get nice and crispy in the oven.

Everyday Light

Preheat the oven to 180°C (fan 160°C/gas mark 4). Grease the flan dish with low-calorie cooking spray.

Place the potato slices in a medium mixing bowl and spray with low-calorie cooking spray. Add the garlic granules and season well with salt and black pepper. Use clean hands to toss the potato slices, so that each one is lightly coated. Line the sides and base of the greased dish with a single layer of overlapping potato slices. Make sure not to leave any gaps.

Sprinkle 30g grated cheese, in an even layer, over the potatoes in the dish. Place on a baking tray and pop into the preheated oven for 15–20 minutes, until the potatoes are just tender and turning lightly golden at the edges. Remove from the oven and set aside while you make the filling.

Reduce the oven temperature to 160°C (fan 140°C/gas mark 3). Spray a small frying pan with low-calorie cooking spray and place over a medium heat. Add the onion, garlic and spring onions and fry gently for 5–10 minutes, until softened.

Place the eggs and milk in a medium mixing bowl, and beat with a balloon whisk until just broken up and evenly mixed. Stir in the cooked onion, garlic and spring onions, plus 60g Cheddar cheese, Parmesan cheese, dill and parsley, and season well with salt and black pepper.

Carefully pour the filling into the potato case, taking care not to dislodge the potatoes. Spray the edge of the potato crust with a little low-calorie cooking spray. Place in the oven on the baking tray and bake for 30 minutes until set, and the potatoes are golden brown around the edges. Serve warm or cold with a mixed salad or other accompaniment of your choice.

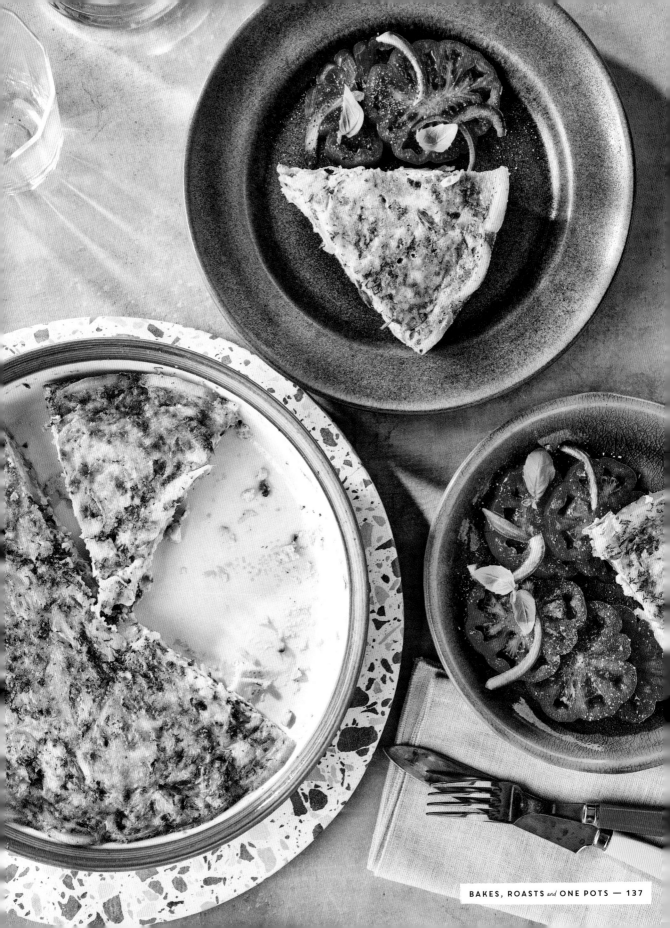

CREAMY VEGETABLE POT PIES

🕐 **15 MINS**　　🗑 **30 MINS**　　✕ **SERVES 4**

PER SERVING:
397 KCAL / 32G CARBS

SPECIAL EQUIPMENT
4 x 10cm (4in) round pie dishes or ramekins

low-calorie cooking spray
2 leeks, trimmed and sliced
1 garlic clove, peeled and crushed
2 medium carrots, peeled and diced
1 celery stick, sliced
100g button mushrooms, sliced
50g green beans, trimmed and sliced into 2cm (¾in) pieces
1 tsp Dijon mustard
½ tsp onion granules
150ml vegetable stock (1 vegetable stock cube dissolved in 150ml boiling water)
150ml light double cream alternative
1 tbsp plain flour
100g low-fat cream cheese
sea salt and freshly ground black pepper
½ sheet of light puff pastry (about 188g)
1 tbsp skimmed milk

TO ACCOMPANY
80g steamed vegetables (+ 38 kcal per serving)

Feeling like some comfort food? Pie is back on the menu! This slimming-friendly twist on a classic pot pie gives you golden pastry and veggies in a silky, rich sauce, all for 397 calories. You don't need to be precious about the filling – just about any vegetables will work, so if there's something you don't fancy in ours, swap it for a different veg!

Weekly Indulgence —————————

Preheat the oven to 180°C (fan 160°C/gas mark 4).

Spray a frying pan with low-calorie cooking spray and place over a medium heat. Add the leeks and fry for 2 minutes until beginning to soften. Add the garlic, carrots, celery and mushrooms and continue to fry for 3 minutes. Add in the green beans, Dijon mustard and onion granules.

Give the pan a stir and pour in the vegetable stock then the double cream alternative, turn down the heat and simmer for 5 minutes.

Put the plain flour into a small bowl and add a little water to make a smooth paste. Add to the pan, along with the low-fat cream cheese, and stir to combine until the pie filling has thickened. Remove the pan from the heat and season with salt and pepper. Leave to one side to cool slightly.

Un-roll the puff pastry and cut four circles around the top of each pie dish.

Spoon the pie mixture into each pie dish and top with a circle of puff pastry. Crimp the edges of the pastry with a fork to seal in the filling, make decorations for the top with any off-cut pastry and brush the top of the pies with the skimmed milk.

Place the pie dishes onto a baking tray and place into the oven for 20 minutes until the puff pastry is golden brown. Serve with steamed vegetables or your choice of accompaniment.

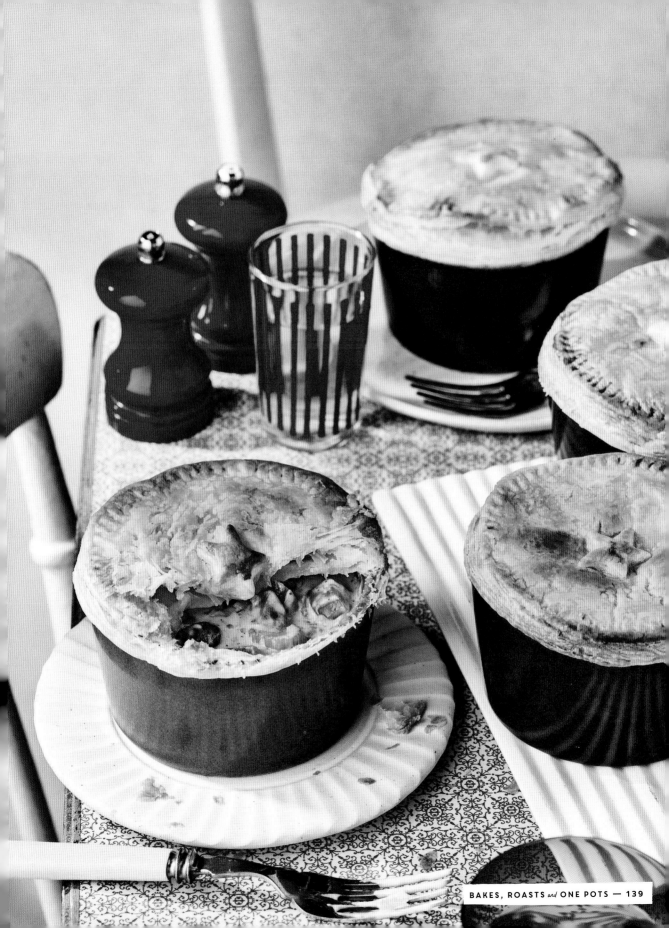

PORK SCHNITZEL

🕐 **10 MINS**   🗑 **VARIABLE** (SEE BELOW)   ✗ **SERVES 4**

PER SERVING:
204 KCAL / 6.6G CARBS

4 pork loin steaks, trimmed
  of fat
½ tsp smoked paprika
½ tsp garlic granules
good pinch of salt
good pinch of black pepper
50g panko breadcrumbs
1 medium egg, lightly beaten
low-calorie cooking spray
lemon wedges, to serve

TO ACCOMPANY
75g mixed salad (+ 15 kcal
  per serving)
225g baked potato wedges
  (+ 173 kcal per serving)

This Pork Schnitzel has far fewer calories than the traditional deep-fried version, without compromising on its crunchy crust – ours is a satisfying, crispy coating of panko breadcrumbs. Fresh from the oven or air fryer in under half an hour, why not serve it with a zesty salad or pair with chunky potato wedges for something a little different at dinner time?

Everyday Light

OVEN METHOD
🗑 **12–15 MINS**

Preheat the oven to 200°C (fan 180°C/gas mark 6).

Take each pork steak and place between two sheets of cling film or greaseproof paper. Using a heavy object such as a rolling pin, mallet or a pan, bash the steaks into an evenly thin escalope, about 5mm (¼in) thick.

Mix together the smoked paprika, garlic granules, salt and pepper, and rub into the pork.

Place the breadcrumbs on a plate. Dip the pork steaks into the beaten egg, and then into the breadcrumbs, making sure you get an even coating.

Spritz both sides of each pork steak with low-calorie cooking spray and place on a baking sheet.

Place into the preheated oven for 12–15 minutes, until crisp and golden. Serve with the lemon wedges and accompanied by a mixed salad and baked potato wedges.

AIR-FRYER METHOD
🗑 **8–10 MINS**

SPECIAL EQUIPMENT Air fryer

Preheat the air fryer to 200°C.

Take each pork steak and place between two sheets of cling film or greaseproof paper. Using a heavy object such

SWAP THIS: You can swap the pork loin steaks for butterflied chicken breasts.

TIP: If your air fryer doesn't have a preheat function, we suggest heating at cooking temperature for a few minutes before cooking your food.

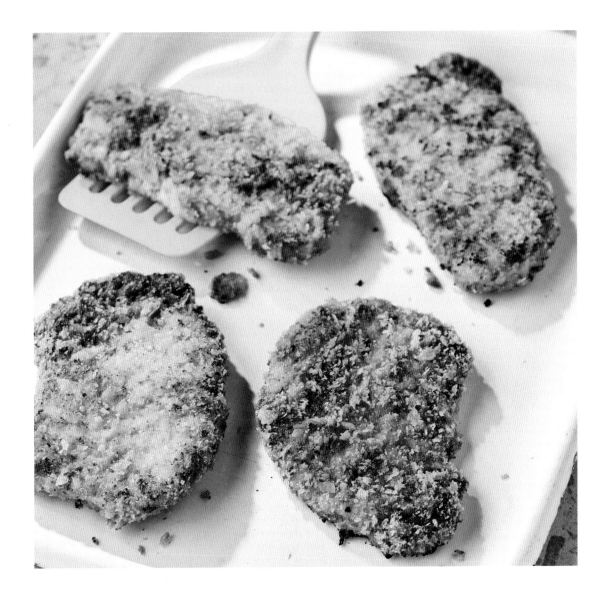

as a rolling pin, mallet or a pan, bash the steaks into an evenly thin escalope, about 5mm (¼in) thick. Mix together the smoked paprika, garlic granules, salt and pepper, and rub into the pork.

Place the breadcrumbs on a plate. Dip the pork steaks into the beaten egg, and then into the breadcrumbs, making sure you get an even coating. Spritz both sides of each pork steak with low-calorie cooking spray.

Place into the preheated air fryer for 8–10 minutes, flipping halfway through, until crisp and golden.

Serve with the lemon wedges and accompanied by a mixed salad and baked potato wedges.

USE GF
BREADCRUMBS

SLOW-COOKED MEATBALLS IN TOMATO SAUCE

🕐 **20 MINS**   🍲 **VARIABLE** (SEE BELOW)   🍴 **SERVES 4**

PER SERVING:
222 KCAL /18G CARBS

FOR THE MEATBALLS
250g 5%-fat minced beef
1 slice wholemeal bread,
  about 30g, made into
  breadcrumbs
½ tsp dried parsley
½ tsp dried oregano
½ tsp dried basil
½ tsp garlic granules
½ tsp onion granules
low-calorie cooking spray

FOR THE SAUCE
low-calorie cooking spray
1 onion, peeled and diced
3 garlic cloves, peeled and
  crushed
100g courgette, diced
100g aubergine, diced
1 x 400g tin chopped
  tomatoes
250g passata
½ tsp dried parsley
½ tsp dried basil
½ tsp dried oregano
½ tsp garlic granules
½ tsp onion granules
1 tsp Henderson's relish
1 tsp balsamic vinegar
sea salt and black pepper

TO SERVE
5 fresh basil leaves, finely
  sliced
20g Parmesan cheese, finely
  grated

TO ACCOMPANY (optional)
4 garlic bread slices (+ 92
  kcal per 26g serving)

We've covered these herby meatballs in a homemade tomato sauce packed with veggie goodness – we won't tell the fussy eaters if you don't! Whether cooked low and slow or left to simmer in the oven, the mince soaks up all the flavour. Pile them on spaghetti or fluffy mashed potato for a midweek warmer that'll go down a storm!

Everyday Light ─────────────────

OVEN METHOD
🍲 **45 MINS**

SPECIAL EQUIPMENT
30 x 20cm (12 x 8in) ovenproof dish
Handheld stick blender

First make the sauce. Spray a saucepan with low-calorie cooking spray and place over a medium heat. Add the onion and fry for 4 minutes, then add the garlic and fry for a further 2 minutes. Next, add the courgette and aubergine and fry for 2 more minutes, stirring every so often.

Pour in the chopped tomatoes and passata and sprinkle over the parsley, basil, oregano, garlic granules and onion granules. Stir through the Henderson's relish and balsamic vinegar. Lower the heat and simmer for 7 minutes.

While the sauce is simmering, preheat the oven to 190°C (fan 170°C/gas mark 5).

To make the meatballs, add the minced beef to a mixing bowl and add in the breadcrumbs, parsley, oregano, basil, garlic granules and onion granules. Give the beef and herbs a really good mix to fully combine – we find it's easier to use our hands.

Divide the mixture into 20 walnut-sized meatballs. Spray a frying pan with low-calorie cooking spray and place over a medium heat. Add the meatballs and lightly brown on all sides for 2 minutes.

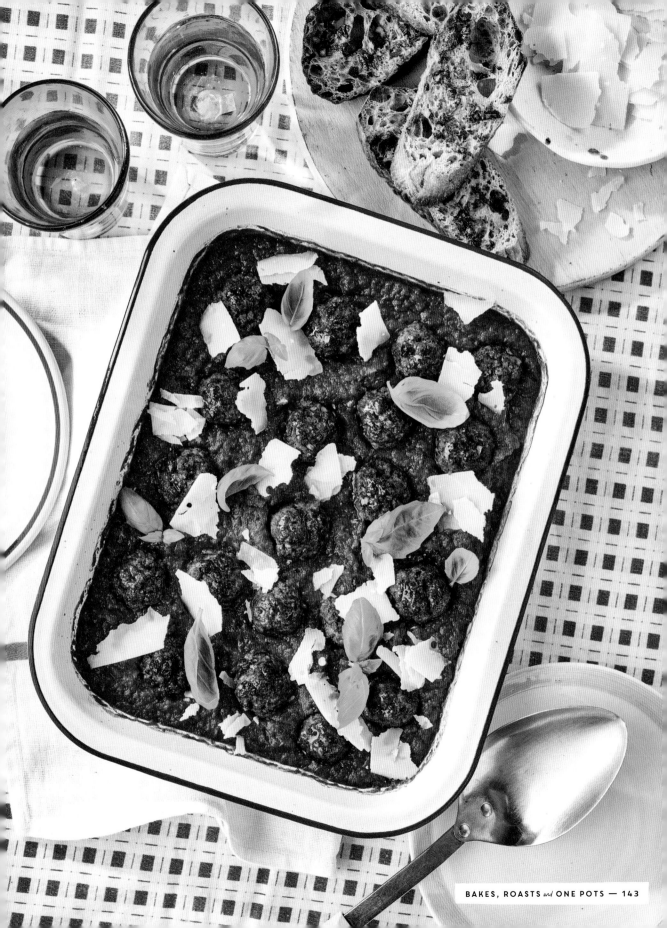

Once the sauce vegetables are soft, use a stick blender to blitz the sauce. We left chunky bits in ours but it's up to you how smooth you would like it. Season to taste with salt and pepper.

Pour the sauce into an ovenproof dish and add the meatballs on top. Cover the dish with foil and pop into the preheated oven for 30 minutes.

Remove from the oven and sprinkle over the sliced basil and Parmesan cheese. Serve with garlic bread or your choice of accompaniment.

SLOW-COOKER METHOD
HIGH: 2 HOURS

SPECIAL EQUIPMENT
Slow cooker
Handheld stick blender

First make the sauce. Spray a saucepan with low-calorie cooking spray and place over a medium heat. Add the onion and fry for 4 minutes, then add the garlic and fry for a further 2 minutes. Next, add the courgette and aubergine and fry for 2 more minutes, stirring every so often.

Pour in the chopped tomatoes and passata and sprinkle over the parsley, basil, oregano, garlic granules and onion granules. Stir through the Henderson's relish and balsamic vinegar. Lower the heat and simmer for 7 minutes.

While the sauce is simmering, add the minced beef to a mixing bowl and add in the breadcrumbs, parsley, oregano, basil, garlic granules and onion granules. Give it all a really good mix to fully combine – we find it's easier to use our hands.

Divide the mixture into 20 walnut-sized meatballs. Spray a frying pan with low-calorie cooking spray and place over a medium heat. Add the meatballs and lightly brown on all sides for 2 minutes.

Once the sauce vegetables are soft, use a stick blender to blitz the sauce. We left chunky bits in ours, but it's up to you how smooth you would like it. Season to taste with salt and pepper.

Pour the sauce into the slow cooker and add the meatballs on top. Cover with the lid and cook on high for 2 hours.

Remove the lid and sprinkle over the sliced basil and Parmesan cheese. Serve with garlic bread or your choice of accompaniment.

SWAP THIS: You can swap the minced beef for 5%-fat minced pork.

"

Thank you for bringing out great cookbooks with low-fat recipes!

— VANESSA

SPICED HADDOCK FISHCAKES

🕐 **20 MINS**　🗑 **VARIABLE** (SEE BELOW)　✗ **SERVES 4**

USE GF
BREADCRUMBS

PER SERVING:
213 KCAL / 24G CARBS

400g skinless, boneless
　smoked haddock
400ml semi-skimmed milk
　(or water, if preferred)
400g potatoes, peeled and
　cut into chunks
50g garden peas, cooked
　according to packet
　instructions
3 spring onions, trimmed and
　thinly sliced
½ tsp garlic granules
2 tsp mild curry powder
1 lemon, half zested and half
　cut into wedges
handful of fresh coriander,
　chopped
salt, to taste
low-calorie cooking spray
1 slice wholemeal bread,
　made into crumbs

TO ACCOMPANY *(optional)*
1 poached egg (+ 143 kcal per
　serving) or 75g mixed salad
　(+ 15 kcal per serving)

TIPS: Poaching the
haddock in milk gives it a
creamy flavour, but you can
poach in water if preferred.

Once you've tried fishcakes with a spice kick, you'll never go back. We've livened this up with some curry powder, and it goes so well with the smoky, salty haddock! Our haddock is poached in milk to give an added sweet, creamy texture, and you can ramp up the indulgence by serving with a soft poached egg on top too.

Everyday Light ───────────────

OVEN METHOD
🍲 **50 MINS**

Place the fish in a shallow pan (a small frying pan is ideal).

Cover with the milk or water and place over a medium to high heat. Bring to the boil, then take off the heat and cover. Allow to sit while you cook the potatoes. The heat from the milk will gently poach the fish.

Cook the potatoes in a saucepan of salted boiling water for around 20 minutes, until soft. Drain well and place back in the hot pan. Leave for 5 minutes to dry out, then mash well.

Place the mash in a large mixing bowl and add the peas, spring onions, garlic granules, curry powder, lemon zest and coriander.

Remove the haddock from the pan using a slotted spoon or fish slice, draining off any excess liquid. Flake the fish into the bowl with the mashed potatoes. Discard the poaching liquid.

Mix well until thoroughly combined. Taste and add a little salt if needed.

Preheat the oven to 200°C (fan 180°C/gas mark 6) and spray a non-stick baking sheet with low-calorie cooking spray.

Roll the fishcake mix into eight evenly-sized balls.

Place the breadcrumbs in a bowl and add a fishcake ball one at a time. Roll around until well-coated, and then flatten slightly into a fishcake shape.

Place on the baking sheet and spray each one well with low-calorie cooking spray.

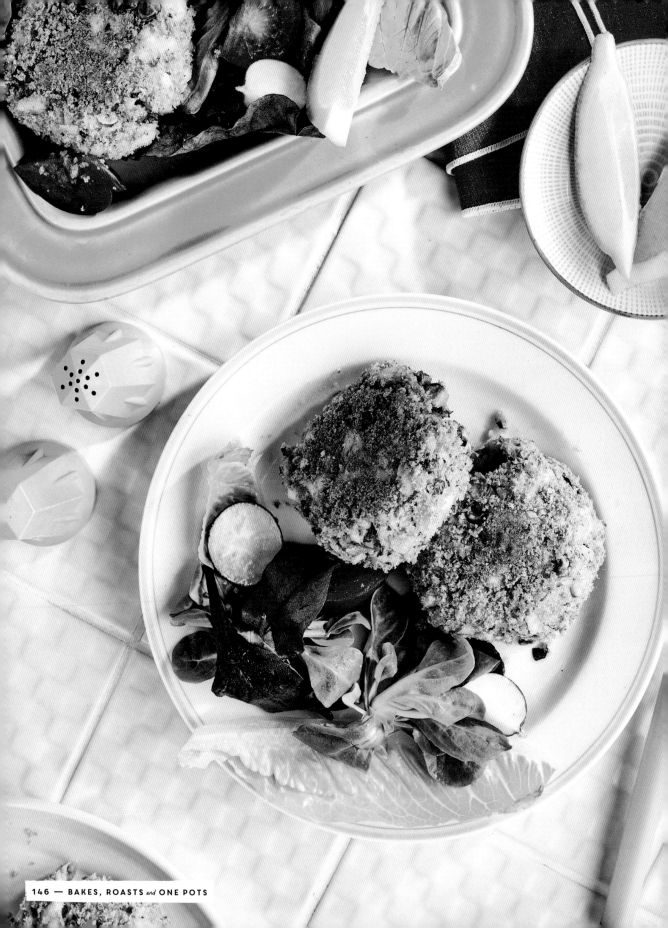

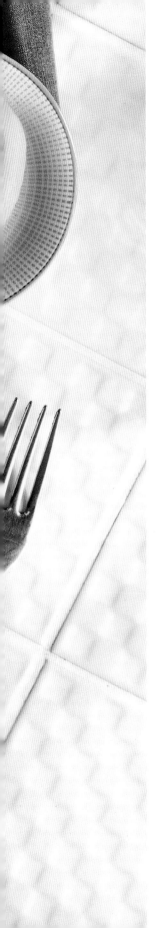

Place in the oven for 25–30 minutes, carefully flipping them over after 15 minutes. The fishcakes are cooked when the breadcrumbs are golden and crispy.

Serve two fishcakes per portion, garnished with the lemon wedges and, if you like, salad or a poached egg on top.

AIR-FRYER METHOD
40 MINS

SPECIAL EQUIPMENT **Air fryer**

Place the fish in a shallow pan (a small frying pan is ideal).

Cover with the milk or water and place over a medium to high heat. Bring to the boil then take off the heat, cover and allow to sit while you cook the potatoes. The heat from the milk will gently poach the fish.

Cook the potatoes in a pan of salted boiling water for around 20 minutes, until soft. Drain well and place back in the hot pan. Leave for 5 minutes to dry out, then mash well.

Place the mash in a large mixing bowl and add the peas, spring onions, garlic granules, curry powder, lemon zest and coriander.

Remove the haddock from the pan and flake the fish into the bowl with the mashed potatoes.

Mix well until thoroughly combined. Taste and add a little salt if needed.

Preheat the air fryer to 200°C.

Roll the fishcake mix into eight evenly-sized balls. Place the breadcrumbs in a bowl and, one at a time, add a fishcake ball. Roll around until well coated, and then flatten slightly into a fishcake shape.

Spray each fishcake well with low-calorie cooking spray. Place in the air fryer basket for 15 minutes, carefully flipping them over halfway through cooking.

The fishcakes are cooked when the breadcrumbs are golden and crispy, so if they are not crispy after 15 minutes continue cooking for a little longer.

Serve two fishcakes per portion, garnished with the lemon wedges and, if you like, salad or a poached egg on top.

SALMON GRATIN

🕐 **15 MINS**   🗑 **35 MINS**   ✕ **SERVES 4**

PER SERVING:
408 KCAL / 44G CARBS

SPECIAL EQUIPMENT
28cm (11in) ovenproof dish

600g potatoes, peeled and
    cut into 2cm (¾in) dice
sea salt and freshly ground
    black pepper
150g tenderstem broccoli
250ml skimmed milk
250ml vegetable stock
    (1 vegetable stock cube
    dissolved in 250ml boiling
    water)
2 tbsp cornflour, mixed to a
    slurry with 2 tbsp water
½ tsp onion granules
½ tsp garlic granules
1 tsp wholegrain mustard
150g reduced-fat spreadable
    cheese
15g Parmesan cheese,
    finely grated
a squeeze of lemon juice
2 skinless, boneless salmon
    steaks, about 220g in total,
    cut into thin slices
15g panko breadcrumbs
lemon wedges, to serve

TO ACCOMPANY *(optional)*
75g mixed salad (+ 15 kcal
    per serving)

We're obsessed with the oh-so-satisfying panko breadcrumb topping on this cheesy salmon bake. If crispy, baked salmon wasn't enough, we've smothered broccoli and potatoes in an irresistible cheese sauce. Perfect for when you fancy a break from meat, you'll be able to count on the winning flavours in this fish dish time and time again. Lemon wedges are a must!

Weekly Indulgence

Preheat the oven to 180°C (fan 160°C/gas mark 4).

Place the potatoes in a pan and cover with cold, salted water.

Bring to the boil and cook for 3 minutes. Add the broccoli and cook for a further 3 minutes. The potatoes should be just cooked and the broccoli should still be crisp and green. Drain well.

While the potatoes are cooking, make the cheese sauce. Add the milk and stock to a saucepan and heat until just boiling, then quickly stir in the cornflour slurry. Allow to bubble for a minute to cook out the cornflour, then reduce the heat.

Stir in the onion and garlic granules, mustard, spreadable cheese, half the Parmesan and the squeeze of lemon juice. Taste and season with some salt and pepper if required. Tip the drained potatoes and broccoli into the ovenproof dish, and mix in the salmon slices.

Pour over the cheese sauce, and top with the remaining Parmesan and the panko breadcrumbs.

Place on a baking sheet and bake in the oven for 25 minutes, until golden brown. Serve with some lemon wedges, and a mixed salad if you like.

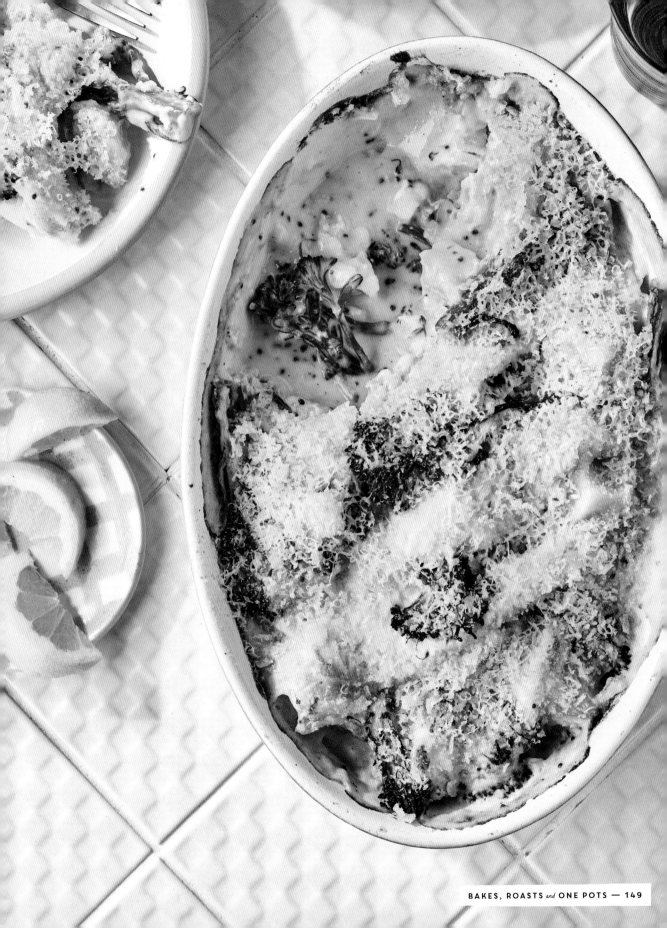

CREAMY MAPLE *and* BACON CHICKEN

🕐 **5 MINS**　🗑 **30 MINS**　🍴 **SERVES 4**

PER SERVING:
296 KCAL /16G CARBS

low-calorie cooking spray
1 onion, peeled and finely
   sliced
4 garlic cloves, peeled and
   crushed
4 smoked bacon medallions,
   diced
680g diced chicken breast
2 tbsp white wine vinegar
1 tbsp Henderson's relish or
   Worcestershire sauce
200ml chicken or pork stock
   (1 chicken or pork stock
   cube dissolved in 200ml
   boiling water)
½ tsp sweet smoked paprika
½ tsp mustard powder
2 tbsp maple syrup
180g low-fat cream cheese
sea salt and freshly ground
   black pepper
a few flat-leafed parsley
   leaves, finely chopped, to
   garnish (optional)

TO ACCOMPANY *(optional)*
80g steamed vegetables
   (+ 38 kcal per serving)

A little bit of maple syrup goes a long way in this indulgent-tasting recipe! The sweet and smoky syrup is the perfect match for savoury, salty bacon and juicy chicken. It all comes together into a rich, creamy dish that we love to pair with the fresh flavour of steamed green veggies.

Everyday Light

Spray a large frying pan with low-calorie cooking spray and place over a medium heat. Add the onion, garlic and bacon to the pan and cook for 5 minutes, or until the onion begins to soften.

Add the chicken, vinegar and Henderson's relish to the pan and cook for another 5 minutes, until the outside of the chicken has coloured.

Add the stock, paprika, mustard and maple syrup to the pan and stir well. Make sure that the stock is bubbling in the pan, increasing the heat if you need to! Keep the chicken and sauce simmering with plenty of movement on the surface, and cook for 15–20 minutes – or until almost all the liquid has evaporated and you are left with a thick glaze.

When the sauce has thickened to a glaze and the chicken is cooked through, take the pan off the heat and stir through the cream cheese, season with salt and pepper, top with the chopped parsley (if using) and serve with steamed vegetables if you like.

TIPS: This dish is also great with mushrooms or peppers added. If it takes a long time to reduce your stock, you may not have the heat high enough or the pan you are using may not be wide enough. Shallower, wider pans like frying pans have a bigger surface area, so the liquid can reduce faster. If you are using a deeper pan like a saucepan, add the stock cube directly to the chicken and add only half of the water, adding more later if you need to.

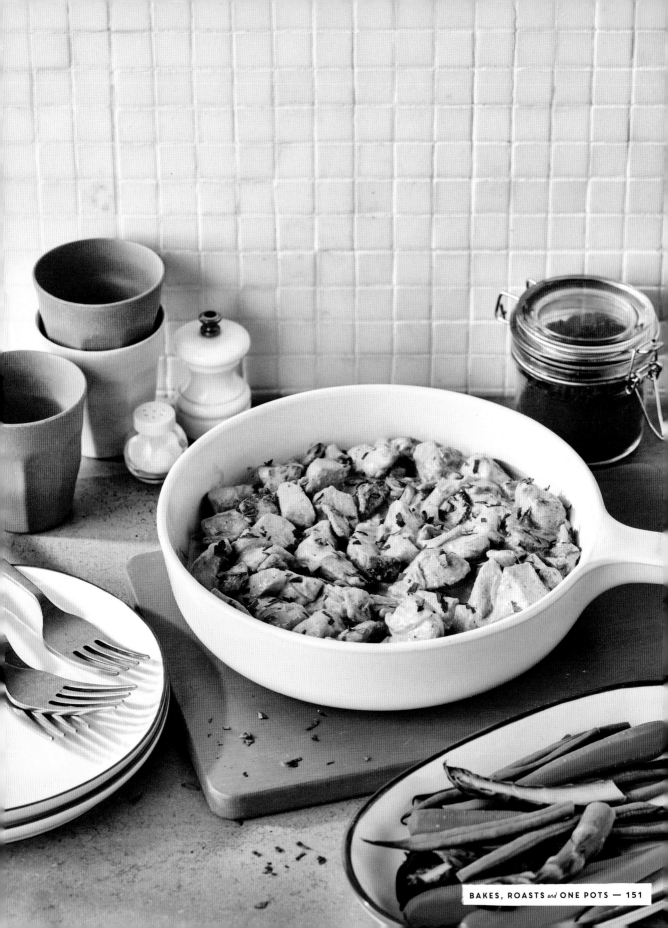

SPICY SALSA CANNELLONI

🕐 **35 MINS**   🗑 **1 HOUR 30 MINS**   ✕ **SERVES 6**

PER SERVING:
303 KCAL / 30G CARBS

SPECIAL EQUIPMENT
20 x 28cm (8 x 11in)
ovenproof dish

FOR THE TOMATO SAUCE
low-calorie cooking spray
1 onion, peeled and finely
   chopped
1 garlic clove, peeled and
   crushed
½ small red chilli, deseeded
   and finely chopped
1 x 400g tin chopped tomatoes
350ml chicken stock
   (1 stock cube dissolved in
   350ml boiling water)
sea salt and black pepper
5g fresh coriander leaves,
   roughly chopped

FOR THE CANNELLONI
low-calorie cooking spray
1 small onion, peeled and
   finely chopped
2 garlic cloves, peeled and
   crushed
1 small red chilli, deseeded
   and finely chopped
½ small red pepper,
   deseeded and finely diced
½ small green pepper,
   deseeded and finely diced
1 tsp mild chilli powder
300g 5%-fat minced beef
1 tbsp Worcestershire sauce
   or Henderson's relish
1 tbsp tomato puree
1 x 400g tin chopped tomatoes
1 x 215g tin red kidney beans
   in water, drained
12 'no precook' cannelloni
   tubes

We've given a twist to this classic Italian-style dish, drawing inspiration from the flavours of Mexico. The cannelloni is stuffed with a spiced beef chilli mixture, and the tomato sauce has the flavours of a salsa, with red chilli and fresh coriander. It's topped with a layer of crispy, golden cheese and is delicious with a mixed salad and a little sliced avocado.

Everyday Light ————————————————

To make the tomato sauce, spray a medium saucepan with low-calorie cooking spray and place over a medium heat. Add the onion and fry for 5 minutes until softening. Add the garlic and red chilli and fry for 1–2 minutes.

Add the tinned tomatoes and chicken stock. Stir, then bring to the boil. Lower the heat and simmer, uncovered, for 15 minutes. Remove from the heat and season with salt and black pepper to taste. Stir in the chopped coriander leaves and set aside.

To make the cannelloni, spray a medium frying pan with low-calorie cooking spray and place over a medium heat. Add the onion and fry for 3–4 minutes until softening.

Add the garlic and red chilli and fry for 1–2 minutes. Then add the red and green peppers and fry for 4–5 minutes, stirring.

Add the chilli powder and minced beef and, breaking up the mince with a wooden spoon, brown on all sides for 3–4 minutes.

Add the Worcestershire sauce or Henderson's relish, tomato puree and tinned tomatoes. Stir and simmer over a low heat for 10 minutes.

Stir in the kidney beans and cook for a further 10 minutes until all liquid has been reduced and you have a moist mixture.

Preheat the oven to 180°C (fan 160°C/gas mark 4). To assemble, place half of the tomato sauce in the base of the ovenproof dish. Spread it out.

Use a teaspoon to fill the cannelloni tubes with the beef mixture. You can pack the mixture down tightly into the tubes using the handle of the teaspoon.

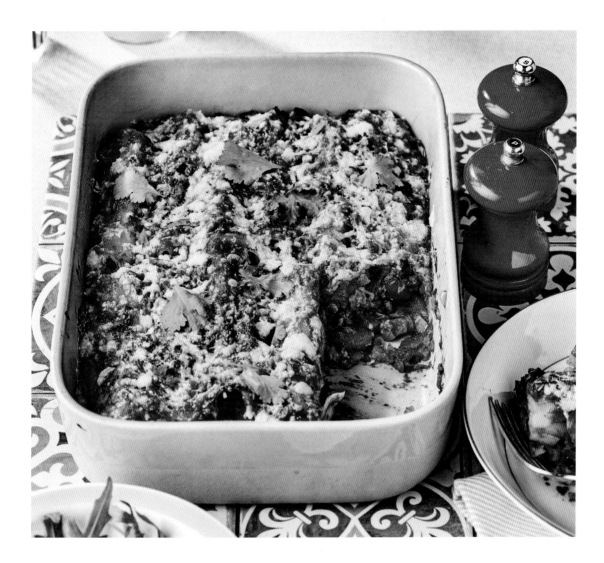

FOR THE TOP
80g reduced-fat Cheddar
  cheese, finely grated
4g fresh coriander leaves,
  roughly chopped

TO ACCOMPANY *(optional)*
75g mixed salad (+ 15 kcal per
  serving)
¼ sliced avocado (about 35g)
  (+ 69 kcal per serving)

Place the filled cannelloni tubes in the dish, on top of the tomato
sauce layer, then pour over the remaining tomato sauce and
spread it over the cannelloni. Sprinkle the grated cheese all over
the top.

Place in the preheated oven for about 30 minutes, until the
pasta is tender, and the top is golden brown.

Sprinkle with the chopped coriander leaves and serve at
once, with a mixed salad and a little sliced avocado.

TIP: This dish is fairly mild.
If you prefer things hot, you
could add another teaspoon
of chilli powder to the beef.

SWAP THIS: You could
swap the beef for minced
turkey or 5%-fat minced
lamb or pork.

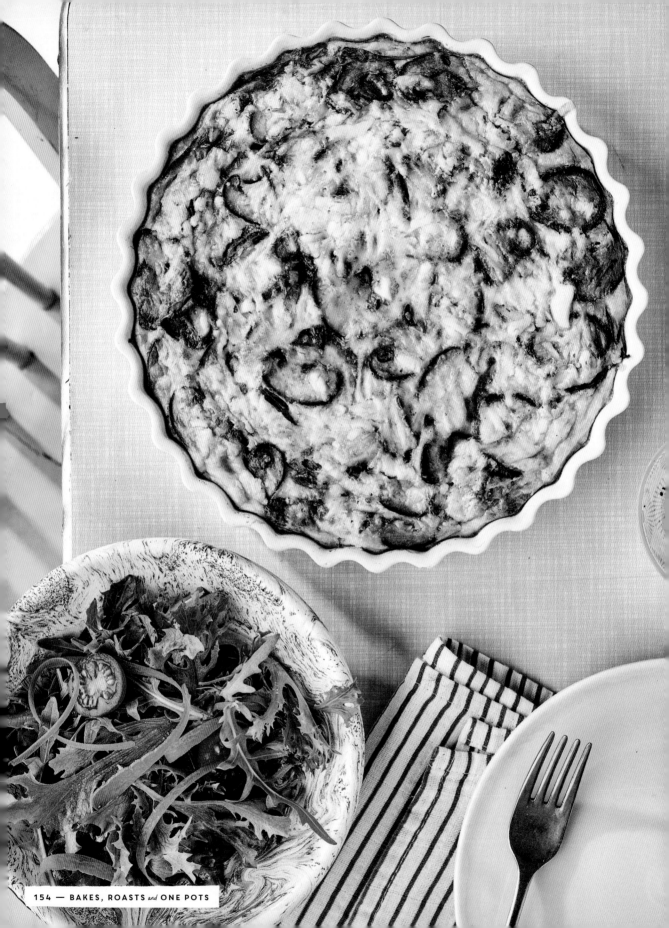

CREAMY GARLIC MUSHROOM QUICHE

🕐 **10 MINS**   🗑 **45 MINS**   ✗ **SERVES 6**

VEGGIE

FREEZE ME

GLUTEN FREE

LOW CARB

PER SERVING:
207 KCAL / 5.3G CARBS

SPECIAL EQUIPMENT
24cm (9½in) quiche dish

low-calorie cooking spray
½ red onion, peeled and finely sliced
4 garlic cloves, peeled and crushed
300g mushrooms (any firm kind), sliced
50g spinach
6 large eggs, beaten
200ml light single cream alternative
120g reduced-fat mature Cheddar, grated
sea salt and freshly ground black pepper

TO ACCOMPANY *(optional)*
75g mixed salad (+ 15 kcal per serving)
225g baked potato (+ 173 kcal per serving)

It's no secret that we love a Crustless Quiche, and this one combines two of our favourite flavours: garlic and mushrooms. So creamy and cheesy, once you taste this, you'll find it hard to believe it's only 207 calories per slice. Served hot or cold, for lunch or dinner, this recipe ticks every box!

Everyday Light ———————————————

Preheat the oven to 170°C (fan 150°C/gas mark 3) and spray a frying pan with low-calorie cooking spray.

Place over a medium heat, add the onion and sauté for 5 minutes until soft.

Add the garlic and mushrooms and continue to cook. After 5 minutes, the mushrooms should start to release moisture. It's important to keep cooking until all this has evaporated. This could take up to another 5 or 6 minutes, depending on the mushrooms and the size of pan you use.

When the mushrooms are cooked, add the spinach and stir for 1–2 minutes, until it has wilted.

In a mixing bowl, beat together the eggs, single cream alternative and Cheddar. Stir in the mushroom mix, and season with salt and pepper to taste.

Pour the mixture into the quiche dish and cook in the oven for 30 minutes, or until the top is golden and the middle is just set.

Cut into six slices and serve, with a mixed salad and a baked potato if liked. This can be eaten warm or can be chilled and served cold.

SWAP THIS: You could swap the light single cream alternative for regular single cream, for additional calories.

MEATBALL LASAGNE

 10 MINS   45 MINS   ✕ SERVES 4

PER SERVING:
308 KCAL /28G CARBS

SPECIAL EQUIPMENT
Handheld stick blender
30 x 20cm (12 x 8in)
lasagne dish

FOR THE MEATBALLS
250g 5%-fat minced beef
1 medium egg
½ tsp garlic granules
½ tsp onion granules
1 tsp dried mixed herbs
sea salt and freshly ground
  black pepper
low-calorie cooking spray

FOR THE LASAGNE
low-calorie cooking spray
1 onion, peeled and diced
1 pepper, deseeded and
  diced
1 carrot, peeled and finely diced
1 courgette, diced
1 garlic clove, peeled and
  crushed
1 beef stock cube
1 x 400g tin chopped
  tomatoes
1 tbsp balsamic vinegar
1 tbsp Henderson's relish or
  Worcestershire sauce
1 tbsp tomato puree
1 tsp dried oregano
6 dried lasagne sheets

FOR THE TOPPING
180g low-fat cream cheese
40g fat-free natural yoghurt
1 tsp Dijon mustard
sea salt and freshly ground
  black pepper
6g reduced-fat Cheddar
  cheese, finely grated

We've used two ultimate comfort foods to create this hearty Meatball Lasagne. Instead of mince, we've layered up herby, homemade meatballs in-between sheets of pasta. Our rich tomato sauce is bursting with chunky vegetables for extra texture, but you can blitz yours into a smoother sauce if you'd prefer.

Weekly Indulgence

Preheat the oven to 190°C (fan 170°C/gas mark 5). In a bowl add the beef mince, egg, garlic granules, onion powder, mixed herbs and a good pinch of salt and pepper. Mix together with your hands until well combined, then roll into 12 equally-sized balls.

Spray a frying pan with low-calorie cooking spray and place over a medium to low heat. Add the meatballs and cook for 5 minutes until golden brown, turning as you cook to get an even colour. Remove from the pan and set aside.

Spray the same frying pan with low-calorie cooking spray and place back over a medium to low heat. Add the onion and pepper, and cook for 5 minutes until they begin to soften.

Add the carrot, courgette and garlic and continue to cook for a further 5 minutes. Crumble in the stock cube then add the chopped tomatoes, balsamic vinegar, Henderson's relish, tomato puree, oregano and mix well. Simmer for 5 minutes. At this stage, we blitzed half the vegetables in the pan with a stick blender to create more of a tomato sauce texture; you can leave it as a chunky vegetable mixture, if you prefer. Once you have blitzed half the vegetables, stir through the rest of the pan.

Add half of the sauce to the bottom of the lasagne dish and spread it out. Lay three of the lasagne sheets on top. Add the meatballs on top and then pour over the rest of the sauce. Place the other three lasagne sheets on top of the meatball and sauce layer.

Add the cream cheese, yoghurt, mustard and a pinch of salt and pepper to a bowl and stir until smooth. Spread the mixture on top of the lasagne sheets. Sprinkle over the grated cheese and loosely cover the top of the dish with foil.

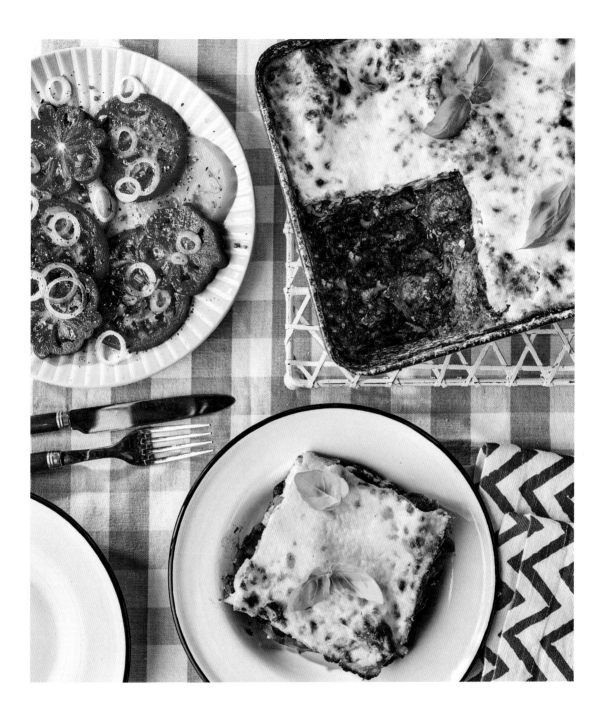

5g torn basil leaves, to garnish (optional)

TO ACCOMPANY *(optional)*
75g mixed salad (+ 15 kcal per serving)

Place the lasagne into the oven for 20 minutes. Remove the foil and cook for a further 10 minutes. The lasagne will be ready when you can push a knife into it and feel that the pasta is soft and not crunchy. If you would like a little more colour on top, you can pop it under the grill for a few minutes until the cheese is bubbly and brown. Top with torn basil leaves if you like, and serve with a mixed salad.

CREAMY BACON, ONION *and* POTATOES

 🕐 **10 MINS**   🗑 **45 MINS**   ✗ **SERVES 4**

PER SERVING:
266 KCAL / 27G CARBS

low-calorie cooking spray
2 onions, peeled and thinly
   sliced
2 garlic cloves, peeled and
   crushed
8 smoked bacon medallions
500g new potatoes,
   unpeeled, cut into 5mm
   (¼in)-thick slices
600ml chicken stock
   (1 chicken stock cube
   dissolved in 600ml boiling
   water)
½ tsp dried mixed herbs
180g low-fat cream cheese
black pepper, to taste
a few flat-leafed parsley
   leaves, finely chopped, to
   garnish (optional)

TO ACCOMPANY *(optional)*
80g steamed vegetables
   (+ 38 kcal per serving)

We've turned cheap and cheerful ingredients into this indulgent-tasting dish that you can make without even turning your oven on. The recipe couldn't be any simpler: everything goes into a pan and, in under an hour, you can be tucking into creamy potatoes and salty bacon.

Everyday Light ──────────────

Spray a large frying pan with low-calorie cooking spray and place over a medium heat. Add the onions and cook gently for 10 minutes until softened and golden.

Add the garlic and whole bacon medallions and cook for 5 minutes. Turn the bacon once and cook until slightly coloured and cooked through.

Add the potatoes in an even layer, pour over the stock and sprinkle over the mixed herbs. Cover the frying pan tightly with a lid or tight-fitting kitchen foil. Simmer over a medium heat for about 20 minutes, or until the potatoes are tender when tested with a sharp knife.

Remove the frying pan from the heat and gently stir in the cream cheese until completely blended, taking care not to break up the potatoes. Return to the heat and simmer, uncovered, for about 10 minutes or until the sauce has reduced and thickened to your liking. If the sauce is too thin, continue to simmer, uncovered, for a bit longer until it has reduced and thickened. If the sauce is too thick, stir in a little water.

Season to taste with black pepper. Serve topped with fresh parsley if you like and with some fresh steamed veggies or an accompaniment of your choice.

SWAP THIS: You could swap the bacon for cooked ham or cooked gammon. Simply add for the final 10 minutes after the cream cheese is stirred in.

TIPS: We recommend a low-fat cream cheese rather than a fat-free one. The result is a little richer and reheats better if you batch cook the recipe. Use new potatoes in this dish as the slices will stay whole and won't break up as easily as floury potatoes. Cut them into uniform 5mm (¼in)-thick slices so that they cook evenly.

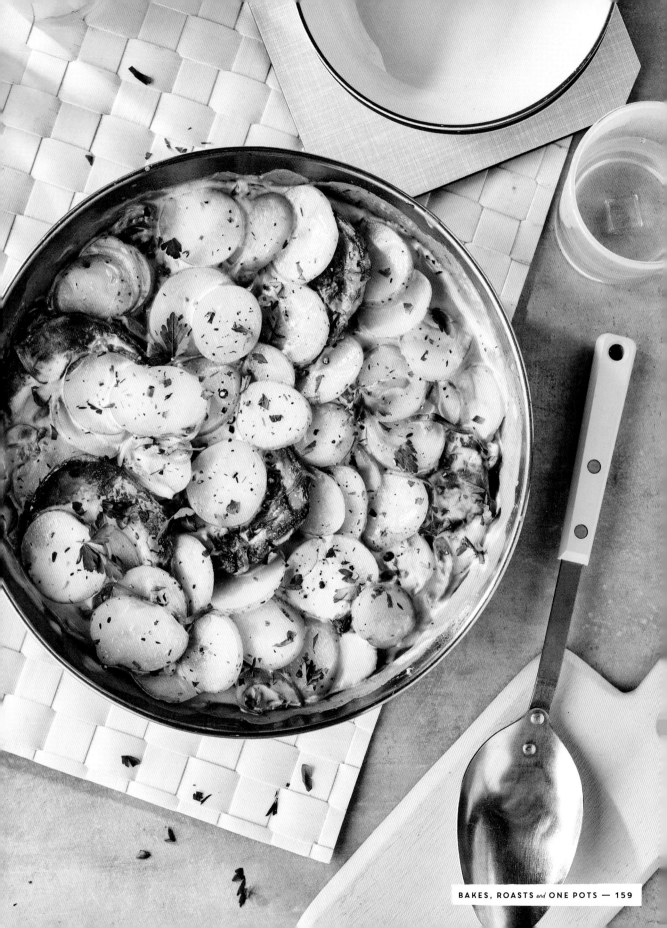

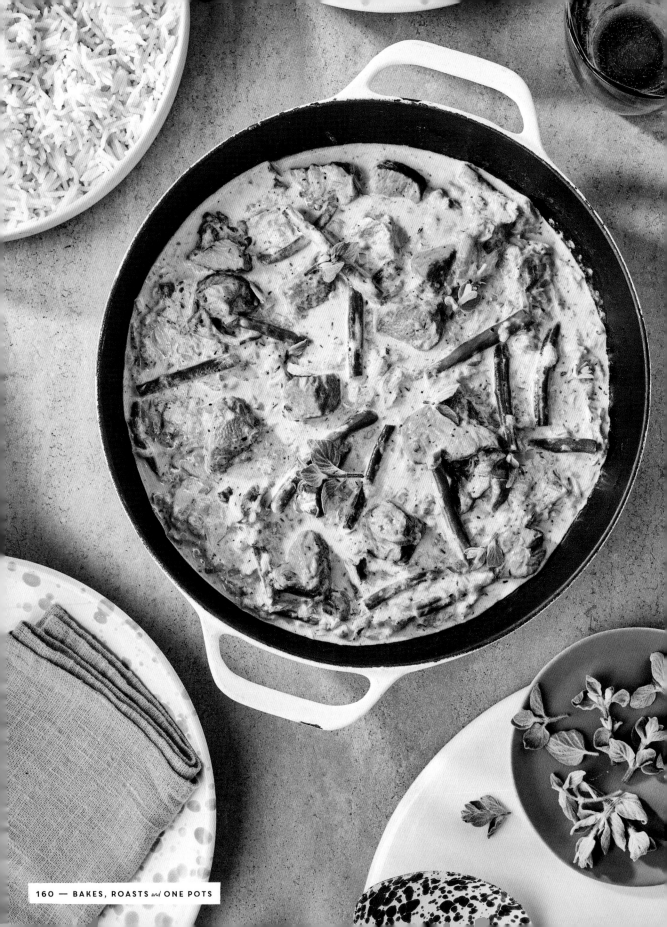

NORMANDY-STYLE CHICKEN

FREEZE ME

GLUTEN FREE

USE GF STOCK CUBE

🕐 **20 MINS**　🗑 **VARIABLE** (SEE BELOW)　✕ **SERVES 4**

low-calorie cooking spray
2 onions, peeled and thinly sliced
3 garlic cloves, peeled and crushed
1 medium leek, trimmed and thinly sliced
2 cooking apples, about 150g each, peeled, cored and thickly sliced
600g diced chicken breast
800ml chicken stock (1 stock cube, dissolved in 800ml boiling water)
2 tbsp Dijon mustard
1 tsp dried thyme
1 tsp dried oregano
100g fine green beans, trimmed and halved
180g low-fat cream cheese
sea salt and black pepper
a few fresh oregano leaves, to garnish (optional)

TO ACCOMPANY
50g uncooked basmati rice per portion, cooked according to packet instructions (+ 173 kcal per 125g cooked serving) or 225g baked potato (+ 173 kcal per serving)

SWAP THIS: You could use wholegrain mustard instead of Dijon mustard in this recipe. Other mustards, such as English mustard, wouldn't be suitable, as they have a much hotter flavour!

It's no secret that we love creamy dishes, and we couldn't wait to put our spin on this rich chicken dinner from Normandy in France. It's the apple, onion, leek and Dijon mustard flavours that make this dish hard to say no to. Whether you stew it low and slow or bake it in the oven, it's bound to impress.

Weekly Indulgence ———————————————————

OVEN METHOD
🍲 **2 HOURS 5 MINS**

Preheat the oven to 180°C (fan 160°C/gas mark 4).

Spray a large frying pan with low-calorie cooking spray and place over a medium heat. Add the onions and cook for 8–10 minutes, until softened and golden.

Add the garlic, leek and apples and cook for a further 5 minutes until golden. Transfer the vegetables to the casserole dish.

Spray the frying pan again with low-calorie cooking spray (there's no need to wash it first; the bits in the frying pan will add flavour and colour to the finished dish). Place over a medium heat and add the chicken when the frying pan is hot.

Fry the chicken for 4–5 minutes to seal on all sides. Once sealed, transfer to the vegetables in the casserole dish. Add the chicken stock, Dijon mustard, dried thyme and dried oregano and stir in. Put the lid on the casserole dish and place in the preheated oven for 1½ hours, stirring halfway through.

After 1½ hours, the liquid in the casserole dish should have reduced and thickened a little. Add the green beans and stir in.

Replace the lid and return to the oven for a further 15 minutes until the beans are tender.

Remove from the oven and stir in the cream cheese, until completely blended. Taste and season with salt and black pepper, if needed.

Serve, sprinkled with a few fresh oregano leaves, if using, and basmati rice or an accompaniment of your choice.

SLOW-COOKER METHOD
🍲 **LOW: 6 HOURS 20 MINS–7 HOURS 20 MINS**
🍲 **HIGH: 4 HOURS 20 MINS–5 HOURS 20 MINS**

SPECIAL EQUIPMENT
Slow cooker

Spray a large frying pan with low-calorie cooking spray and place over a medium heat. Add the onions and cook for 8–10 minutes, until softened and golden.

Add the garlic, leek and apples and cook for a further 5 minutes until golden. Transfer to the slow cooker.

Spray the frying pan again with low-calorie cooking spray (there's no need to wash it first; the bits in the frying pan will add flavour and colour to the finished dish).

Place over a medium heat and add the chicken when the frying pan is hot. Fry the chicken for 4–5 minutes on all sides. Once sealed, transfer to the vegetables in the slow cooker.

Add the chicken stock, Dijon mustard, dried thyme, dried oregano and stir in.

Put the lid on the slow cooker and turn on. Cook on high for 4–5 hours or on low for 6–7 hours, adding the green beans for the last 30 minutes of the cooking time.

Stir in the cream cheese until completely blended. If you think the sauce is too runny for your liking, you can simmer with the lid off until reduced to a consistency you prefer.

Taste and season with salt and black pepper, if needed.

Serve, sprinkled with a few fresh oregano leaves, if using, and basmati rice or an accompaniment of your choice.

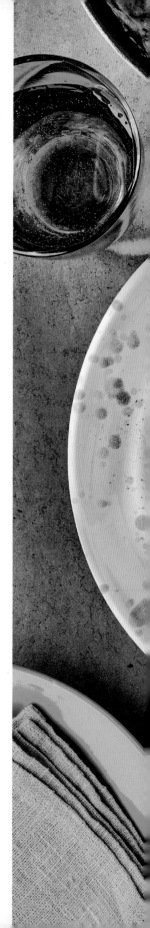

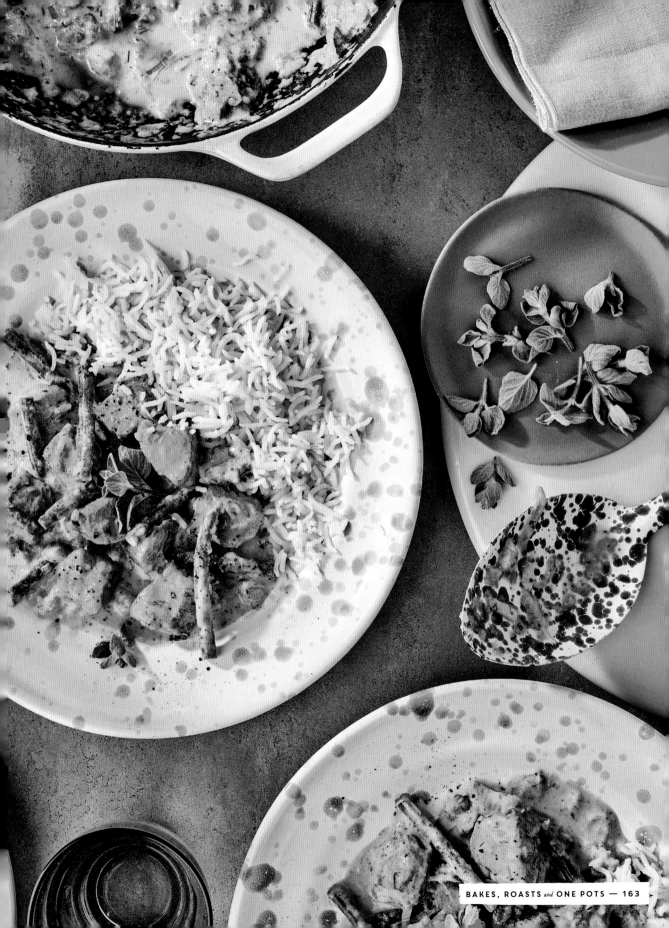

FREEZE ME

DAIRY FREE

BATCH FRIENDLY

GLUTEN FREE

USE GF STOCK CUBE AND SAUSAGES

SOMERSET SAUSAGES

🕐 **10 MINS**   🗑 **50 MINS**   ✕ **SERVES 4**

PER SERVING:
356 KCAL /26G CARBS

low-calorie cooking spray
8 reduced-fat sausages
1 small onion, peeled and sliced
1 small leek, trimmed and sliced
2 carrots, peeled and sliced
2 garlic cloves, peeled and crushed
2 tsp tomato puree
200ml dry cider
400ml chicken stock
  (1 chicken stock cube dissolved in 400ml boiling water)
2 tsp wholegrain mustard
1 dessert apple, cored and cut into 12 wedges
1 x 400g tin butter beans, drained and rinsed
6 sage leaves (or 1 tsp dried sage)

TO ACCOMPANY *(optional)*
100g green beans (+ 24 kcal per serving)

Our Somerset Sausages have all the flavours of a West Country orchard, and they're so light on calories! We're all about hearty, fuss-free meals, and this one leaves you with hardly any washing up. Cider adds a subtle sweetness to our gravy, while the butter beans bring a silky, substantial texture.

Everyday Light ———————————————

Spray a large saucepan or casserole dish with low-calorie cooking spray and place over a medium heat.

When hot, add the sausages and cook for 4–5 minutes, turning frequently until all sides are browned. Remove from the pan and set to one side.

Wipe out the pan with some kitchen towel and spray again with low-calorie cooking spray. Add the onion, leek and carrots. Fry for 5 minutes until soft.

Add the garlic and tomato puree and cook for another minute.

Add the cider, stock and mustard and then the apple wedges and return the sausages to the pan.

Bring to the boil, then turn the heat down to low. Cover and allow to simmer for 30 minutes.

Add the butter beans and continue to cook for 10 minutes, uncovered.

Stir in the sage and serve with green beans or another accompaniment of your choice.

SWAP THIS: If you aren't keen on using cider, you can swap it out for apple juice! You can also swap the pork sausages for chicken or veggie alternative ones.

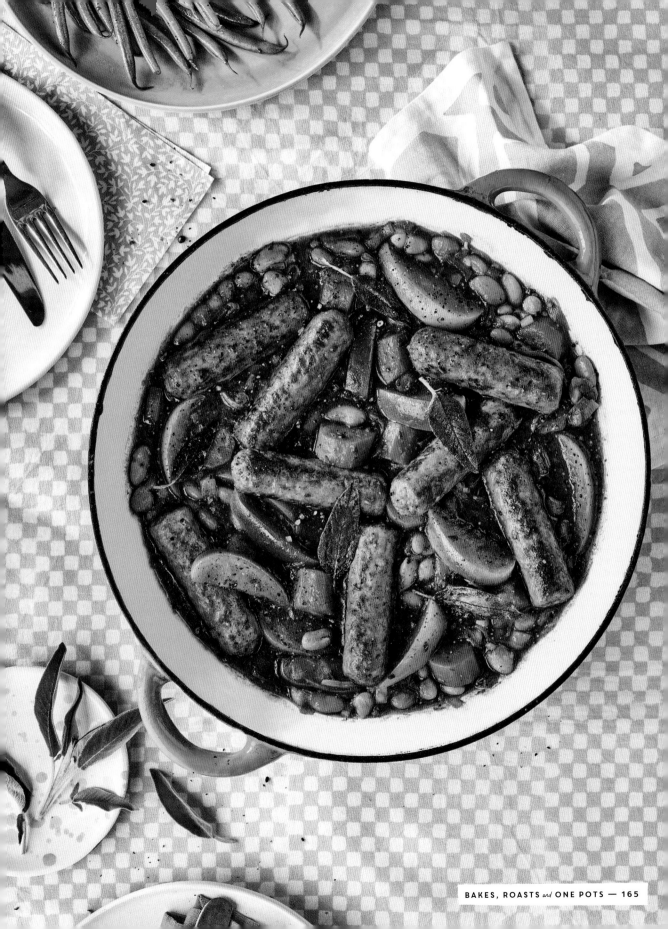

FREEZE ME

BATCH FRIENDLY

DAIRY FREE

USE A DF
ALTERNATIVE FOR
CREAM CHEESE

GLUTEN FREE

USE GF
STOCK POTS

LOW CARB

CHICKEN SUPREME

 10 MINS   **40 MINS**   ✕ **SERVES 4**

PER SERVING:
225 KCAL / 8.8G CARBS

low-calorie cooking spray
1 onion, peeled and thinly
  sliced
2 garlic cloves, peeled and
  crushed
4 smoked bacon medallions,
  cut into 1cm (½in) dice
4 medium, skinless chicken
  breasts, about 130g each
2 white wine stock pots,
  dissolved in 400ml boiling
  water
180g low-fat cream cheese
freshly ground black pepper,
  to taste
a few flat-leafed parsley
  leaves, finely chopped, to
  garnish (optional)

TO ACCOMPANY *(optional)*
Creamy Mashed Potatoes
  from the Pinch of Nom
  website (+ 176 kcal per
  serving)
80g steamed vegetables
  (+ 38 kcal per serving)

This is one of those recipes that you'll find yourself making time and time again. It's our version of the classic and indulgent Chicken Supreme, but instead of a glug of white wine and lashings of cream, we've made some low-calorie swaps to lighten it. The result is a dish that tastes decadent, and is far kinder to your waistline.

Weekly Indulgence

Spray a large frying pan with low-calorie cooking spray and place over a low to medium heat. Add the onion and fry gently for 10–15 minutes, or until the onion is soft, golden and starting to caramelise.

Add the garlic, bacon and chicken breasts. Cook the chicken breasts for 2–3 minutes on each side until lightly golden and the bacon is cooked.

Pour in the white wine stock, stir in, partially cover with a lid or kitchen foil, and simmer over a medium heat for 10 minutes.

Uncover, turn the chicken breasts over and continue to simmer for a further 10 minutes until the chicken is cooked through. There should be no signs of pinkness and the juices should run clear.

Take the frying pan off the heat and add the cream cheese. Stir in until completely blended and the sauce is smooth. If the sauce is too thin, return to the heat and continue to simmer until reduced to your liking. If the sauce is too thick, stir in a little water.

Taste and season with black pepper, garnish with a few flat-leafed parsley leaves, if using, and serve with mash and steamed vegetables or an accompaniment of your choice.

MAKE IT VEGGIE:
For a vegetarian meal, swap the chicken breasts for Quorn fillets.

TIPS: Taste before seasoning. We found the bacon provides saltiness, so you are unlikely to need to season this dish with salt. Use a low-fat cream cheese rather than a fat-free one in this dish. The result is a little richer and stands up better to reheating if you plan to batch cook this recipe.

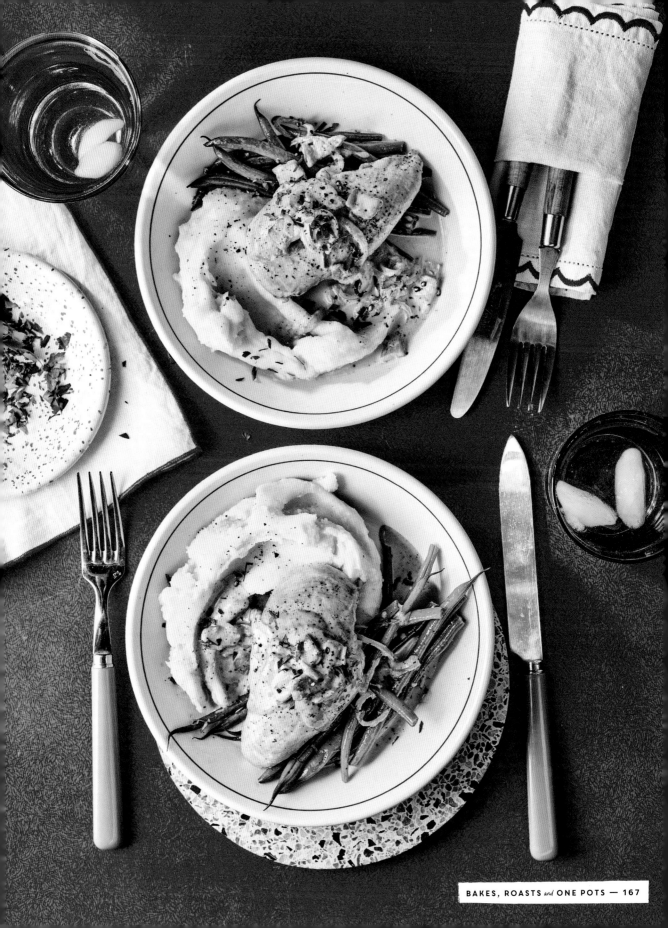

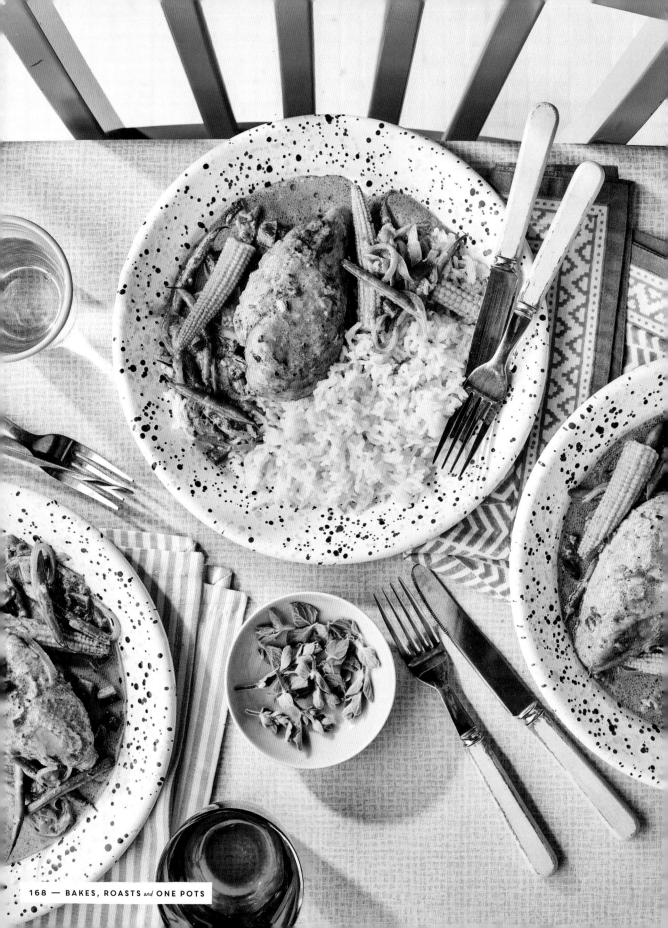

CREAMY CAJUN-STYLE CHICKEN

🕐 **10 MINS**　　🗑 **35 MINS**　　✕ **SERVES 4**

FREEZE ME

BATCH FRIENDLY

GLUTEN FREE

USE GF STOCK CUBE

PER SERVING:
224 KCAL /14G CARBS

low-calorie cooking spray
2 onions, peeled and thinly
  sliced
4 garlic cloves, peeled and
  crushed
1 small red chilli, deseeded
  and finely chopped
4 medium, skinless chicken
  breasts, about 130g each
½ red pepper, deseeded and
  cut into 1cm (½in) dice
½ green pepper, deseeded
  and cut into 1cm (½in) dice
2 tbsp Cajun seasoning
500ml chicken stock
  (1 chicken stock cube
  dissolved in 400ml boiling
  water)
100g baby corn
100g fine green beans,
  trimmed and halved
180g low-fat cream cheese
sea salt and freshly ground
  black pepper
a few fresh oregano leaves,
  to garnish (optional)

TO ACCOMPANY *(optional)*
50g uncooked basmati
  rice per portion, cooked
  according to packet
  instructions (+ 173 kcal per
  125g cooked serving)

Gather everyone around the table to tuck into this creamy chicken dish! If you like your food with a little heat, you'll love cooking with Cajun spices. To balance the chilli kick we've used low-fat cream cheese to make a silky, rich sauce. We'd say this turns out medium-hot, but if you're brave, just throw in some extra chillies!

Everyday Light ——————————————

Spray a large frying pan with low-calorie cooking spray and place over a medium heat. Add the onions, garlic and red chilli, and fry gently for 5 minutes until softened a little.

Add the chicken breasts, red pepper, green pepper and Cajun seasoning. Stir, then cook for 4 minutes, turning the chicken breasts over halfway through. The chicken breasts should be lightly golden.

Add the chicken stock and simmer, uncovered, for 10 minutes.

Turn the chicken breasts over and loosely cover with a lid or with kitchen foil.

Simmer for a further 10 minutes, or until the chicken is cooked and white throughout. Use a small, sharp knife to cut into the thickest part of the chicken to check. There should be no pinkness and the juices should run clear.

Add the baby corn and green beans and simmer, uncovered, for 5–6 minutes, until tender but not soft.

Remove from the heat and stir in the cream cheese until completely blended. If the sauce is too thin, continue to simmer, uncovered, for a little longer until the sauce has reduced and thickened to your liking. If the sauce is too thick, add a little water to loosen it.

Season to taste with salt and black pepper, top with oregano leaves (if liked) and serve with basmati rice or an accompaniment of choice.

 SWAP THIS: You could swap the baby corn for 100g tinned sweetcorn, well drained.

TIP: Use a low-fat cream cheese rather than a fat-free one. This will give a richer, creamier sauce, and will stand up to reheating better if you're going to batch cook this recipe.

CHEESY MEATBALL PARMENTIER

 30 MINS   **1 HOUR 10 MINS**   ✕ **SERVES 4**

PER SERVING:
502 KCAL / 46G CARBS

SPECIAL EQUIPMENT
Handheld stick blender
30 x 25cm (12 x 10in)
ovenproof dish

FOR THE SAUCE
low-calorie cooking spray
1 carrot, peeled and finely
   diced
1 small onion, peeled and
   diced
1 courgette, diced
1 tsp garlic granules
1 x 400g tin chopped
   tomatoes
90g reduced-fat spreadable
   cheese

FOR THE MEATBALL BAKE
700g potatoes, peeled and
   cut into 5mm (¼in) slices
500g 5%-fat minced beef
1 small onion, finely chopped
25g panko breadcrumbs
1 tbsp Henderson's relish or
   Worcestershire sauce
1 medium egg, beaten
80g reduced-fat Cheddar
   cheese, finely grated
salt and freshly ground black
   pepper
a few basil leaves, to garnish
   (optional)

TO ACCOMPANY *(optional)*
75g mixed salad (+ 15 kcal
   per serving)

We aren't too sure where we got the idea for this dish, but how could we resist the sound of a cheesy meatball and potato bake? This is super family-friendly because, as well as being delicious, we've packed the creamy sauce with loads of hidden veg. Oooh, just look at that golden cheesy topping! Serve with a mixed salad.

Special Occasion ──────────────

Make the sauce first. Spray a saucepan with low-calorie cooking spray and place over a medium heat. Sauté the carrot, onion and courgette for 5 minutes until beginning to soften. Add the garlic granules and tomatoes. Bring to a bubble and lower the heat. Simmer the sauce for 25 minutes, stirring occasionally, until the carrots are cooked through. If it looks like it's drying out too much, add a little water.

While the sauce simmers, put the potato slices in a pan of cold salted water and bring to the boil. Reduce the heat and simmer for 5 minutes but no longer as they will be too soft. Drain and leave until they are cool enough to handle.

While the potatoes cool, mix together the rest of the meatball ingredients, reserving the grated cheese, and season well with salt and pepper. Roll into 12 evenly-sized meatballs.

When the vegetables in the sauce are cooked, stir in the spreadable cheese and then blitz with a stick blender until smooth. Preheat the oven to 180°C (fan 160°C/gas mark 4).

Now, assemble the bake. Spray the ovenproof dish with low-calorie cooking spray and place a layer of potatoes on the bottom. Arrange the meatballs on top, then smother in the tomato sauce. Tuck the remaining potato slices around the meatballs, leaving the top half of each slice above the sauce. Spray the top with low-calorie cooking spray, then sprinkle over the cheese.

Place in the oven and cook for 40 minutes, until the meatballs are cooked through and the potatoes are crispy. Top with basil (if you like) and serve with salad or your choice of accompaniment.

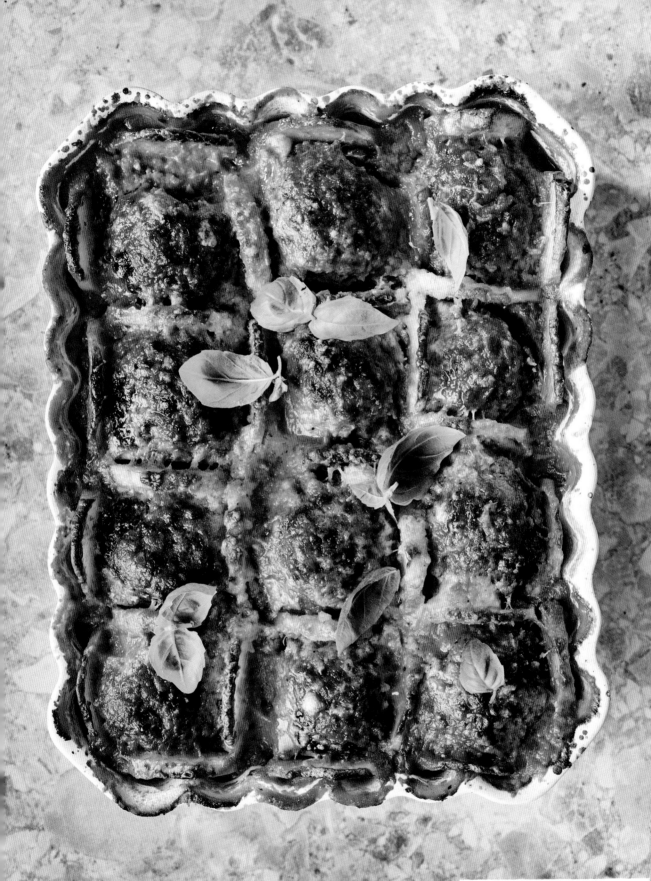

POULTRYMAN'S PIE

 10 MINS   **55 MINS**   ✗ **SERVES 4**

PER SERVING:
391 KCAL /42G CARBS

SPECIAL EQUIPMENT
30 x 20cm (12 x 8in)
shallow ovenproof dish

low-calorie cooking spray
1 large onion, peeled and
   diced
2 large carrots, peeled and
   diced
2 garlic cloves, peeled and
   crushed
500g 2%-fat minced turkey
½ tsp dried thyme
½ tsp dried tarragon
1 tbsp white wine vinegar
2 tbsp Henderson's relish or
   Worcestershire sauce
300ml chicken stock
   (2 chicken stock cubes
   dissolved in 300ml boiling
   water)
600g potatoes, peeled and
   quartered
sea salt and freshly ground
   black pepper
¼ tsp mustard powder
90g low-fat cream cheese
150g frozen peas

TO ACCOMPANY *(optional)*
80g steamed vegetables
   (+ 38 kcal per serving)

While Shepherd's Pie is a classic British dish that's pretty perfect as it is, we couldn't resist playing with new flavours to create this slimming-friendly Poultryman's Pie! We've baked traditional peas and carrots with the mince in our rich, creamy sauce. You'll know your potato-topped pie is ready when the cheesy topping is golden brown and there's a tussle for first dibs!

Weekly Indulgence ─────────────────

Spray a large frying pan with low-calorie cooking spray and place over a medium heat. Add the onion, carrots and garlic and cook for 5 minutes, until the onion begins to soften.

Add the minced turkey, thyme, tarragon, white wine vinegar and Henderson's relish to the pan. Cook for 5 minutes, breaking up the mince with a wooden spoon, until the mince has browned.

Add the stock, bring to the boil and cover and simmer for 20 minutes, removing the lid for the final 5 minutes. You want there to be a little liquid left so that the pan looks glossy, but it shouldn't be swimming in stock.

While this is cooking, cook the potatoes in a pan of boiling salted water. When they are soft, remove from the heat, drain off the water and mash with a little salt and pepper and the mustard powder.

Stir the cream cheese and the frozen peas in with the mince mixture and season with salt and pepper, to taste.

Preheat the oven to 200°C (fan 180°C/gas mark 6).

Pour the mince mixture into the ovenproof dish and allow to cool slightly. If you don't, the mash may sink through the mince. Spoon the mashed potato on top and run a fork over it to completely cover the mince and give it some texture. Give the top of the mash a little spritz with low-calorie cooking spray.

Place in the oven and cook for 20 minutes until golden brown on top. Serve with steamed vegetables, if you like.

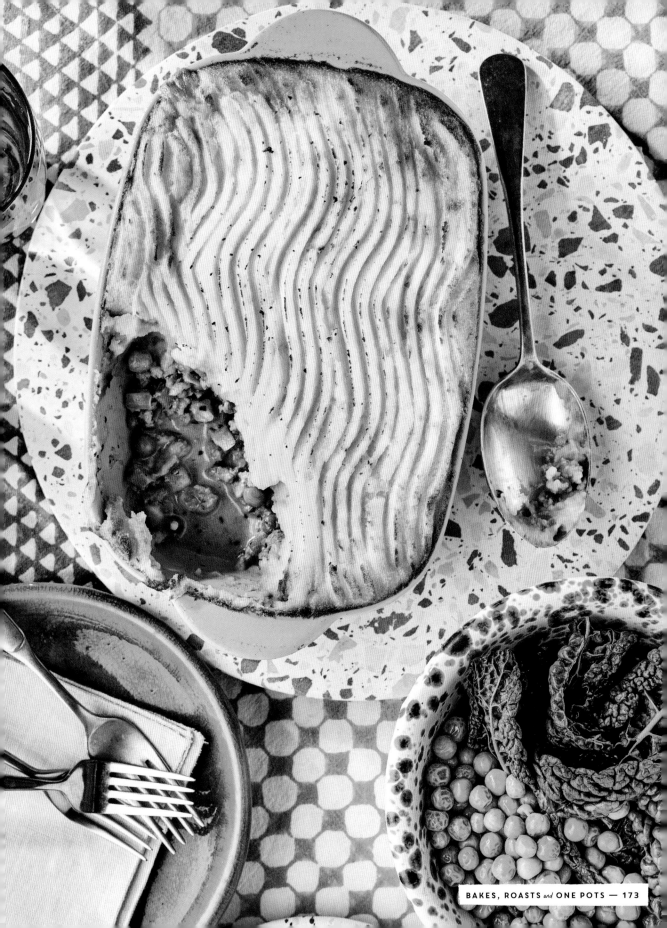

VEGGIE

USE
VEGETARIAN
FETA

FREEZE
ME

GLUTEN
FREE

USE GF
STOCK CUBES

SWEETCORN RISOTTO

🕐 **5 MINS**   🍲 **25 MINS**   🍴 **SERVES 4**

PER SERVING:
404 KCAL / 72G CARBS

low-calorie cooking spray
1 onion, peeled and finely
    chopped
2 garlic cloves, peeled and
    crushed
300g Arborio rice
1 tbsp white wine vinegar
1 tsp dried chilli flakes (more
    or less depending on your
    liking for spice!)
1.2 litres vegetable stock
    (2 vegetable stock cubes
    dissolved in 1.2 litres boiling
    water)
2 x 200g tins of sweetcorn,
    drained (or 300g of cooked
    sweetcorn)
juice of ½ lemon
100g reduced-fat feta
    cheese, crumbled
sea salt and freshly ground
    black pepper (optional)
a few chopped chives, to
    garnish (optional)

TO ACCOMPANY *(optional)*
75g mixed salad (+ 15 kcal
    per serving)

This non-traditional risotto doesn't keep you cooped up in the kitchen stirring for 30 minutes (and we promise, no one will taste the difference). Combining budget-friendly tinned sweetcorn with fresh feta, garlic and onion, this rich dish is good for your bank and even better for your calorie count. We love it with cheesy garlic bread, green beans or salad!

Weekly Indulgence

Spray a large saucepan with low-calorie cooking spray and place over a medium heat.

Add the onion and the garlic and sauté for 5 minutes until soft but not coloured.

Stir in the rice and cook for a minute, until well coated. Add the white wine vinegar, chilli flakes and the hot stock.

Stir until the stock comes to the boil, then reduce the heat to a simmer. Allow to cook, uncovered for 15 minutes. No need to keep stirring.

After 15 minutes, most of the stock should have been absorbed but there should be some remaining. If it has dried out too much, you may have had your heat turned up a little high – don't worry! Just add a splash of hot water.

Add the sweetcorn and lemon juice and stir for 5 minutes, or until the remaining stock has been absorbed.

Stir in three-quarters of the crumbled feta, taste and then add some salt and pepper if needed.

Serve garnished with the remaining feta and a few chopped chives (optional) and, if you like, a mixed salad.

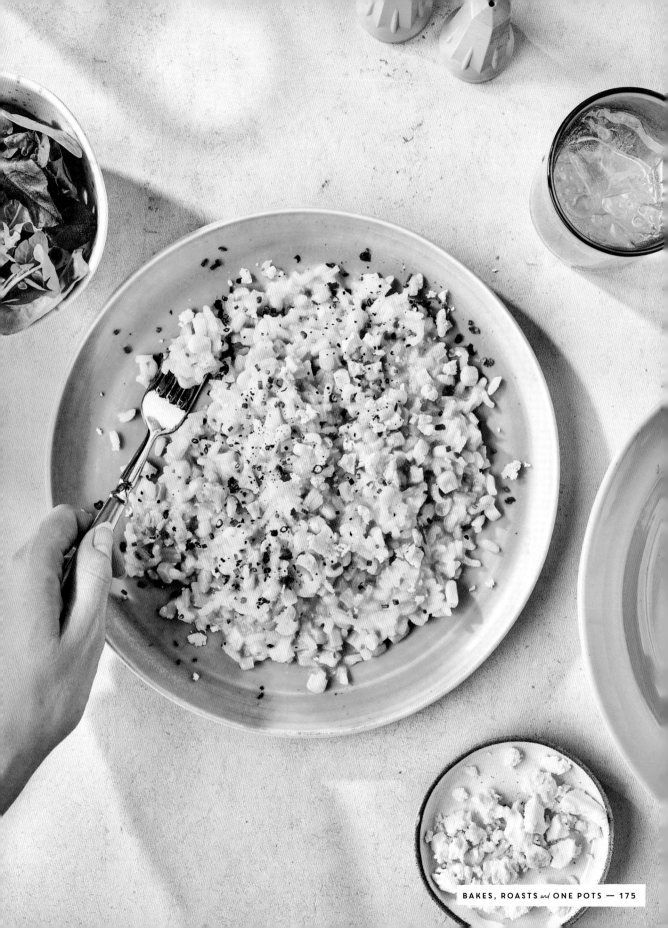

SNACKS
AND SIDES

CHICKEN TIKKA NAANWICH

🕐 **20 MINS*** 🗑 **10 MINS** ✕ **SERVES 4**

***PLUS 10 MINS PROVING**

PER SERVING:
357 KCAL /56G CARBS

FOR THE NAAN BREAD
250g white self-raising flour,
  plus extra for dusting
1 tsp caster sugar
½ tsp salt
½ tsp baking powder
250g fat-free natural yoghurt
10g reduced-fat spread, plus
  a little extra for greasing

FOR THE RAITA
125g fat-free natural yoghurt
80g cucumber, very finely
  chopped
4g fresh coriander leaves,
  finely chopped
4g fresh mint leaves, finely
  chopped
1 small garlic clove, peeled
  and crushed
sea salt and freshly ground
  black pepper

FOR THE FILLING
200g ready-cooked chicken
  tikka slices
20g baby spinach leaves

SWAP THIS: You could
swap the chicken for
any other ready cooked
chicken such as Peri Peri
or BBQ chicken slices.

Why make a sandwich when you can have a Naanwich?
If you are bored of the same old lunches, this is guaranteed
to spice up your midday meal! Our Naan Breads freeze
really well, so stock your freezer for days just like today. The
slimming-friendly raita in the Naanwich filling is not
to be missed – it's so light and refreshing.

Everyday Light ―――――――――――――――――

For the naan bread, sift the flour, sugar, salt and baking
powder into a medium mixing bowl. Make a well in the
centre and add the yoghurt. Using clean fingertips, gradually
draw in the flour, mixing to form a ball of soft dough.

Place the dough on a lightly floured surface and knead for
5 minutes until the dough forms a smooth ball. Place in a
lightly greased bowl and cover. Set aside for 10 minutes.

Preheat the oven to 200°C (fan 180°C/gas mark 6).

Turn the dough out onto a lightly floured surface and, using
a sharp knife, cut into four pieces. If the dough is sticky,
dust with a little more flour.

Form the pieces of dough into four oval-shaped balls, then
roll out into ovals of about 11 x 22cm (4 x 8½in). Place on
two lightly greased baking trays and prick with a fork.
Bake in the oven for about 8 minutes until golden and puffy.

Place the reduced-fat spread in a small saucepan over a
very low heat until just melted. Brush over the naan breads
and leave to cool.

Combine all the raita ingredients in a small bowl and mix.
Season to taste with salt and pepper.

Split one side of each naan bread open using a small
serrated knife. Fill each naan bread with some of the
cooked chicken tikka slices, baby spinach leaves and the
raita. Serve at once.

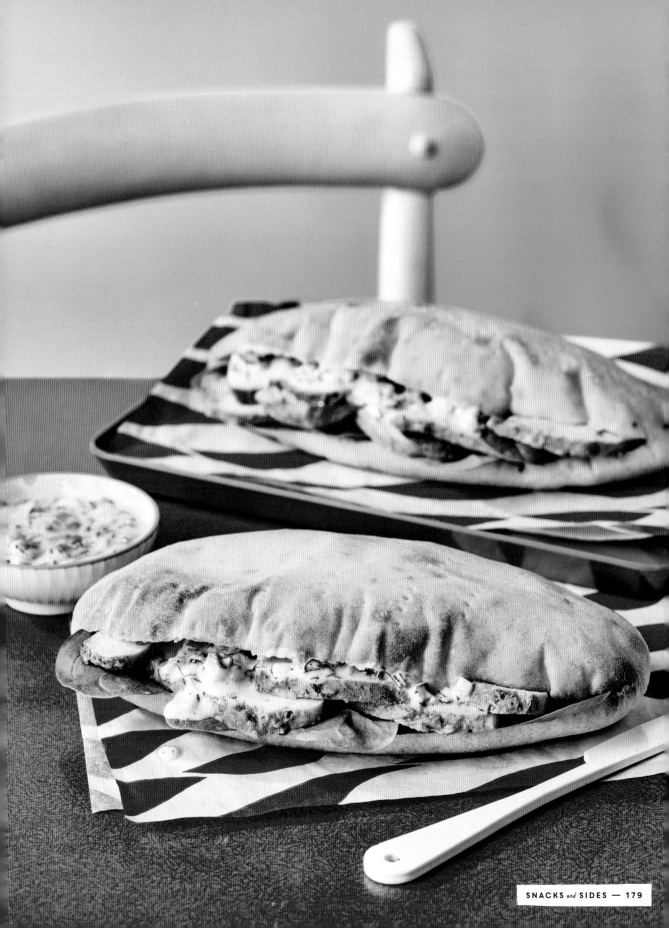

FREEZE ME

DAIRY FREE

GLUTEN FREE

USE GF PLAIN FLOUR

CHICKEN TIKKA PAKORAS

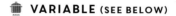 🕐 **15 MINS*** 🗑 **VARIABLE** (SEE BELOW) ✕ **SERVES 4**

*PLUS 30 MINS MARINATING

PER SERVING:
180 KCAL / 17G CARBS

400g skinless chicken
breasts, cut into 3cm
(1¼in) chunks
1 medium egg, beaten
50g cornflour
25g plain flour
low-calorie cooking spray
2g coriander and/or mint
leaves, chopped, to garnish
(optional)

FOR THE TIKKA SPICE MIX
1½ tsp paprika
1 tsp ground coriander
1 tsp ground cumin
1 tsp garam masala
½ tsp ground turmeric
½ tsp ground ginger
½ tsp garlic powder
½ tsp salt
pinch of ground black
pepper
pinch of cayenne pepper

TO ACCOMPANY *(optional)*
Raita (see Tips on page 182)
(+ 33 kcal per serving) and
75g green salad (+ 15 kcal
per serving)

MAKE IT VEGGIE:
For vegetarian pakoras,
swap the chicken for
Quorn fillets.

TIP: Use non-stick
baking paper rather than
greaseproof paper. It
works really well, and
the chicken pakoras will
not stick to it.

Snacks don't get much better than succulent chicken, covered in a crispy, mildly spiced tikka coating. Chicken Tikka Pakoras from the takeaway are usually deep-fried, so we created our own slimming-friendly version, and they're just as tasty. Once you realise how easy it is to make this Indian-style snack or starter at home, it'll be fakeaway night every night at your house!

Weekly Indulgence —————————————————

OVEN METHOD
🗑 **25 MINS**

Place all the dry tikka spice mix ingredients in a mixing bowl and stir until well combined. Add the chicken chunks and mix well until completely coated in the dry spice mix. Cover and place in the fridge for 30 minutes to marinate.

Preheat the oven to 200°C (fan 180°C/gas mark 6). Line a baking tray with non-stick baking paper.

Remove the chicken from the fridge and stir in the beaten egg until completely coated.

Mix together the cornflour and plain flour and add to the bowl containing the chicken and egg. Mix with a wooden spoon until evenly coated. Stir in 2 tablespoons of water and mix well until the chicken is covered in a thick, sticky coating.

Place the coated chicken pieces on the lined baking tray, spacing them out so they don't stick together.

Spray the chicken pakoras with low-calorie cooking spray and place in the preheated oven for 10 minutes. Remove from the oven and turn over. Spray again with low-calorie cooking spray and return to the oven for a further 10–15 minutes until golden and crispy. The chicken should show no sign of pinkness and the juices should run clear.

Sprinkle with chopped coriander and/or mint leaves, if using, and with raita and salad (if you like).

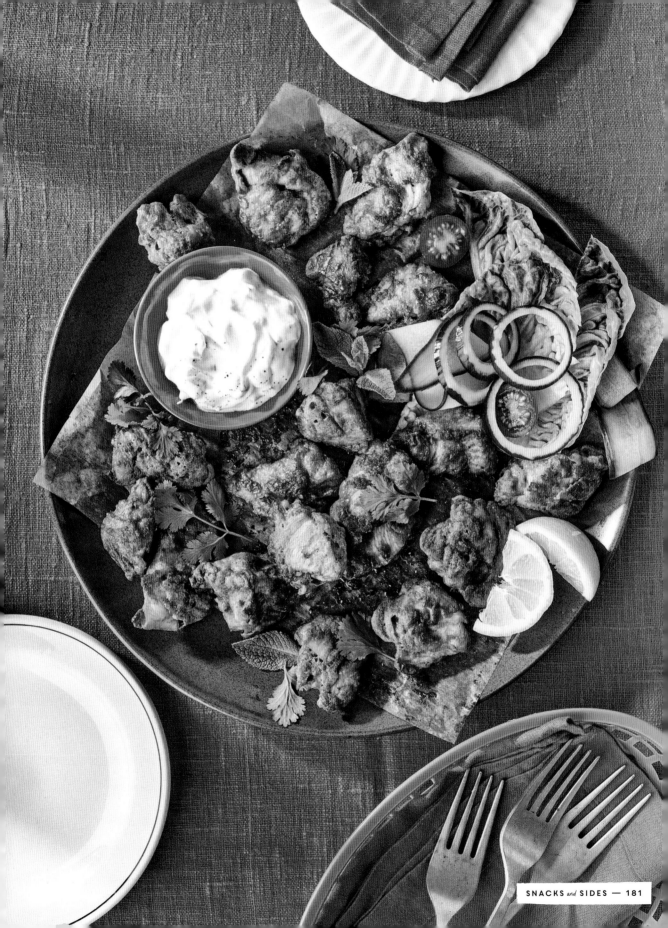

AIR-FRYER METHOD
🍲 30 MINS

SPECIAL EQUIPMENT
Air fryer

Place all the dry tikka spice mix ingredients in a medium mixing bowl and stir until well combined. Add the chicken chunks and mix well until completely coated in the dry spice mix. Cover and place in the fridge for 30 minutes to marinate.

Preheat the air fryer to 200°C.

Remove the chicken from the fridge and stir in the beaten egg until completely coated.

Mix together the cornflour and plain flour and add to the bowl containing the chicken and egg. Mix with a wooden spoon until evenly covered. Stir in 2 tablespoons water and mix well until the chicken is covered in a thick, sticky coating.

Place the coated chicken pieces in the preheated air fryer, spacing them out so they don't stick together. Depending on the size of your air fryer, you may need to cook in batches.

Spray the chicken pakoras with low-calorie cooking spray and cook for 12–15 minutes, turning or shaking halfway through, until golden and crispy. The chicken should show no sign of pinkness and the juices should run clear.

Sprinkle with chopped coriander and/or mint leaves, if using, and serve with raita and salad (if you like).

TIPS: Add the water carefully: the coating needs to be thick and sticky. We found 2 tablespoons was the perfect amount. If your air fryer doesn't have a preheat function, we suggest heating at cooking temperature for a few minutes before cooking your food. To serve with raita, mix 150g fat-free natural yoghurt with ½ cucumber, deseeded and thinly sliced, 10 mint leaves, finely chopped, and 1 teaspoon of granulated sweetener. Cover and chill until needed.

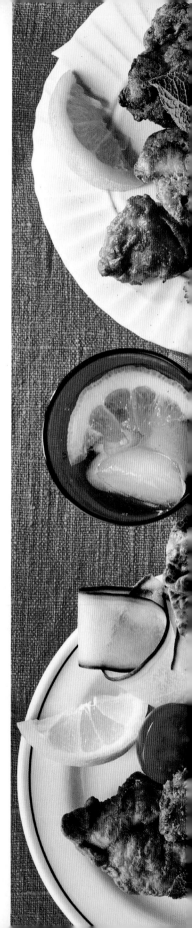

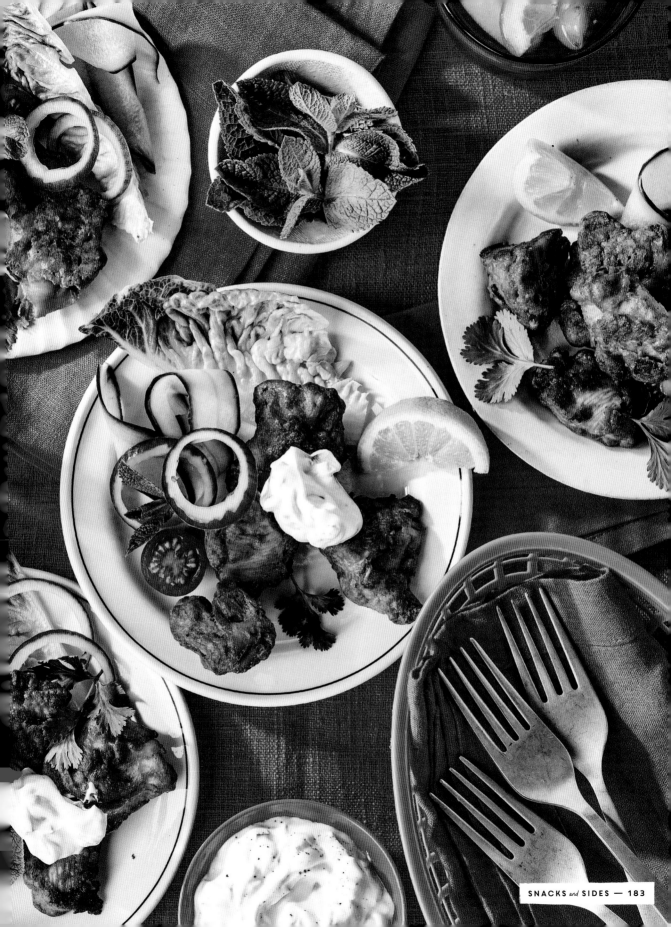

KEEMA NAAN PASTIES

🕐 **30 MINS**   🗑 **40 MINS**   ✕ **SERVES 4**

PER SERVING:
389 KCAL / 58G CARBS

FOR THE NAAN BREAD
250g white self-raising flour,
  plus extra for dusting
1 tsp caster sugar
½ tsp salt
½ tsp baking powder
250g fat-free natural yoghurt
1 medium egg, beaten

FOR THE KEEMA FILLING
low-calorie cooking spray
200g 5%-fat minced beef
½ onion, peeled and finely
  chopped
1 medium red pepper,
  deseeded and cut into 1cm
  (½in) dice
1 medium carrot, peeled and
  cut into 1cm (½in) dice
1cm (½in) piece root ginger,
  peeled and finely grated
1 tsp garlic granules
1 tbsp mild curry powder
1½ tbsp tomato puree
225ml beef stock (½ beef
  stock cube dissolved in
  225ml boiling water)
1 tbsp lemon juice
40g frozen peas
sea salt and freshly ground
  black pepper

TO ACCOMPANY *(optional)*
75g mixed salad (+ 15 kcal
  per serving)

SWAP THIS: You can
swap the minced beef
for 5%-fat minced turkey,
lamb or pork.

Ready for meaty pasties with a Pinch of Nom twist? Keema provides the perfect filling for our Indian-inspired pasties! Instead of traditional pastry, we've used dough from our Simple Naan Bread recipe to create our crispy casing and the softer 'bready' texture is a real treat.

Weekly Indulgence

For the naan bread, sift the flour, sugar, salt and baking powder into a large bowl. Make a well in the centre and add the yoghurt. Use your clean fingertips to draw the flour into the yoghurt, mixing to form a ball of soft dough.

Place the dough on a lightly floured surface and knead well for 5 minutes until the dough forms a smooth ball. Set aside as you make the filling.

Spray a large frying pan with low-calorie cooking spray and place over a medium heat. Add the mince and cook for 1–2 minutes to seal and lightly brown, stirring well. Add the onion, red pepper and carrot and cook for 3–4 minutes, stirring. Add the ginger, garlic granules and curry powder and stir well. Add the tomato puree, beef stock and lemon juice, stir and bring to the boil.

Reduce the heat to low and simmer gently, uncovered, for 20–25 minutes until the carrot is tender. The stock should have reduced completely, and the mixture should be thick. Stir in the peas until completely mixed in and season to taste with salt and black pepper. If the stock hasn't completely reduced, simmer uncovered, for a little longer.

Remove the keema from the heat, transfer to a large plate and spread out thinly to cool. Preheat the oven to 200°C (fan 180°C/gas mark 6). Spray a baking tray with low-calorie cooking spray and use to grease thoroughly.

Turn the dough onto a lightly floured surface and, using a sharp knife, cut into four equal pieces. Shape into oval balls, then roll out into four ovals about 22 x 16cm (8½ x 6in) in size.

When the keema mixture has cooled, divide it between the dough ovals, placing it in the centre of the top half. Leave a 2cm (¾in) gap around the edge. Brush the beaten egg around the edge of the dough ovals.

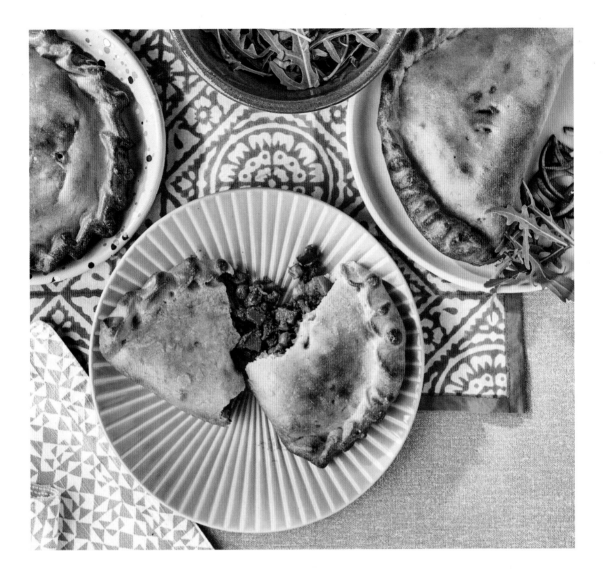

Fold the lower half of the dough ovals over the keema filling to make semicircular pasties. Press the edge to seal and then crimp the edge with your fingers, or use a fork to press down around the edge.

Use a fish slice to lift the pasties off the surface and place them on the prepared baking tray, leaving a gap between each. Brush all over with the remaining beaten egg and cut a couple of small slits in the top of each pasty, to allow steam to escape.

Place in the preheated oven and bake for about 10 minutes until golden. To check if the dough is cooked, lift and check the underside of the pasties. The underside should sound hollow when tapped and will no longer look doughy. Serve with a salad or an accompaniment of your choice.

TIP: We used mild curry powder, but if you prefer things a bit hotter you can try medium curry powder instead.

VEGGIE

GLUTEN FREE

CHECK THE CHOCOLATE

LOW CARB

SALTED CARAMEL *and* CHOCOLATE POPCORN BITES

🕐 **10 MINS***   🗑 **8 MINS**   ✕ **MAKES 16**

*PLUS 25 MINS CHILLING

PER POPCORN BITE:
69 KCAL / 9.9G CARBS

SPECIAL EQUIPMENT
18cm (7in) square cake tin

low-calorie cooking spray
100g popcorn kernels
100g plain dark chocolate,
  broken into pieces
13 x sugar-free creamy
  chewy toffees (80g)
80g ¼ tsp sea salt flakes

Bring the whole family together around a shareable treat with these tasty popcorn bites. Bound with sticky caramel, we've made these chocolate-covered popcorn pieces extra-delicious with a light sprinkling of sea salt on top (which you can omit if you prefer). Budget-friendly, lower in calories than most shop-bought alternatives (just 69 calories a pop!) and super easy to make – give them a go!

Everyday Light ───────────────────

Spray the square tin with a couple of sprays of low-calorie cooking spray. Use to grease the base and sides of the tin thoroughly. Line the base and sides of the tin with non-stick baking paper.

Place the popcorn kernels in a large bowl suitable for use in the microwave. Cover with a plate and microwave on high for 4–5 minutes, checking on the popcorn halfway through to see how much has popped. Cover and continue cooking until most of the popcorn has popped but take care not to let any unpopped kernels burn in the bottom of the bowl. You will need 50g of popped popcorn at the end of cooking.

Discard any unpopped kernels and place the 50g of popped popcorn in a clean large bowl.

Place the chocolate pieces in a small bowl suitable for the microwave. Microwave, uncovered, for 1–1½ minutes on high, until just melted, stirring halfway through and taking care not to overheat. Remove from the microwave and continue to stir until completely melted and immediately pour over the popcorn, stirring to coat. The chocolate will not completely coat the popcorn but mix as evenly as you can.

Working quickly, scrape the mixture into the lined tin and spread out evenly. Lightly press the mixture down with the back of a spoon. Place in the fridge for about 15 minutes until set completely.

TIP: We use sugar-free chewy creamy toffees such as Werther's Original Sugar-free Creamy Toffees, not hard butter candies.

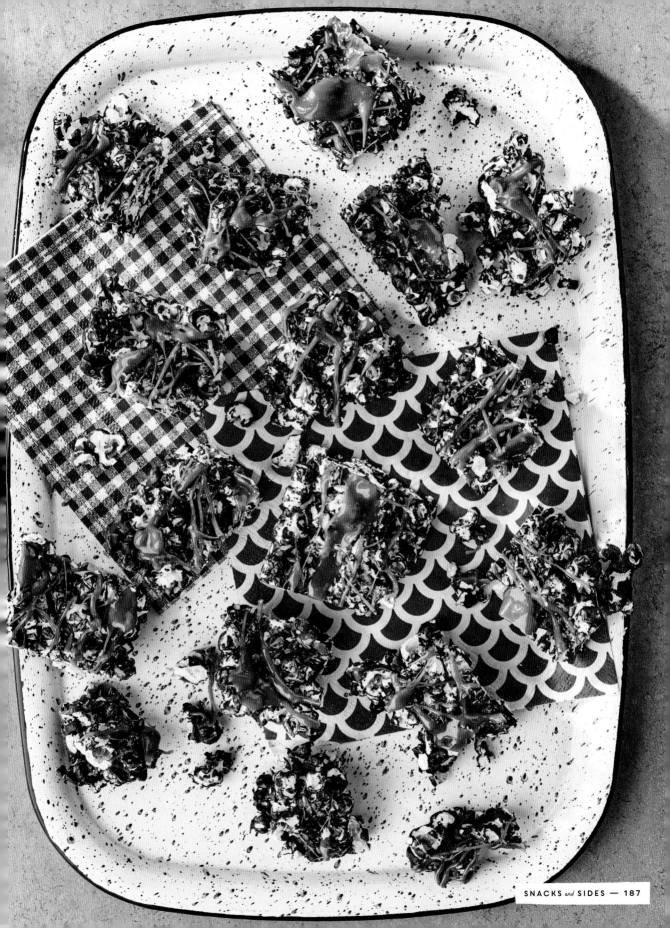

Place the chewy toffees in a small bowl and microwave, uncovered, for about 30–40 seconds on high, stirring halfway through, until just melted. Take care not to overheat.

Remove from the microwave and continue stirring until just melted. Remove the chocolate popcorn from the fridge and immediately drizzle the melted toffee evenly over the top.

Sprinkle evenly with the sea salt flakes and place in the fridge for a further 10 minutes or until completely set.

Lift out of the tin using the non-stick paper to help you and place it on the work surface. Cut into 16 pieces using a large sharp knife. The pieces will have rough edges due to the texture of the popcorn.

Serve alone or as part of a selection of teatime treats!

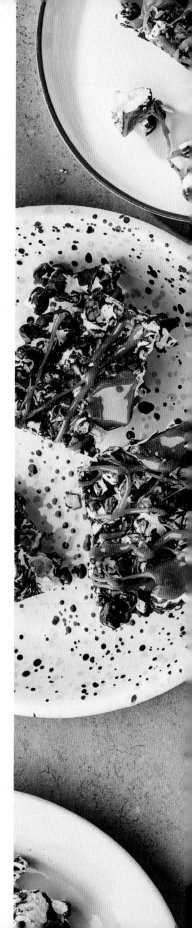

TIP: The wattage and power output of different microwaves varies. These timings were tested in an 800-watt microwave and are a guide only, so you may need to adjust the timings slightly depending on the power of your microwave.

SWAP THIS: To make these with shop-bought ready-made popcorn rather than popping your own kernels, you will need 50g of ready-made popcorn. Try a lightly salted type to add a bit more saltiness to the salted caramel flavour or you may wish to omit the sea salt flakes on the top, depending on your taste. Alternatively, if you like things sweet, use lightly sweetened ready-made popcorn and add the sea salt flakes. Popcorn coated in butter or caramel may make the bites too sweet.

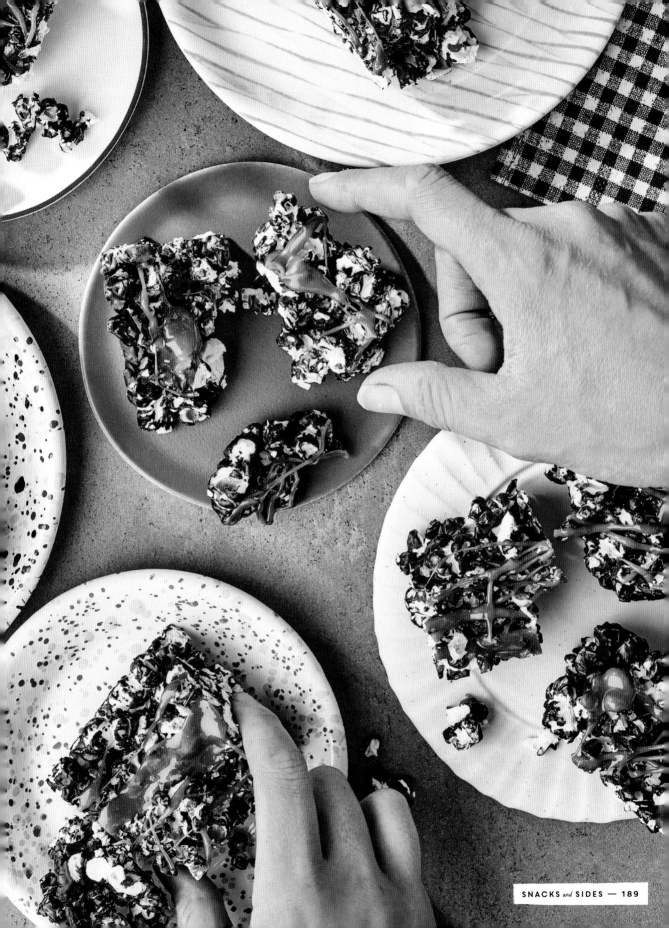

VEGGIE

USE A
VEGETARIAN
ITALIAN HARD
CHEESE

VEGAN

USE A
DF CHEESE

DAIRY
FREE

USE A
DF CHEESE

GLUTEN
FREE

USE CIDER NOT
MALT VINEGAR

LOW
CARB

POTATO PEEL CRISPS

🕐 **5 MINS**   🗑 **20 MINS**   🍴 **SERVES 2**

PER SERVING:
READY SALTED
45 KCAL / 9.1G CARBS

SALT AND VINEGAR
46 KCAL / 9.2G CARBS

CHEESE AND ONION
67 KCAL / 9.4G CARBS

100g potato peelings, from
   4 medium washed and
   dried potatoes
light olive oil spray

FOR READY SALTED
½ tsp sea salt, crushed

FOR SALT AND VINEGAR
2 tsp malt vinegar
½ tsp sea salt, crushed

FOR CHEESE AND ONION
10g Parmesan cheese, finely
   grated
½ tsp onion salt

Help do away with food waste and turn your potato peelings into these tasty crisps! These are so quick and easy to make and are lower in calories than shop-bought crisps. We've given you three popular flavours to choose from. Enjoy alone or with other snacks of your choice!

Everyday Light ─────────────────────

Preheat the oven to 180°C (fan 160°C/gas mark 4). Place the potato peelings in a medium bowl and spray with light olive oil spray.

For Ready Salted, add the sea salt and toss well to coat.

For Salt and Vinegar, add the malt vinegar and sea salt and toss well to coat.

For Cheese and Onion, add the Parmesan cheese and onion salt; toss well to coat.

Place the potato peelings in a single layer on a baking tray and place in the preheated oven. Bake for 15–20 minutes until crisp and golden.

Serve at once, alone or with other snacks of your choice.

TIPS: Make sure to wash and dry your potatoes well first. Remove any eyes or bruised parts from the potato peelings. We used light olive oil spray rather than low-calorie cooking spray as we found this made crispier crisps. Eat freshly made as these can soften over time.

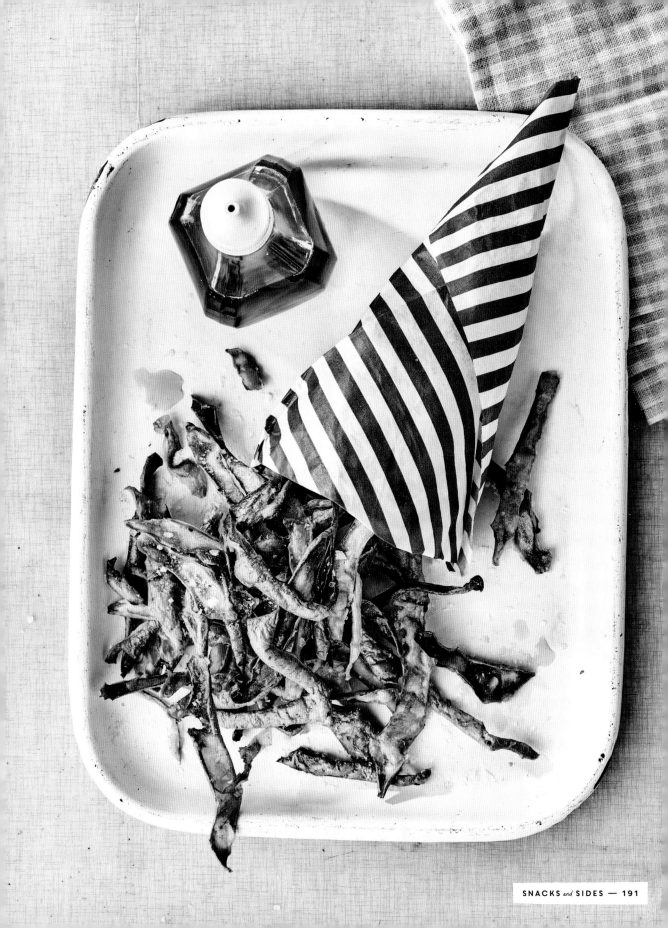

GREEK-STYLE BAKED BEANS

🕐 **10 MINS**   🗑 **55 MINS**   ✗ **SERVES 6**

PER SERVING:
175 KCAL /22G CARBS

low-calorie cooking spray
2 onions, peeled and finely
   chopped
2 garlic cloves, peeled and
   crushed
2 x 400g tins chopped
   tomatoes
2 tbsp tomato puree
2 tbsp fresh oregano leaves,
   chopped
sea salt and freshly ground
   black pepper
2 x 400g tins butter beans,
   rinsed and drained
90g reduced-fat feta cheese,
   crumbled into large pieces
pinch of white granulated
   sweetener (optional)
1 tbsp roughly chopped flat-
   leafed parsley, to garnish

TO ACCOMPANY *(optional)*
75g mixed salad (+ 15
   kcal per serving) and
   4 wholemeal folded
   flatbreads (+ 114 kcal per
   serving)

With rich tomato sauce and tangy feta cheese, these Greek-style Baked Beans always remind us of holidays. Enjoy this rustic, flavour-packed recipe as a protein-rich snack or a side dish. Give beans on toast a Pinch of Nom twist and try serving a portion on a slice of crusty bread; proper hearty, wholesome food.

Special Occasion ———————————————————

OVEN METHOD

SPECIAL EQUIPMENT
**Large ovenproof frying pan or
18 x 27cm (7 x 10½in) ovenproof dish**

Preheat the oven to 160°C (fan 140°C/gas mark 3).

Spray a large frying pan with low-calorie cooking spray and place over a medium heat. Add the onions and cook for 10–15 minutes, until softened and golden.

Add the garlic and cook for a further 1–2 minutes.

Add the tomatoes, tomato puree and oregano, then season to taste with salt and black pepper. Stir well and bring to a simmer.

Add the drained butter beans and stir in. Taste the mixture and if the tomatoes taste a little sharp, add a pinch of granulated sweetener.

If your frying pan isn't ovenproof, transfer the mixture to a medium ovenproof dish (around 18 x 27cm/7 x 10½in in size) and cover with a lid or foil.

Place in the preheated oven for 25–30 minutes.

Remove the lid or foil and sprinkle with feta cheese. Return to the oven for a further 5 minutes, until the cheese begins to soften a little. Sprinkle with parsley and serve with a mixed salad and flatbreads, or an accompaniment of your choice.

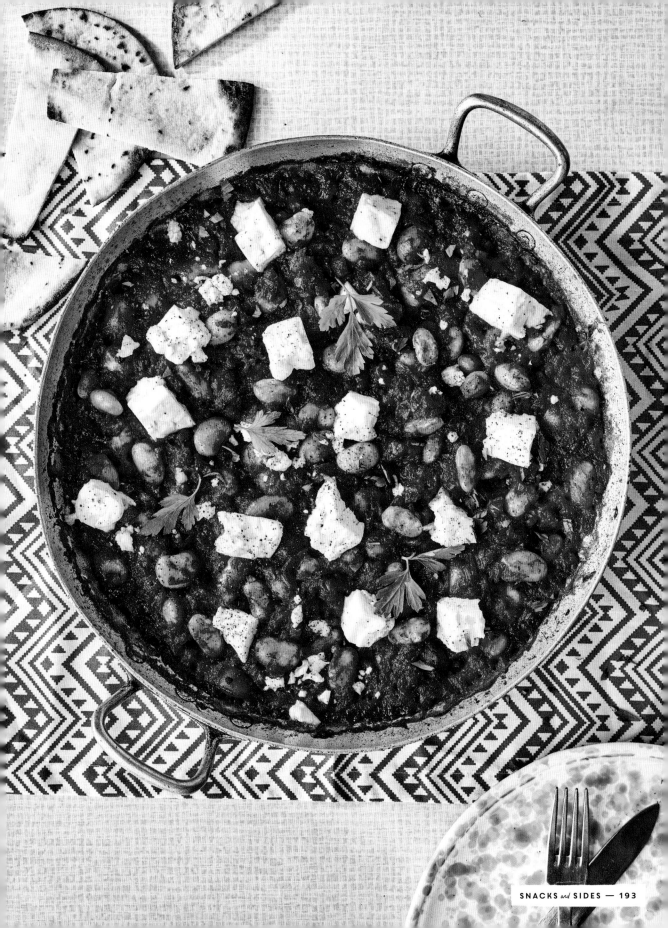

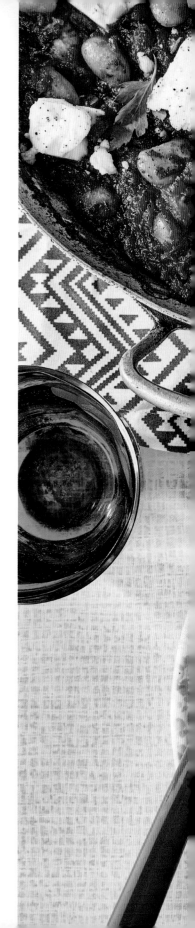

HOB-TOP METHOD

SPECIAL EQUIPMENT
**Large ovenproof frying pan or
18 x 27cm (7 x 10½in) ovenproof dish**

Spray a large frying pan with low-calorie cooking spray and place over a medium heat. Add the onions and cook for 10–15 minutes, until softened and golden.

Add the garlic and cook for a further 1–2 minutes.

Add the tomatoes, tomato puree and oregano, then season to taste with salt and black pepper. Stir well and bring to a simmer.

Add the drained butter beans and stir in. Taste the mixture and if the tomatoes taste a little sharp, add a pinch of granulated sweetener.

Lower the heat and cover tightly with a lid or kitchen foil. Simmer gently for 25–30 minutes, stirring occasionally. Preheat the grill on the medium setting. Remove the lid or foil from the frying pan and sprinkle with feta cheese.

If your frying pan isn't ovenproof, transfer the mixture to a medium ovenproof dish (around 18 x 27cm/7 x 10½in in size). Place the pan or dish under the grill for about 5 minutes, until the cheese begins to soften a little.

Sprinkle with parsley and serve with a mixed salad and flatbreads, or an accompaniment of your choice.

SWAP THIS: You could swap the butter beans for two tins of cannellini beans.

TIP: Use good-quality tinned tomatoes as they have a rich depth of flavour. Cheaper brands can sometimes be a bit acidic and this will affect the finished dish.

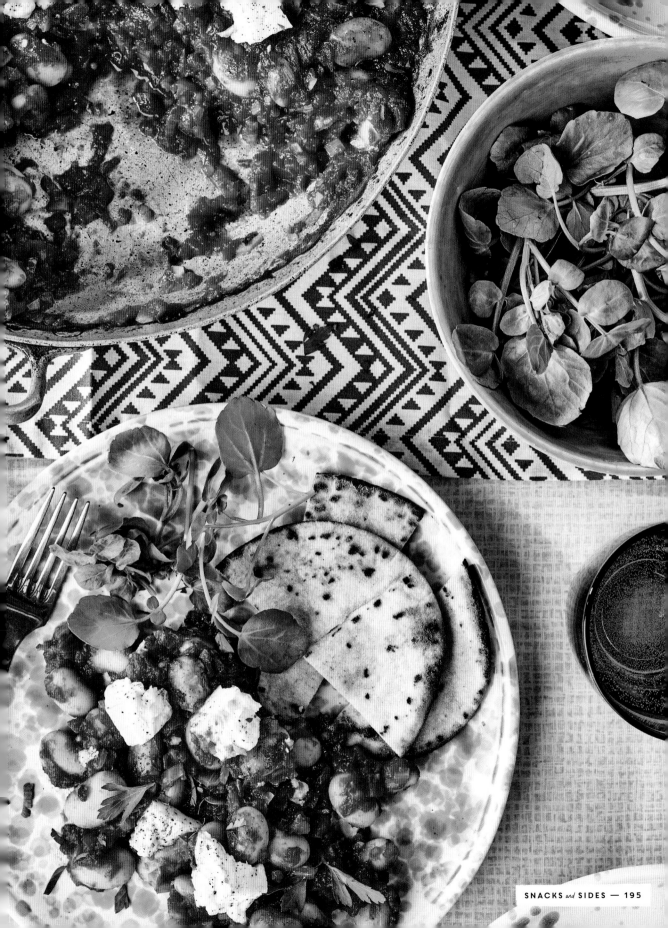

VEGETABLE SPRING ROLLS *with* SWEET CHILLI DIPPING SAUCE

🕐 **15 MINS**   🗑 **VARIABLE** (SEE BELOW)   ✕ **MAKES 8 ROLLS**

PER ROLL:
114 KCAL / 20G CARBS

6 spring onions, trimmed and cut into fine matchsticks, about 3cm (1¼in) long
2 garlic cloves, peeled and crushed
2cm (¾in) piece root ginger, peeled and grated
1 small red chilli, deseeded and finely chopped
1 medium carrot, peeled and cut into fine matchsticks, about 3cm (1¼in) long
¼ small red pepper, deseeded and cut into fine matchsticks, about 3cm (1¼in) long
¼ small green pepper, deseeded and cut into fine matchsticks, about 3cm (1¼in) long
70g fresh beansprouts
1 tbsp dark soy sauce
pinch of Chinese five-spice powder
24 squares of filo pastry measuring 12 x 12cm (5 x 5in) (see Tips opposite)
1 small egg, beaten
¼ tsp sesame seeds (optional)
low-calorie cooking spray

A Chinese-inspired fakeaway spread isn't complete without the crunchy satisfaction of spring rolls! Traditionally deep-fried, we've kept ours light by baking them in the oven (or air fryer). Why not invite everybody to have a go at wrapping their veggies in a light filo pastry package? Whether you enjoy them as a snack, starter or side, don't forget to dip!

Everyday Light ─────────────

OVEN METHOD
🗑 **25 MINS**

To make the spring rolls, preheat the oven to 180°C (fan 160°C/gas mark 4). Line a baking tray with non-stick baking paper.

Spray a large frying pan with low-calorie cooking spray and place over a medium heat. Add the spring onions, garlic, ginger and red chilli. Stir-fry for 1 minute. Add the carrot, red pepper and green pepper and stir-fry for 3 minutes. Add the beansprouts, soy sauce and five-spice powder. Stir-fry for another minute, taking care not to overcook the vegetables. Transfer to a plate and leave to cool for a few minutes.

Place three of the filo pastry squares on top of each other on the work surface – the three squares will create the casing for one of your spring rolls. Turn the square so that the square now looks like a diamond shape with one corner facing downwards towards you.

Divide the vegetable filling into eight portions on the plate. Place one portion of the vegetable filling into the centre of the filo square, placing it across the centre, from one corner to the opposite corner, leaving a small gap at the edges. Brush the beaten egg around all sides of the square.

Fold the bottom corner that is facing towards you upwards to overlap the vegetable filling. Fold in both ends of the filo square a little, to just overlap the filling. You should

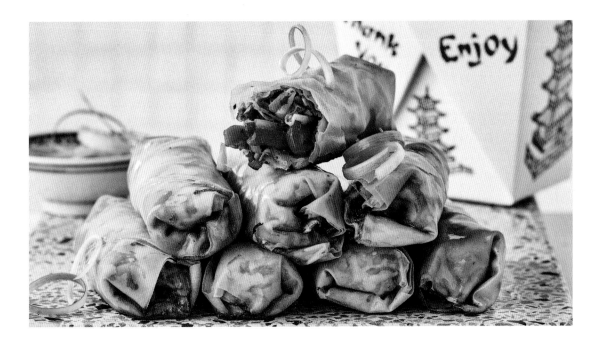

FOR THE SWEET CHILLI DIPPING SAUCE

low-calorie cooking spray
2 garlic cloves, peeled and crushed
1 small red chilli, deseeded and finely chopped
80ml white wine vinegar
2½ tbsp white granulated sweetener
1 tsp salt
2 tsp tomato puree
1 tsp clear honey
2 tsp cornflour

TIPS: You will need to measure and cut the 24 squares of filo pastry. The number of full, ready-rolled sheets you need will depend on the brand you use as the sheet size can vary. Cover the filo pastry with a clean, damp tea towel to stop it drying out as you make the spring rolls. Make sure to cut the vegetables neatly into fine matchsticks so that they will fit well into the spring rolls.

have a shape that now looks like an open envelope. Roll up the spring roll starting from the side nearest to you, finishing with the seam side down. Repeat this process to make the remaining spring rolls.

Once all eight spring rolls are on the lined baking tray, spray them liberally with low-calorie cooking spray and sprinkle with sesame seeds, if using. Place in the oven for 15–18 minutes, or until crisp and golden brown.

To make the dipping sauce, spray a small saucepan with low-calorie cooking spray and place over a medium heat. Add the garlic and red chilli and fry for 1–2 minutes until lightly coloured.

Add the white wine vinegar, 80ml cold water, white granulated sweetener, salt and tomato puree. Stir well and bring to the boil. Stir in the honey, simmer for 1 minute and remove from the heat.

In a small bowl, mix the cornflour with 2 teaspoons of cold water until smooth. Return the saucepan to the heat and stir in the cornflour and water mixture. Simmer, stirring constantly, for 1–2 minutes or until thickened and glossy. Taste the sauce and add a little more granulated sweetener to suit your taste if needed. Pour into a small serving dish and set aside while the spring rolls cook. Serve the dipping sauce alongside the spring rolls.

AIR-FRYER METHOD
🕐 20 MINS

SPECIAL EQUIPMENT
Air fryer

Preheat the air fryer to 160°C and line the basket with non-stick baking paper.

Spray a large frying pan with low-calorie cooking spray and place over a medium heat. Add the spring onions, garlic, ginger and red chilli. Stir-fry for 1 minute. Add the carrot, red pepper and green pepper and stir-fry for 3 minutes. Add the beansprouts, soy sauce and five-spice powder. Stir-fry for another minute, taking care not to overcook the vegetables. Transfer to a plate and leave to cool for a few minutes.

Place three of the filo pastry squares on top of each other on the work surface – the three squares will create the casing for one of your spring rolls. Turn the square so that the square now looks like a diamond shape with one corner facing downwards towards you.

Divide the vegetable filling into eight portions on the plate. Place one portion of the vegetable filling into the centre of the filo square, placing it across the centre, from one corner to the opposite corner, leaving a small gap at the edges. Brush the beaten egg around all sides of the square.

Fold the bottom corner that is facing towards you upwards to overlap the vegetable filling. Fold in both ends of the filo square a little, to just overlap the filling. You should have a shape that now looks like an open envelope. Roll up the spring roll starting from the side nearest to you, finishing with the seam side down. Repeat this process to make the remaining spring rolls.

Once all eight spring rolls are made, place them into the air-fryer basket seam side down. Depending on the size of your air fryer, you may need to cook them in batches. Spray liberally with low-calorie cooking spray and sprinkle with sesame seeds, if using.

Place into the air fryer for 12–15 minutes until crisp and golden brown.

To make the dipping sauce, sray a small saucepan with low-calorie cooking spray and place over a medium heat. Add the garlic and red chilli and then fry for 1–2 minutes until lightly coloured.

Add the white wine vinegar, 80ml cold water, white granulated sweetener, salt and tomato puree. Stir well and bring to the boil.

Stir in the honey, simmer for 1 minute and remove from the heat.

In a small bowl, mix the cornflour with 2 teaspoons of cold water until smooth. Return the saucepan to the heat and stir in the cornflour and water mixture. Simmer, stirring constantly, for 1–2 minutes or until thickened and glossy. Taste the sauce and add a little more granulated sweetener to suit your taste if needed. Pour into a small serving dish and set aside while the spring rolls cook.

Serve the dipping sauce alongside the spring rolls.

SWAP THIS: You can swap some of the vegetables with some cooked shredded duck, cooked chicken or cooked prawns.

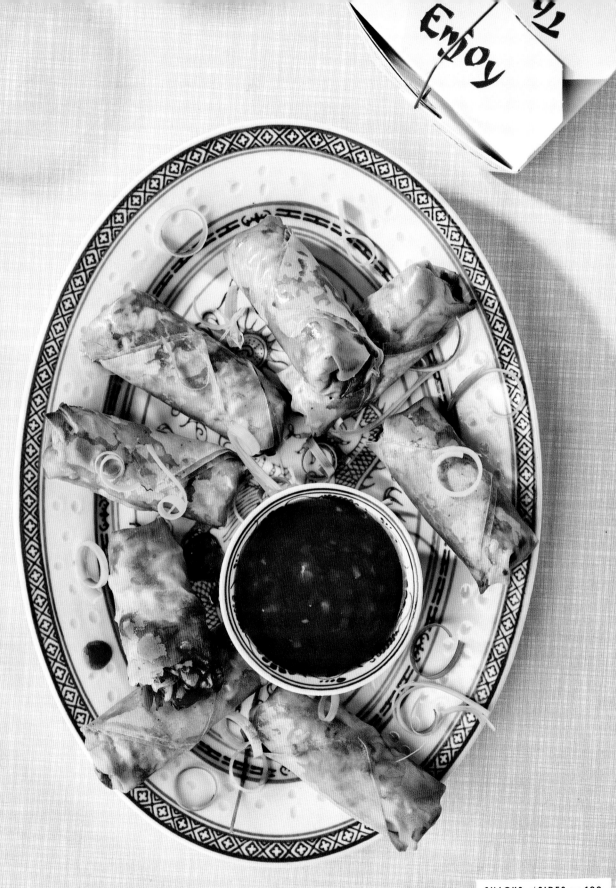

VEGAN

FREEZE ME

DOUGH BALLS ONLY

DAIRY FREE

USE A DF REDUCED-FAT SPREAD

GARLIC DOUGH BALLS

🕐 **25 MINS***   🗑 **10 MINS**   ✕ **16 DOUGH BALLS**

*PLUS 1 HOUR PROVING

PER DOUGH BALL:
78 KCAL / 12G CARBS

FOR THE GARLIC 'BUTTER'
50g reduced-fat spread
2 garlic cloves, peeled and crushed
2g flat-leafed parsley, stalks removed and leaves finely chopped
sea salt and freshly ground black pepper

FOR THE DOUGH BALLS
250g strong white bread flour, plus extra for dusting
2 tsp (5g) easy-blend dried yeast
½ tsp caster sugar
½ tsp salt
150ml warm water
low-calorie cooking spray

Forget going out to a restaurant – we promise there's nothing more irresistible than the smell of these homemade Garlic Dough Balls baking in your oven. They take a bit of effort, but the process is so satisfying! Once you've perfected making your dough from scratch, you'll want to make these every time you're having Italian-style meals.

Everyday Light

First, make the garlic 'butter'. Place the reduced-fat spread, garlic, parsley, salt and black pepper in a small micowave-safe bowl. Stir until well mixed, then place in the fridge while you make the dough balls.

For the dough balls, line a baking tray with non-stick baking paper.

Sift the flour into a large mixing bowl. Stir in the yeast, caster sugar and salt until evenly mixed.

Add the warm water and mix with a round-bladed knife until the dough starts to come together. Use clean hands to press the dough into a ball. Dust the work surface with a little of the extra flour. Turn the dough out onto the floured surface.

Knead the dough for 10 minutes, until smooth and elastic. Spray a clean, mixing bowl with a little low-calorie cooking spray and use it to thoroughly grease the bowl. Place the dough, seam side down in the greased bowl and cover with a plate. Place somewhere warm to prove for 1 hour until the dough has at least doubled in size and feels puffy when pressed. After the dough has been proving for 45 minutes, preheat the oven to 200°C (fan 180°C/gas mark 6).

Turn the dough out onto the work surface and lightly knead just four or five times. Form into a smooth ball, placing seam side down on the surface.

Cut the ball of dough into 16 equal-sized pieces. Shape the pieces into 16 small, smooth balls and place them seam side down on the lined baking tray, leaving space between each. Place in the preheated oven for 8–10 minutes until golden. The dough balls should sound hollow when tapped on the bottom.

SWAP THIS:
You could swap the flat-leafed parsley for chopped fresh chives or curly parsley.

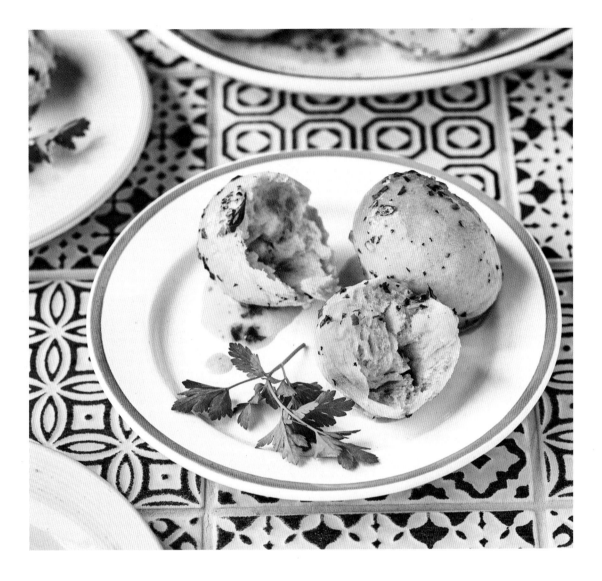

Remove from the oven and tip the dough balls into a large bowl.

Remove the garlic 'butter' from the fridge and microwave for about 20 seconds, or until just melted. Pour over the dough balls and toss to coat. Serve while still warm.

TIPS: Make sure you measure the yeast accurately (2 level teaspoons), using measuring spoons. The water must be warm, as this will help activate the yeast. Water that is too hot or too cold will not work. The caster sugar in this recipe helps activate the yeast, so do not replace the caster sugar with artificial sweetener. Kneading the dough for a full 10 minutes will ensure the gluten in the dough becomes elastic enough to get a good rise when cooked. It's worth timing the 10 minutes, as it's longer than you think when kneading! Make sure to place the dough somewhere warm when proving it. An airing cupboard would be the ideal temperature; anywhere hotter or colder may inactivate the yeast. If your oven has a built-in proving or warming drawer, use that.

HONEY GARLIC POTATOES

🕐 **5 MINS**   🗑 **VARIABLE** (SEE BELOW)   ✕ **SERVES 6**

PER SERVING:
130 KCAL / 27G CARBS

1kg new potatoes, chopped
  to be roughly the same size
low-calorie cooking spray
1 tsp garlic granules
sea salt and freshly ground
  black pepper
1 tbsp honey

Ever thought of drizzling honey over your roasties? Well, we tried it and it's completely delicious! This faff-free side dish uses new potatoes, so there's no need for peeling or chopping (the recipe will work just as well if you want to use larger potatoes though).

Everyday Light

OVEN METHOD
🍲 **35 MINS**

Preheat the oven to 200°C (fan 180°C/gas mark 6).

Add the potatoes to an ovenproof dish and coat well with low-calorie cooking spray. Sprinkle over the garlic granules and toss well so the potatoes are evenly coated. Season with salt and pepper to taste.

Place the potatoes in the preheated oven and cook for 30–35 minutes. When they are cooked, the outsides will be golden and crispy and the insides will be soft. Poke with a fork to check before removing them from the oven. Drizzle over the honey and toss until they're well coated. Serve alongside a main meal of your choice.

AIR-FRYER METHOD
🍲 **30 MINS**

SPECIAL EQUIPMENT Air fryer

Preheat the air fryer to 180°C.

Add the potatoes to a bowl and coat well with low-calorie cooking spray. Sprinkle over the garlic granules and toss well so the potatoes are evenly coated. Season with salt and pepper to taste.

Add the potatoes into the preheated air fryer basket and cook for 25–30 minutes, shaking the basket halfway through cooking. When they are cooked, the outsides will be golden and crispy and the insides will be soft. Poke with a fork to check. Once ready, transfer the potatoes to a bowl and toss with honey as described above.

TIPS: Runny honey works best in this recipe. If yours has crystallised, sit the jar in warm water for a few minutes to loosen it up. If your air fryer doesn't have a preheat function, we suggest heating at cooking temperature for a few minutes before cooking your food.

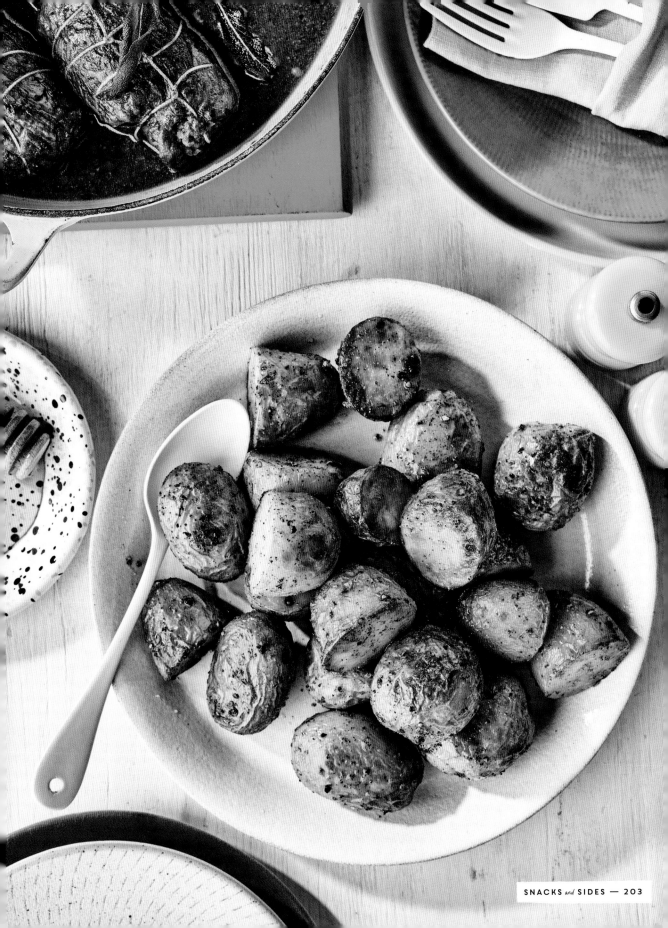

CHEESY MARMITE MASH

 VARIABLE (SEE BELOW)   **VARIABLE** (SEE BELOW)   ✕ **SERVES 4**

PER SERVING:

239 KCAL / 39G CARBS

800g potatoes, peeled and
   cut into 5cm (2in) chunks
150g reduced-fat spreadable
   cheese
1 tbsp Marmite
sea salt and freshly ground
   black pepper
a few snipped chives
   (optional)

If you love savoury flavours, you'll want to serve this Cheesy Marmite Mash with just about everything. It goes well as an accompaniment to any meat or veggie dishes, and we love using it instead of regular mash to top a cottage pie. Make sure you use spreadable cheese, not cream cheese – it won't give quite the right flavour!

Weekly Indulgence —————————————————————

HOB-TOP METHOD
🕐 **5 MINS**
🍲 **20 MINS**

Place the potatoes in a pan of cold, salted water and place over a high heat. Bring to the boil and then reduce the heat and simmer for 15–20 minutes until soft. You should be able to easily insert a knife into the centre of a chunk of potato.

Drain well and return to the pan. Add the spreadable cheese and Marmite. Mash thoroughly until you have no lumps and the spreadable cheese and Marmite are evenly combined with the potatoes.

Season with some black pepper. You probably won't need to add any salt as the Marmite and spreadable cheese are both salty. Garnish with fresh chives if using, and serve!

ELECTRIC PRESSURE-COOKER METHOD
🕐 **10 MINS**
🍲 **9 MINS**

SPECIAL EQUIPMENT

Electric pressure cooker

Place the potatoes into the pressure cooker and cover with cold water and a pinch of salt.

Place the lid onto the pressure cooker and set the valve to sealing. Select manual pressure and set a time of 9 minutes.

Once the pressure cooker has reached pressure, the timer will begin to count down.

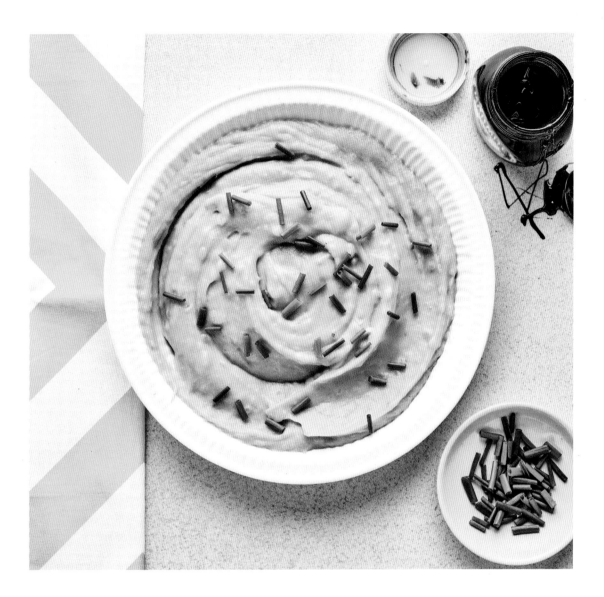

Once 9 minutes is complete, press cancel on the pressure cooker and turn the valve to 'venting' to manually release the pressure.

Once pressure has released, drain thoroughly and place the potatoes in a bowl.

Add the spreadable cheese and Marmite. Mash thoroughly until you have no lumps and the spreadable cheese and Marmite are evenly combined with the potatoes.

Season with some black pepper. You probably won't need to add any salt as the Marmite and spreadable cheese are both salty. Garnish with fresh chives if using, and serve!

PEA *and* BROCCOLI RICE

🕐 **15 MINS**   🗑 **25 MINS**   ✗ **SERVES 4**

PER SERVING:
205 KCAL / 34G CARBS

SPECIAL EQUIPMENT
Blender or food processor

120g basmati rice
2 vegetable stock cubes,
   crumbled
1 head of broccoli, florets
   only, about 250g
low-calorie cooking spray
1 large onion, peeled and
   diced
2 garlic cloves, peeled and
   minced
1 tbsp white wine vinegar
2 tbsp lemon juice
150g frozen peas
40g spinach, any large
   stalks removed, leaves
   finely chopped
8g mint leaves, stalks
   removed, finely chopped
sea salt and freshly ground
   black pepper

Say hello to your new favourite way to liven up rice! We love the vibrant, fun shades of green from all these summery veggies. With added garlic, onion, spinach and mint, there's no shortage of flavour here. Delicious all on its own, or a half a portion served up with your favourite main to brighten up your plate in an instant!

Weekly Indulgence ────────────

Cook the rice according to the packet instructions, adding the crumbled stock cubes to the water. This will take about 20 minutes. Drain well, cover and set aside.

While the rice is cooking, place the broccoli florets into a blender and pulse until it is the consistency of rice. Set aside.

Spray a large frying pan with low-calorie cooking spray and place over a medium heat. Add the onion and garlic and cook gently for 10 minutes to soften the onion – the aim is for them to be soft and glossy. If they are browning too much, lower the heat a little.

Add the vinegar, lemon juice, broccoli and peas to the frying pan, stir in and cook for 5 minutes over a medium heat.

Add the cooked rice, spinach and mint to the pan and stir in. Spray with some more low-calorie cooking spray and cook for another 5 minutes.

Season with salt and black pepper to taste and serve.

SWAP THIS: If you aren't vegetarian, chicken stock cubes are also great in this dish!

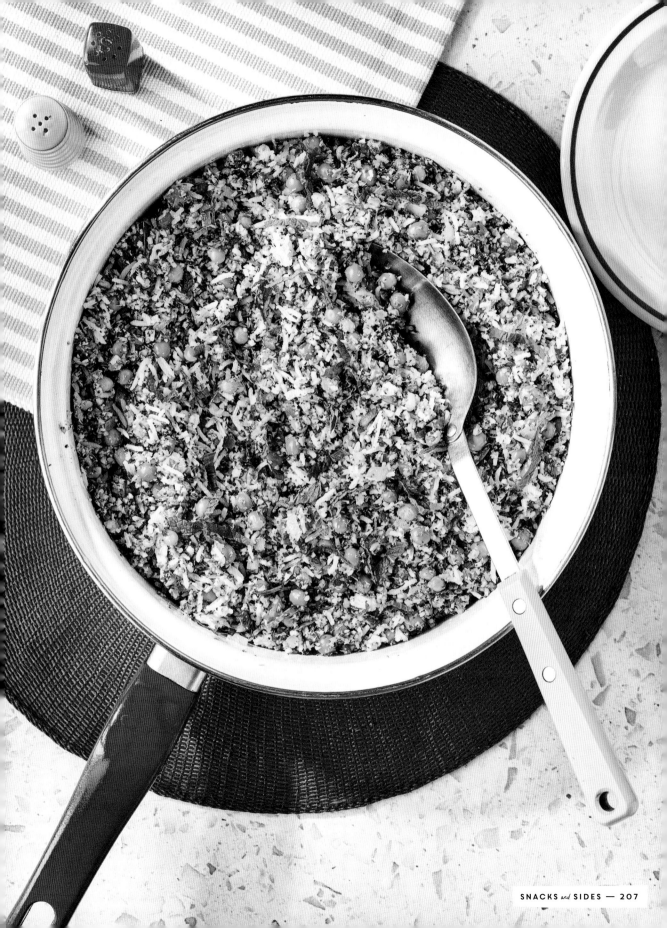

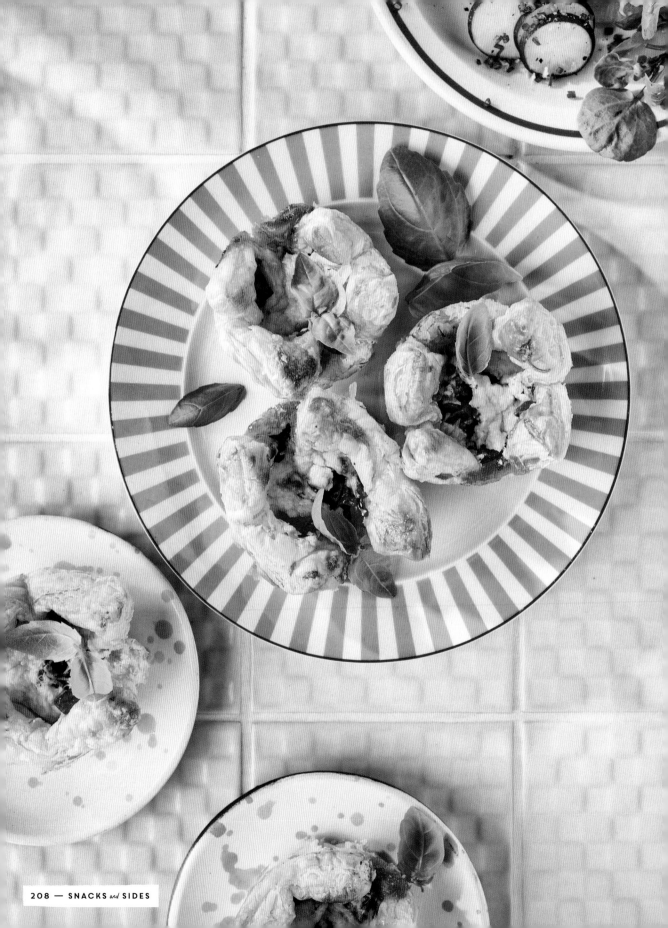

PIZZA PUFFS

🕐 **10 MINS**   🗑 **20 MINS**   ✕ **MAKES 8 PUFFS**

PER PUFF:
184 KCAL / 20G CARBS

SPECIAL EQUIPMENT
12-hole muffin tin

low-calorie cooking spray
2 tbsp tomato puree
½ tsp Italian mixed dried
   herbs
½ tsp Henderson's relish or
   Worcestershire sauce
320g ready-rolled light puff
   pastry sheet
30g pepper of your choice,
   deseeded and diced
3 cherry tomatoes, diced
3 slices pepperoni, about 15g,
   diced
20g reduced-fat Cheddar
   cheese, finely grated
pinch of ground black
   pepper
a few basil leaves, to garnish
   (optional)

These golden nibbles pack pizza flavours into a tasty bite. With light puff pastry and just a few other simple ingredients, you can have all the cheesy, tomato flavours puffed up and ready to enjoy with a crisp salad in just 30 minutes. Why not try them with oven chips for a slimming-friendly midweek pizza night?

Everyday Light

Preheat the oven to 190°C (fan 170°C/gas mark 5) and spray eight of the holes in the muffin tin with a little low-calorie cooking spray.

Add the tomato puree, mixed herbs, Henderson's relish and half a teaspoon of water to a small bowl and mix until smooth.

Roll the puff pastry sheet out flat and cut in half lengthways. Cut each half into four sections, giving you eight pieces. Press each section of puff pastry into a hole in the muffin tin.

Add a little of the tomato puree mix into the bottom of each puff pastry cup. Split the pepper, cherry tomatoes and pepperoni between the eight cups. Sprinkle over the cheese and season with a little black pepper.

Use a pastry brush to spread half a teaspoon of water onto the edges of the pastry. Pop into the oven for 20 minutes until the pastry is golden and cheese is melted.

Garnish with basil leaves, if you like, and serve alone or with your choice of accompaniment.

SWAP THIS: You can swap the pepperoni for diced wafer-thin ham, or for a vegetarian option, use meat-free cooked sausage.

VEGGIE

FREEZE ME

LOW CARB

CHEESE *and* MARMITE SWIRLS

🕐 **6 MINS**   🗑 **15 MINS**   ✗ **MAKES 16 SWIRLS**

PER SWIRL:
89 KCAL / 9.5G CARBS

320g ready-rolled light puff
  pastry sheet
40g reduced-fat mature
  Cheddar cheese, finely
  grated
3 tsp Marmite
2 tsp boiling water

If you're a Marmite lover, you've just found your new favourite snack. You only need four ingredients to make this recipe, which gives it a big thumbs up from us! The light puff pastry is stuffed with a moreish cheesy filling and baked to perfection. From buffets and picnics to cheeseboards, you'll want to take every opportunity to make these.

Everyday Light

Preheat the oven to 220°C (fan 200°C/gas mark 7) and line a baking tray with non-stick baking paper.

Unroll the pastry sheet, leaving it on its greaseproof paper packaging, and place it on your work surface.

Add the Marmite to a small bowl with the boiling water and mix until smooth. Spread the Marmite in an even layer onto the puff pastry, leaving a 1cm (½in) gap on each of the short edges. Sprinkle over the Cheddar cheese.

Roll up the pastry, starting with one of the long edges, using the greaseproof paper packaging to help you. Keep rolling until you have made a 'Swiss roll'. When you have finished rolling up the pastry, make sure it is seam side down.

Use a large serrated knife, such as a bread knife, to carefully cut into 16 spiral-shaped slices. Place the swirls onto the lined baking tray, leaving gaps between each swirl.

Place the tray in the oven and bake for 15–20 minutes, until golden and crisp. Place on a wire rack to cool or serve warm fresh from the oven.

TIP: If you find the pastry difficult to slice, wrap the roll up in the greaseproof paper and pop back in the fridge to chill for 10 minutes. The pastry will firm up and be easier to slice.

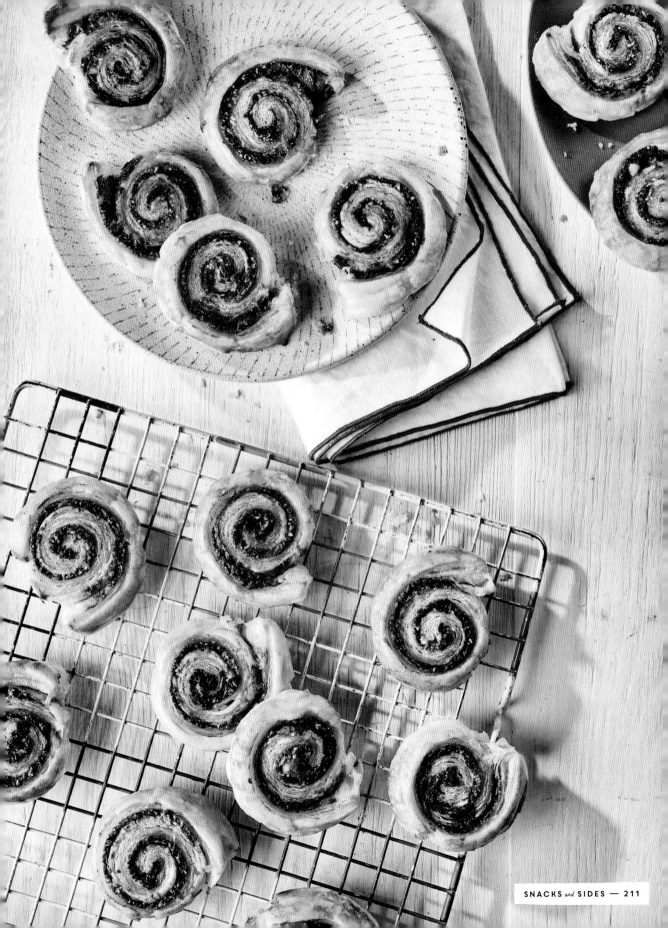

DAIRY FREE
USE DF CREAM CHEESE AND CHEDDAR CHEESE

GLUTEN FREE
USE GF WHOLEMEAL BREAD

TUNA MELT TOASTS

🕐 **10 MINS**　🍳 **10 MINS**　✕ **SERVES 4**

PER SERVING:
184 KCAL / 13G CARBS

SPECIAL EQUIPMENT
Grill pan and rack

1 x 145g tin tuna chunks in brine, well drained
¼ small red onion, peeled and finely diced
¼ medium red pepper, deseeded and finely diced
2 spring onions, trimmed and finely chopped
4 cherry tomatoes, finely diced
1 tsp lemon juice
25g low-fat cream cheese
pinch of sea salt and freshly ground black pepper
4 small, thin slices of wholemeal bread, about 28g per slice
80g reduced-fat mature Cheddar cheese, finely grated

TO ACCOMPANY *(optional)*
75g mixed salad (+ 15 kcal per serving)

Is it just us or is everything better toasted? Change your lunchtime sandwich routine with a simple tuna melt treat that you can have ready in minutes. A joyful combination of tuna, crunchy veggies and cheese makes this satisfying, slimming-friendly melt a total crowd-pleaser. It's filling as a standalone snack or add a salad to the side for lunch!

Everyday Light ────────────────

Place all the ingredients except the wholemeal bread and Cheddar cheese in a small bowl and stir well to make a spreadable mixture.

Preheat the grill to medium. Place the bread slices on the grill-pan rack and place under the preheated grill for a couple of minutes to lightly toast on one side.

Turn the bread slices over and spread the tuna mixture evenly over the untoasted side, right to the edges.

Sprinkle the Cheddar cheese over the tuna mixture and place under the grill for 4–5 minutes, or until melted and golden. Serve at once with a crisp mixed salad or accompaniment of your choice.

SWAP THIS: You can swap the bread for a halved wholemeal bread roll, ciabatta, flatbread or other bread base of choice – but don't forget to adjust the calories accordingly.

TIP: For a spicy kick you could try adding a small pinch of mild chilli powder, chilli flakes or a few drops of hot pepper sauce to the tuna and cheese mixture.

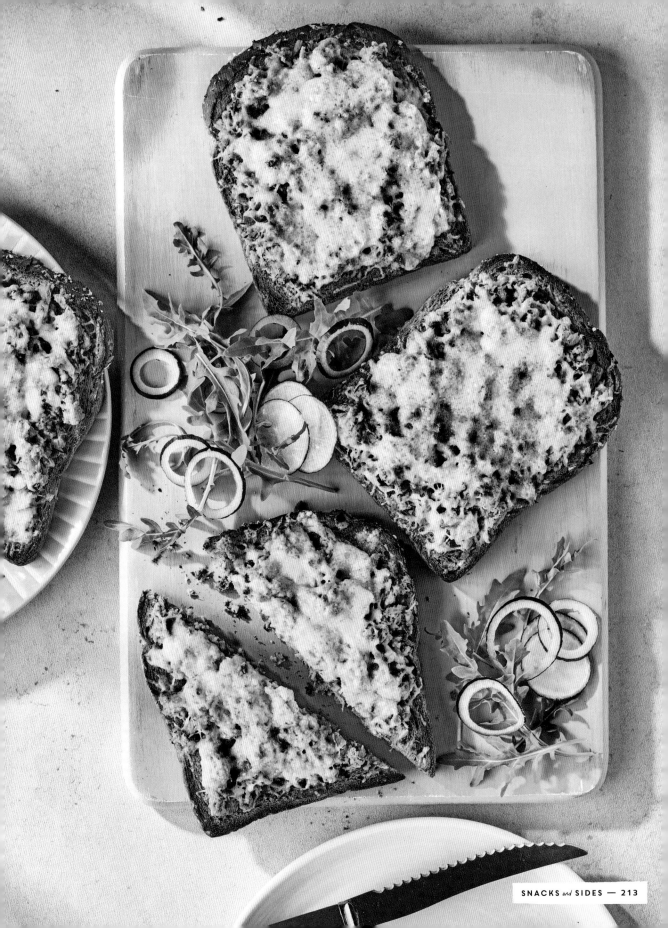

VEGGIE

USE VEGETARIAN
GREEK SALAD
CHEESE

FREEZE
ME

GLUTEN
FREE

USE GF STOCK
CUBE

GREEK-STYLE SPINACH *and* RICE

🕐 **5 MINS**   🍲 **15 MINS**   ✕ **SERVES 4**

PER SERVING:
224 KCAL / 43G CARBS

low-calorie cooking spray
1 onion, peeled and finely
  diced
1 small leek, trimmed and
  finely sliced
½ tsp dried oregano
1 tsp garlic granules
200g basmati rice
grated zest and juice of
  1 lemon
350ml vegetable stock
  (1 vegetable stock cube
  dissolved in 350ml boiling
  water)
150g spinach, roughly
  chopped
small handful of fresh dill,
  chopped
sea salt and freshly ground
  black pepper
50g reduced-fat feta cheese

Lemony, garlicky and tangy from the feta cheese, this rice is almost too good to be a side dish! Inspired by punchy Greek flavours, it's so simple and quick to make, you'll want to serve it with everything. Spoon onto the side of fish or meat dishes, or crumble extra feta on the top and enjoy as a lovely light lunch.

Weekly Indulgence

Spray a saucepan with low-calorie cooking spray and place over a medium heat. Add the onion and leek to the pan and sauté for 5 minutes until softened but not coloured.

Stir in the oregano and garlic granules.

Give the rice a quick rinse, then add to the pan and cook for 1 minute.

Add the lemon zest, stock and stir.

Bring to the boil, then reduce the heat to low. Add the spinach to the pan (no need to stir it in) then cover with a lid and cook for 10 minutes.

Remove from the heat. Stir in the lemon juice and dill. Season with salt and pepper, then replace the lid and allow it to stand for 5 minutes.

Crumble over the feta and serve.

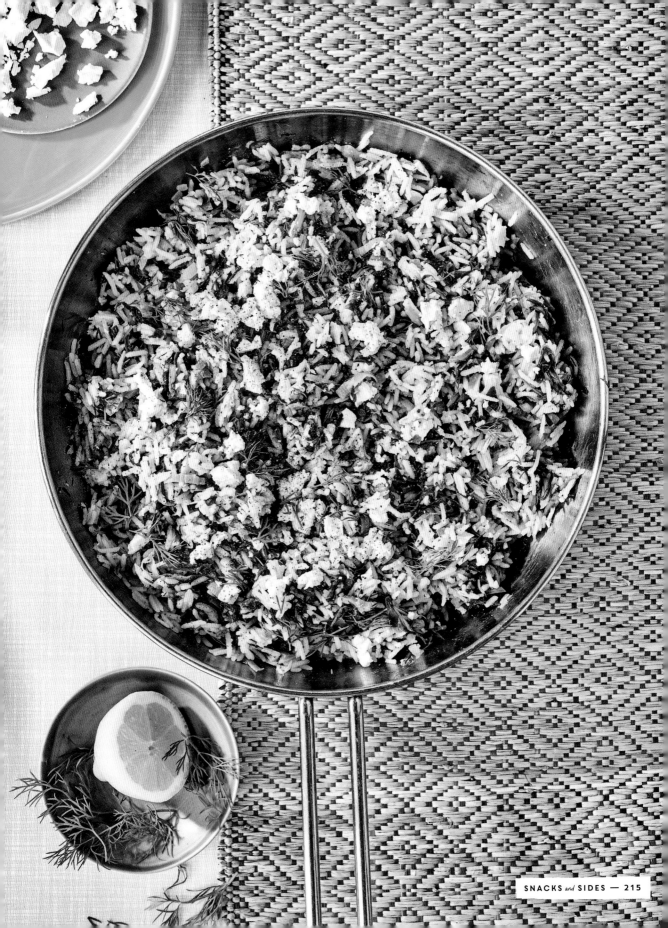

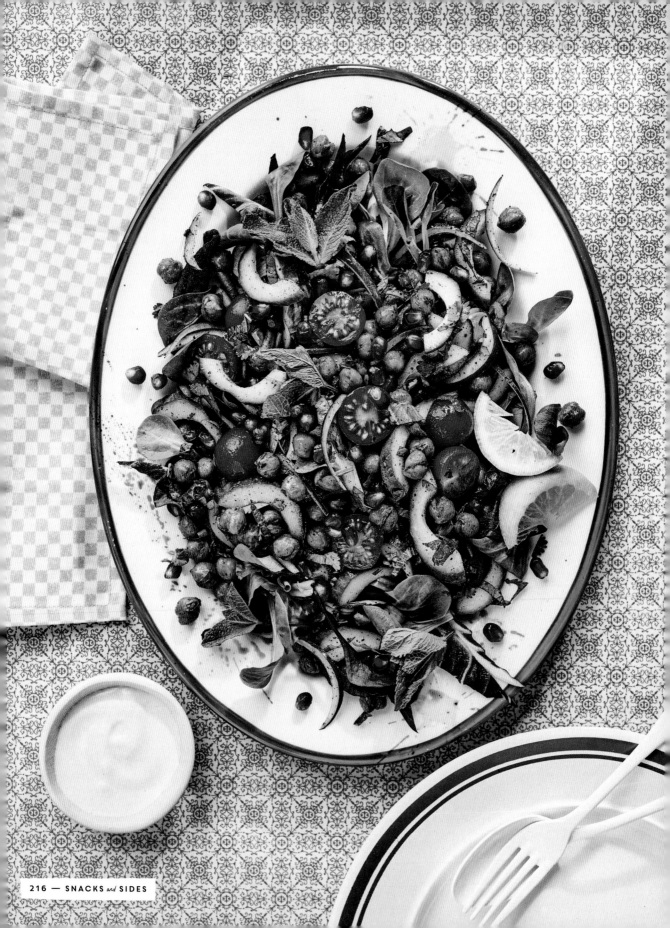

CHICKPEA SALAD

🕐 **15 MINS**   🗑 **5 MINS**   ✕ **SERVES 2**

PER SERVING:
300 KCAL / 30G CARBS

SPECIAL EQUIPMENT
**Small food processor
or blender**

low-calorie cooking spray
1 x 400g tin chickpeas,
  drained and rinsed
2 tsp sumac
½ tsp chilli powder (more if
  you like heat)
1 garlic clove, peeled and
  crushed
sea salt and freshly ground
  black pepper
10 cherry tomatoes, halved
½ medium red onion, peeled
  and finely sliced
½ cucumber, about 300g,
  cut in half lengthways,
  deseeded and sliced into
  half-moon shapes
handful of fresh coriander,
  roughly chopped
a few mint leaves, chopped
2 good handfuls of mixed
  salad leaves
2 tbsp pomegranate seeds
lemon wedges (optional)

FOR THE FETA DRESSING
75g fat-free Greek-style
  yoghurt
50g reduced-fat feta cheese,
  crumbled
squeeze of lemon juice

We've loaded this refreshing recipe with a balance of sharp, zingy and savoury flavours – the citrus hint of the sumac really brings the chickpeas to life. You won't believe how quickly it comes together! This makes a tasty and filling packed lunch and it's even better if you leave the flavours to mingle in the fridge overnight.

Special Occasion ─────────────────

Spray a frying pan with low-calorie cooking spray and place over a medium to low heat.

Pat the chickpeas dry with some kitchen towel and then add to the pan along with the sumac, chilli powder and garlic. Gently fry for around 5 minutes to toast the spices and cook the garlic. Taste and season with some salt and pepper if needed. Leave to cool, while you make the dressing.

To make the dressing, place the yoghurt, feta and a squeeze of lemon juice in a small food processor or blender and blitz. Add a tablespoon or two of water until you get a smooth consistency.

Add the tomatoes, onion, cucumber, chickpeas and chopped herbs to a bowl and toss together.

Place a handful of mixed leaves on two plates and top with the chickpea salad.

Drizzle over the feta and yoghurt dressing, scatter over the pomegranate seeds and serve with a lemon wedge, if using.

MEXICAN-STYLE
STREET CORN SALAD

🕙 **10 MINS**　　🗑 **NO COOK**　　✗ **SERVES 4**

PER SERVING:
206 KCAL / 22G CARBS

5 ripe salad tomatoes
1 x 340g tin sweetcorn,
　drained
1 x 400g tin black beans,
　rinsed and drained
70g reduced-fat feta cheese,
　crumbled
1 large handful of fresh
　coriander, stalks removed
　and finely chopped
1 tbsp lime juice, plus lime
　slices to serve
1 tsp smoked paprika
½ tsp chilli powder
sea salt and freshly ground
　black pepper

TO ACCOMPANY *(optional)*
30g individual bag of tortilla
　chips (+ 38 kcal per serving)

We love corn on the cob, so we've borrowed the fresh, hot and zingy flavours from street corn to create this super-colourful salad. You can't get much closer to eating a rainbow for lunch than this! Quick and simple to throw together, the bold flavours will brighten even the sunniest of days.

Weekly Indulgence

Cut your tomatoes in half and use a spoon to scoop out the seeds from the centre and discard. Dice the remaining tomato flesh and add to a large bowl.

Add the rest of the ingredients to the bowl and toss to coat.

Add salt and black pepper to taste, and serve with a few tortilla chips, if you like.

TIP: Using good-quality, ripe salad tomatoes will make a big difference in this dish. It is especially tasty with on-the-vine varieties.

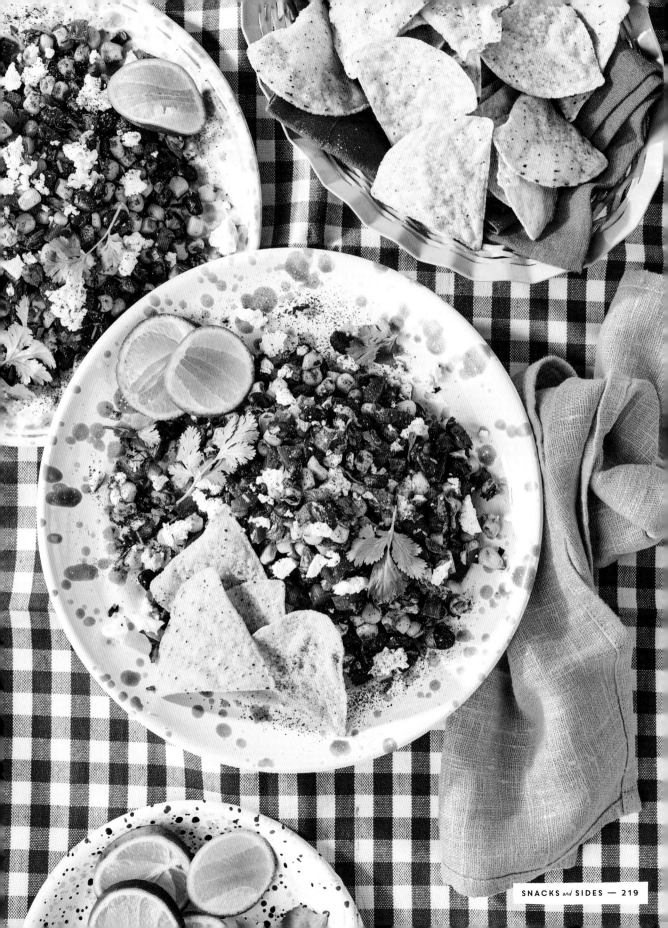

VEGAN

DAIRY
FREE

GLUTEN
FREE

USE GF SOY
SAUCE

LOW
CARB

ROASTED SOY *and* GINGER BROCCOLI

🕐 **5 MINS**   🗑 **18 MINS**   ✕ **SERVES 4**

PER SERVING:
56 KCAL /5G CARBS

2 tbsp light soy sauce
1 garlic clove, peeled and
  crushed
1cm (½in) piece root ginger,
  peeled and finely grated
1 head of broccoli, about
  350g
low-calorie cooking spray
1 tsp white sesame seeds

Who says broccoli has to be boring? We love a good oven-baked broccoli recipe, and the Asian-inspired flavours we've used to coat our florets are bound to impress even the pickiest eaters at the table. We love how well the charred flavours complement the garlicky coating of ginger and soy sauce, and there's room to experiment with added dried chilli flakes too!

Everyday Light

Preheat the oven to 200°C (fan 180°C/gas mark 6).

Mix the soy sauce, garlic and ginger together in a large mixing bowl.

Trim the woody stem off the broccoli, cut into bite-sized florets and place in the bowl with the soy sauce mixture. Toss to coat the florets.

Spray a baking sheet with low-calorie cooking spray. Scatter the florets evenly across the tray, making sure you don't overcrowd the tray. This will ensure even cooking. Spray with more low-calorie cooking spray and sprinkle over the sesame seeds.

Place in the oven for 12–18 minutes. Check regularly, as the broccoli can catch and become bitter. When cooked, the broccoli should be brown and crispy around the edges while remaining tender in the middle.

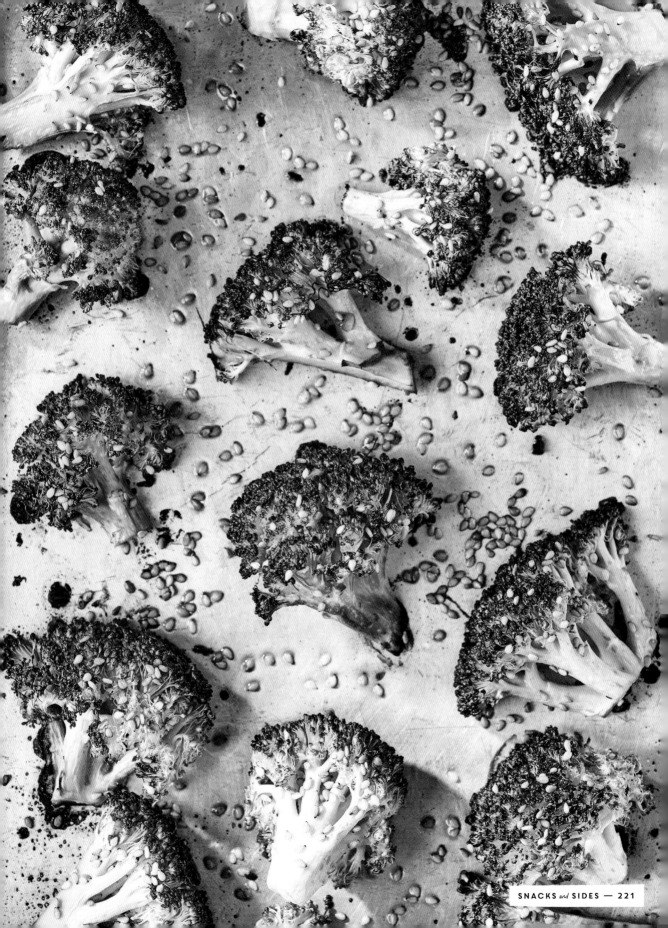

CHEESY GARLIC SWEET POTATO

🕐 **5 MINS**   **25 MINS**   ✕ **SERVES 4**

PER SERVING:
190 KCAL / 27G CARBS

SPECIAL EQUIPMENT
Large roasting tin

500g sweet potato, peeled
  and cut into 3cm (1¼in)
  chunks
low-calorie cooking spray
1 small onion, peeled and
  diced
3 garlic cloves, peeled and
  crushed
1 tsp dried parsley
sea salt and freshly ground
  black pepper
20g Parmesan cheese, finely
  grated
40g reduced-fat mature
  Cheddar cheese, finely
  grated
30g reduced-fat mozzarella,
  finely grated
2 tsp chopped fresh chives

Calling all cheese lovers – this dish is topped with not one, not two, but three different cheeses. Baked until everything is golden and melty, we can't get enough of these garlicky, cheesy spuds. Spoon them onto your Sunday roast or serve them instead of plain chips.

Everyday Light ─────────────────────────

Preheat the oven to 180°C (fan 160°C/gas mark 4).

Add the sweet potato to a saucepan and cover with cold water. Bring to the boil, then reduce the heat to medium and cook for 4 minutes until the sweet potato is softened but still holding its shape. Drain well.

While the sweet potato is cooking, spray a frying pan with low-calorie cooking spray and place over a medium heat. Add the onion and fry for 4 minutes. Add the garlic and continue to fry for a further 2 minutes.

Add the sweet potato, onion and garlic to the large roasting tin. Sprinkle over the parsley and season with salt and pepper and stir well.

Sprinkle over the Parmesan, Cheddar and mozzarella cheese and pop into the oven for 20 minutes.

When the cheese is golden and melted, remove from the oven, sprinkle over the chives and serve.

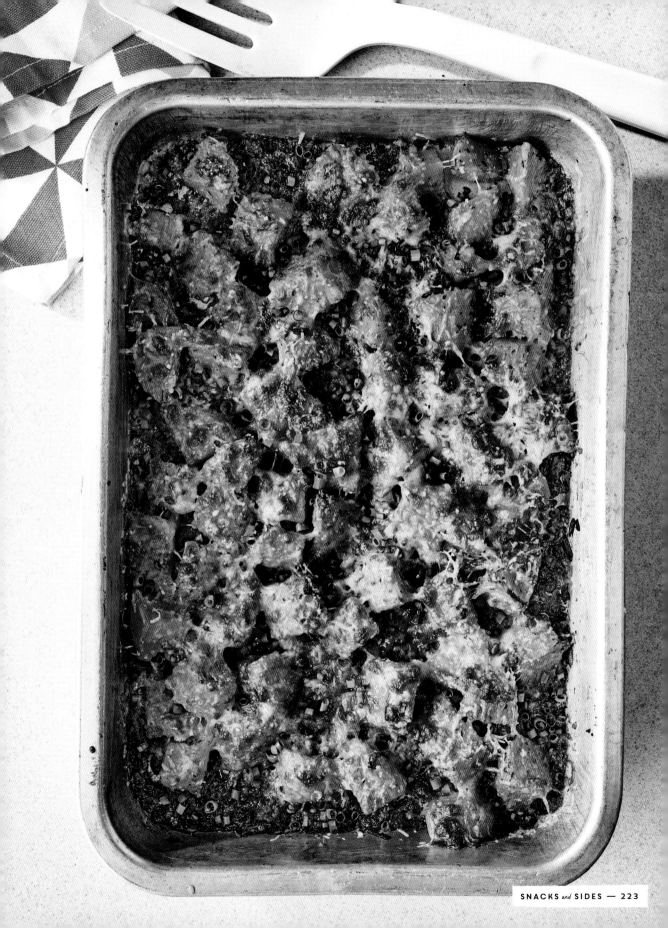

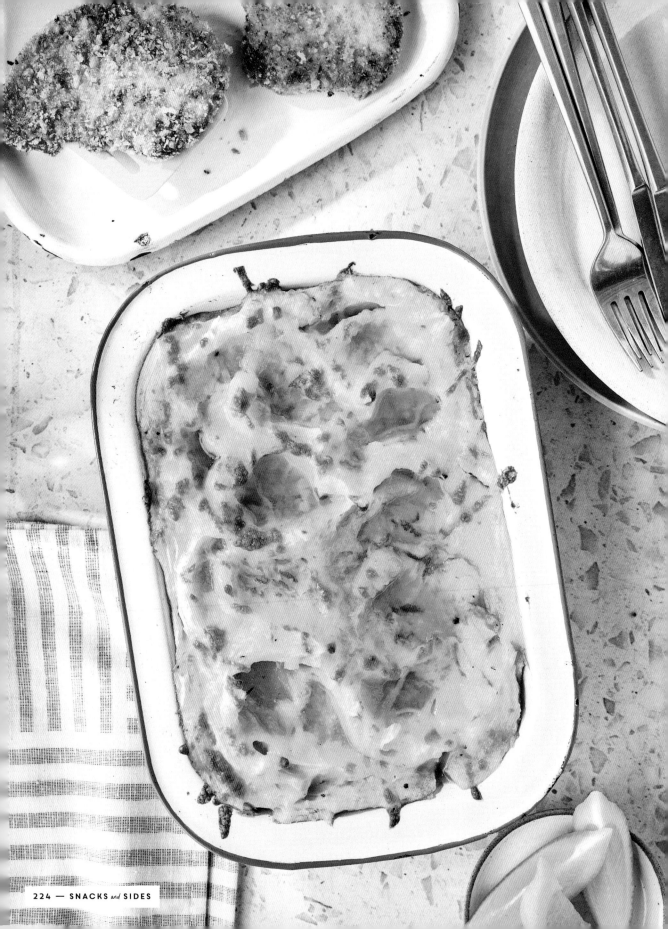

ROASTED GARLIC MASHED POTATO

🕐 **10 MINS** 🗑 **VARIABLE** (SEE BELOW) ✕ **SERVES 4**

PER SERVING:
249 KCAL / 47G CARBS

SPECIAL EQUIPMENT
18 x 27cm (7 x 10½in) ovenproof dish

1 whole head of garlic, made up of about 8 cloves
1kg potatoes, peeled and cut into large chunks
sea salt and freshly ground black pepper
100ml skimmed milk
a little reduced-fat spread, for greasing
20g reduced-fat Cheddar cheese, finely grated

Our Roasted Garlic Mashed Potato recipe is so rich, creamy and low in calories, there's really no reason to say no! As if having garlicky flavours in each and every spoonful wasn't enough, the melty golden cheese topping really seals the deal. This one's ideal to rustle up if you want to add an extra-special side dish to a midweek meal.

Weekly Indulgence ───────────────

HOB-TOP METHOD
🍲 **1 HOUR 10 MINS**

Preheat the oven to 180°C (fan 160°C/gas mark 4).

Wrap the whole head of garlic in foil and place in the oven to bake for about 45 minutes, until softened.

Remove the garlic from the foil and set aside.

Place the potatoes in a large saucepan of salted water, partially cover with a lid and bring to the boil. Lower the heat and simmer for 20 minutes until the potatoes are tender.

Drain the potatoes in a colander and return them to the saucepan.

Squeeze each of the softened roasted garlic cloves into the potatoes and discard the skins.

Add the milk and some salt and pepper to the potatoes and garlic and mash together until smooth.

Preheat the grill on the medium setting. Lightly grease the ovenproof dish with a little reduced-fat spread and add the mashed potato mixture. Roughly spread out and sprinkle with grated cheese.

Place under the grill for about 5 minutes until golden brown.

Serve with a meal of your choice.

TIPS: We used one whole head of garlic, which contains around 8 individual cloves. This may sound like a lot, but the flavour of garlic mellows when it's roasted. You may even want to use two whole heads if you're a big fan of strong garlic flavours! Why not put your potato peelings in the oven with the garlic and make a batch of Potato Peel Crisps (see page 190)?

ELECTRIC PRESSURE-COOKER METHOD
🍲 **54 MINS**

SPECIAL EQUIPMENT
Electric pressure cooker

Preheat the oven to 180°C (fan 160°C/gas mark 4).

Wrap the whole head of garlic in foil and place in the preheated oven to bake for about 45 minutes, until softened.

Remove the garlic from the foil and set aside.

Around 10 minutes from the end of the garlic cooking time, place the potatoes into the pressure cooker and cover with cold water.

Place the lid onto the pressure cooker and set the valve to sealing. Select manual pressure and set a time of 9 minutes. Once the pressure cooker has reached pressure, the timer will begin to count down.

Once the time is complete, press cancel on the pressure cooker. Carefully set the valve to 'venting' to manually release pressure. Once all pressure has released, remove the lid and drain the potatoes well.

Squeeze each of the softened roasted garlic cloves into the potatoes and discard the skins.

Add the milk and salt and pepper to the potatoes and garlic and mash together until smooth.

Preheat the grill on the medium setting. Lightly grease the ovenproof dish with a little reduced-fat spread and add the mashed potato mixture. Roughly spread out and sprinkle with grated cheese.

Place under the grill for about 5 minutes until golden brown.

Serve with a meal of your choice.

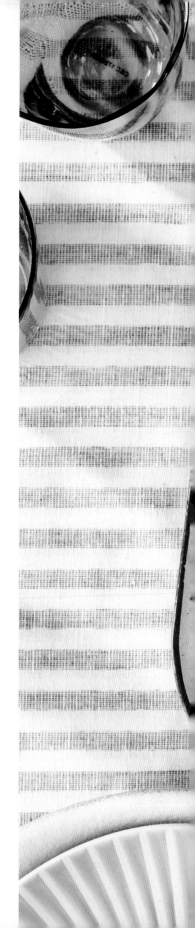

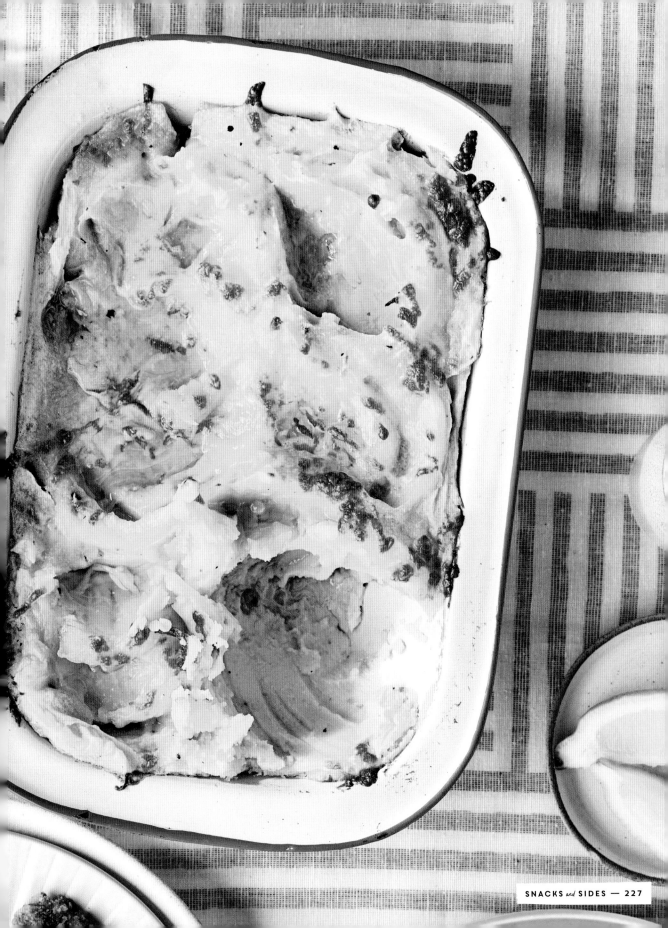

Sweet
Treats

BANANA BREAD BROWNIES

🕐 **10 MINS**   🗑 **16 MINS**   ✕ **MAKES 16 SQUARES**

PER SQUARE:
128 KCAL / 20G CARBS

SPECIAL EQUIPMENT
20cm (8in) square cake tin

50g reduced-fat spread, plus
  extra for greasing
100g golden granulated
  sweetener
200g self-raising flour
3 tbsp cocoa powder
1 tsp baking powder
3 medium eggs, beaten
3 medium bananas
20g white chocolate chips

Why choose between your two favourite sweet treats when you can combine them into one dreamy bake? These Banana Bread Brownies just make so much sense. This recipe is lighter than a traditional brownie, and you get to enjoy the heavenly pairing of banana and chocolate. We can't think of a better way to use up spare bananas.

Everyday Light

Preheat the oven to 170°C (fan 150°C/gas mark 3) and grease the cake tin with a little reduced fat-spread. Line the base and sides with greaseproof paper and leave to one side.

Add the reduced-fat spread and sweetener to a bowl and beat with a wooden spoon until fluffy. In a separate bowl, stir together the flour, cocoa and baking powder. Add the dry mixture to the wet ingredients with the eggs and mix thoroughly until fully combined.

Add two of the bananas to a small bowl and mash with a fork until smooth. Stir into the brownie mixture.

Pour the brownie mixture into the lined tin and spread out the top until smooth. Slice the last banana lengthways into four slices and arrange on top of the brownie, pushing them into the mixture slightly.

Sprinkle with the chocolate chips and bake in the oven for 16 minutes until the mixture is just set. Leave to cool in the tin and slice into 16 squares. These will keep tor up to 3 days in an airtight container.

TIP: When these brownies are left to cool in the tin they will carry on cooking a little, so undercooking them slightly in the oven will result in a perfect brownie!

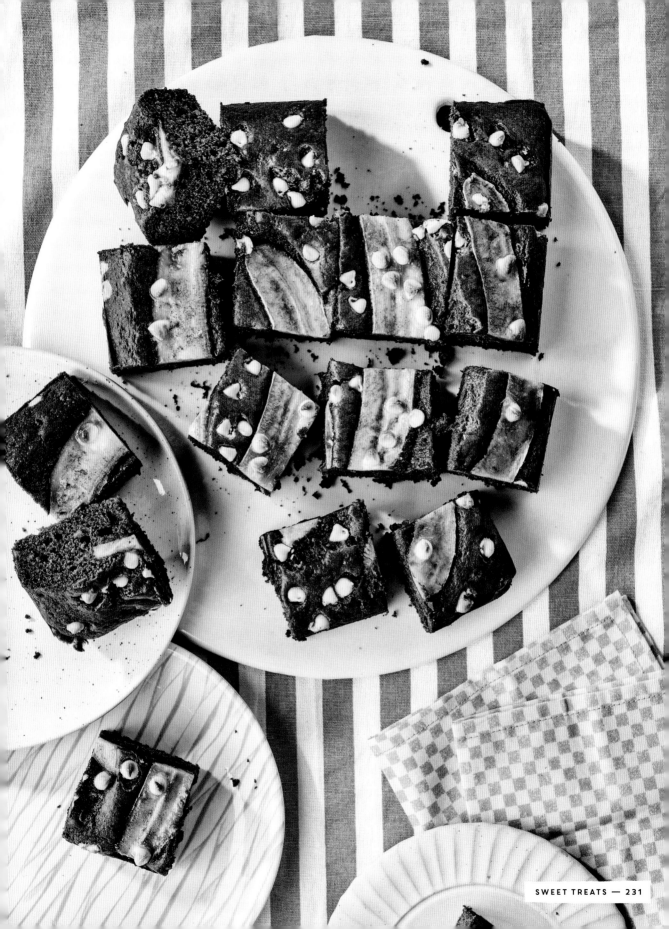

BAKED PINEAPPLE CHEESECAKE

🕐 **20 MINS*** 🗑 **1 HOUR** ✕ **SERVES 10**

*PLUS MINIMUM 3 HOURS CHILLING

PER SERVING:
270 KCAL / 31G CARBS

SPECIAL EQUIPMENT
**20cm (8in) round,
loose-bottomed cake tin**

FOR THE CHEESECAKE
50g reduced-fat spread,
  melted, plus a little extra for
  greasing
175g ginger nut biscuits,
  crushed
400g lightest cream cheese
400g fat-free Greek-style
  yoghurt
1 tbsp white granulated
  sweetener
grated juice and zest
  of 1 lime
2 tbsp cornflour
2 medium eggs

FOR THE TOP
½ tsp ground ginger
2 tbsp honey
2 tbsp white granulated
  sweetener
juice of 1 lime
5 slices fresh pineapple rings
  (about 200g)
low-fat aerosol cream
1 ginger nut biscuit, crushed
10 cherries

▌ **TIP:** Add the aerosol
cream just before you
are about to serve as
it will lose its shape
and melt.

You can't go wrong with a cheesecake, and with a tropical twist, this is a total showstopper. Cheesecakes can be a little heavy, but we've lightened this up with a few low-calorie swaps. The crumbly gingernut biscuit base adds the perfect crunch; and you'll love the pineapple rings caramelised in zesty syrup for the top. Well worth the effort!

Weekly Indulgence ─────────────────

Preheat the oven to 140°C (fan 120°C/gas mark 1). Grease the cake tin with a little reduced-fat spread and line the base with some greaseproof paper.

Add the crushed biscuits to a bowl and stir in the melted reduced-fat spread. Press into the base of the tin. Pop into the fridge while you make the cream cheese mixture.

In a large mixing bowl, beat together the cream cheese, yoghurt, sweetener, lime juice, lime zest, cornflour and eggs. Pour the mixture onto the biscuit base and place the tin onto a baking tray.

Place on a low shelf in the oven and bake for 50–60 minutes until it's set around the edges but still has a wobble in the centre.

Remove from the oven and leave to cool for 1 hour. Once cooled, place in the fridge to chill for a minimum of 2 hours. Remove the cheesecake from the tin and peel away the greaseproof paper. Place onto your serving plate.

In a small bowl, add the ground ginger, honey, sweetener and lime juice. Add the pineapple rings to a small frying pan and place over a low heat. Pour over the honey mixture. Cook the pineapple for 8 minutes, flipping the rings over halfway through. The honey and lime should have reduced and become syrupy and thick. Allow to cool completely.

Cut the pineapple rings in half and arrange around the top of the cheesecake, followed by any syrup left in the pan. Just before you serve, squirt 10 swirls of cream into each hole in the pineapple rings, sprinkle the crushed biscuit over the top and add a cherry to each swirl of cream.

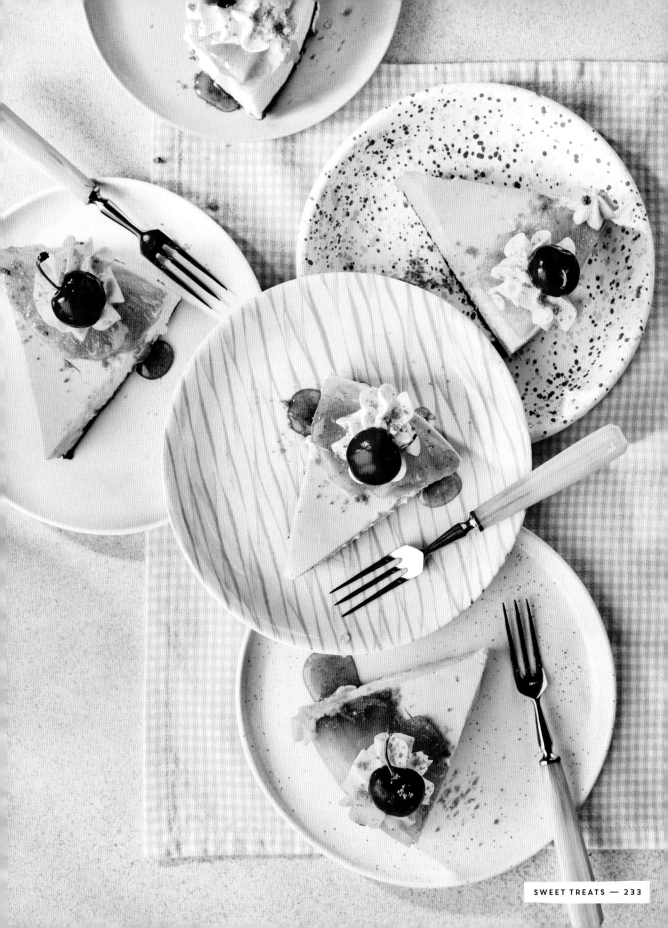

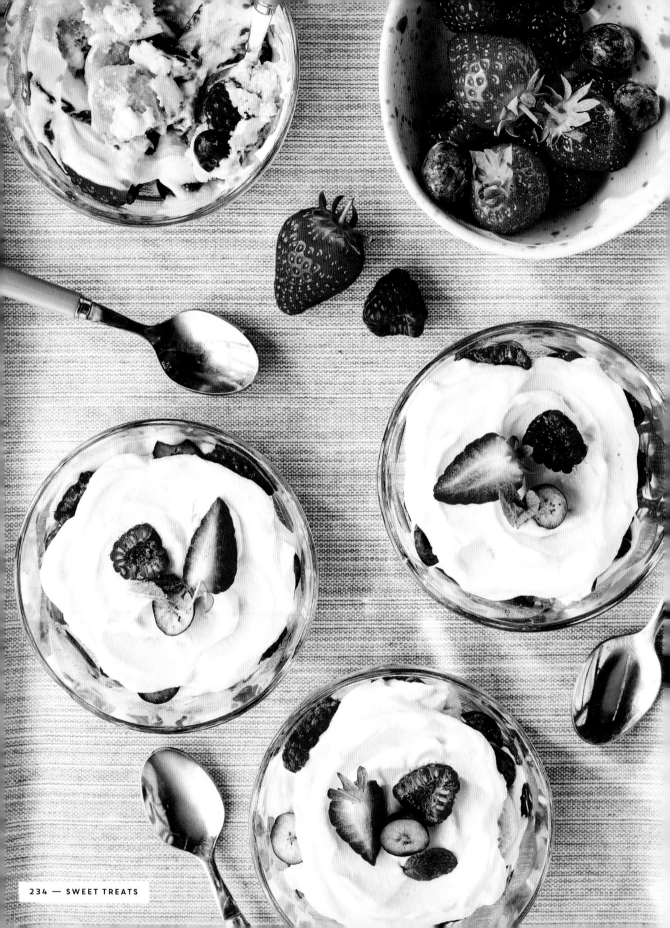

SUMMER BERRY *and* PROSECCO TIRAMISU

USE GF SPONGE
FINGERS

🕐 **15 MINS**   🗑 **NO COOK**   ✕ **SERVES 4**

*PLUS 2 HOURS CHILLING

PER SERVING:
192 KCAL / 19G CARBS

SPECIAL EQUIPMENT
**4 x 200ml individual
dessert dishes**

250g ricotta
3 tsp granulated white
   sweetener (or sugar)
juice of ½ lemon
200g fresh berries (we used
   a mix of strawberries,
   raspberries and blueberries)
100ml prosecco
8 sponge fingers, broken
   in half
mint leaves, to decorate

We've given the traditionally coffee-infused pud a summer berry makeover! By using ricotta cheese instead of mascarpone for our creamy layers, we've made this dessert scrumptious and slimming friendly at only 192 calories per serving. We've added a cheeky glug of prosecco for a merry hint of fizz, or you can use apple juice to keep the flavours alcohol-free.

Everyday Light ―――――――――――――――――

Place the ricotta, sweetener and lemon juice in a mixing bowl and beat together until smooth.

Slice the berries into evenly-sized pieces, saving a few to decorate the top.

Pour the prosecco into a bowl and dip in the sponge fingers. Allow them to soak up some prosecco, but don't allow them to become mushy.

Place two sponge finger halves in the bottom of each dish, divide half of the berries between the dishes, then spread over half of the ricotta mix.

Place another two sponge finger halves in each dish, layer up with the remaining sliced berries and top with the remaining ricotta mix.

Cover and chill for 2 hours. Before serving, decorate with the reserved berries and a mint leaf.

VEGAN

FREEZE ME

DAIRY FREE

GLUTEN FREE

FROZEN PINEAPPLE WHIP

🕐 **10 MINUTES***   🗑 **NO COOK**   ✕ **SERVES 4**

*PLUS 5–6 HOURS FREEZING

PER SERVING:
61 KCAL /12G CARBS

SPECIAL EQUIPMENT
Blender or food processor
Freezer-proof container
with a lid
4 x 125ml serving dishes
Piping bag and star nozzle

400g fresh ripe pineapple,
skinned, cored, eyes
removed and cut into small
chunks
50ml coconut dairy-free milk
alternative
1 tbsp lemon juice
maraschino cherries, to serve
(optional)

Zingy and refreshing, this fruity whip is perfect for a hot day, or any time you fancy something sweet yet light. You could serve in dishes or divide into little paper cones. You can't go wrong with a swirl of this served in an ice-cream cone – it tastes like sunshine!

Everyday Light ────────────────────

Place the pineapple chunks in a freezer-proof container and spread them out as much as you can. Cover with the lid and place in the freezer for a minimum of 5–6 hours, or overnight.

Remove the frozen pineapple from the freezer 5 minutes before you want to make the whip.

Place the frozen pineapple, coconut milk alternative and lemon juice in a food processor or blender. Blitz until smooth and creamy.

Quickly pipe into a swirl in each of the serving dishes using a piping bag and star nozzle. Only fill the bag with one portion at a time, otherwise you may find the heat from your hand melts the frozen whip. Alternatively, just spoon into the dishes when ready to serve. Serve at once, decorated with a cherry, if liked.

SWAP THIS: You can swap the fresh pineapple for tinned pineapple chunks in natural juice (well drained) or frozen pineapple chunks.

TIPS: You may find you need to blitz the ingredients in two batches depending on the size of your blender or food processor. We found a handheld stick blender was not suitable for blitzing the ingredients. If you like to prepare ahead, make sure your dishes are suitable to place in the freezer and pipe or spoon into them, then place in the freezer and serve later. Take out of the freezer 5 minutes before serving to soften a little.

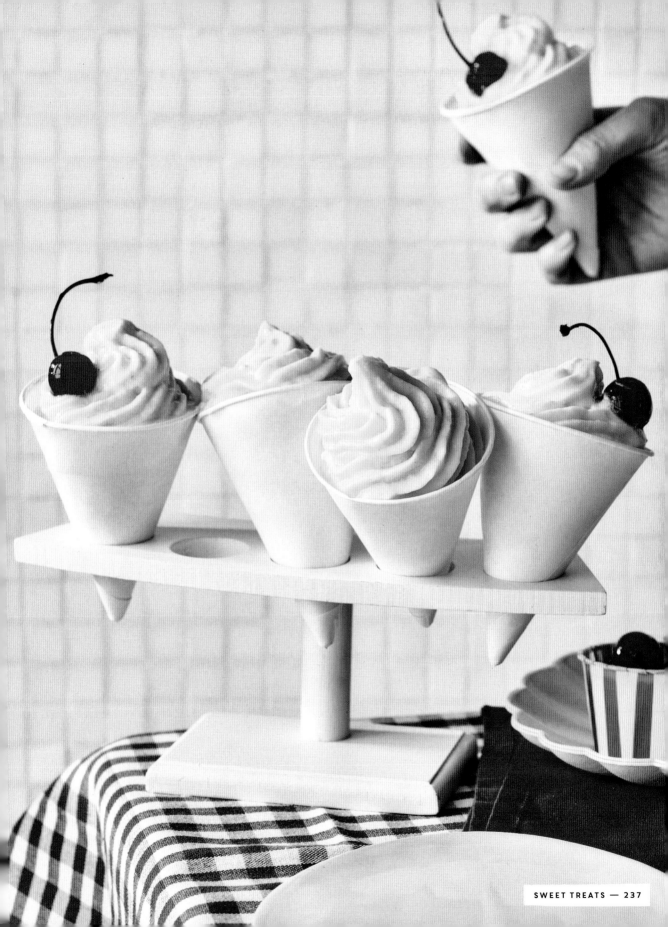

VEGGIE

FREEZE ME

SHORTCAKES ONLY

STRAWBERRY SHORTCAKE TRIFLES

🕐 **20 MINS*** 🗑 **10 MINS** ✕ **SERVES 4**

*PLUS 2 HOURS CHILLING

PER SERVING:
251 KCAL / 34G CARBS

SPECIAL EQUIPMENT
4 x 250ml glass serving dishes
5cm (2in) cookie cutter

FOR THE JELLY LAYER
11.5g sachet strawberry
   sugar-free jelly crystals
140ml boiling water
50g strawberries, sliced

FOR THE SHORTCAKES
100g self-raising flour, plus
   extra for dusting
1 tsp baking powder
25g reduced-fat spread
25g white granulated
   sweetener
50ml skimmed milk

TO ASSEMBLE
150g fat-free Greek-style
   yoghurt
150g light custard
100g strawberries, sliced,
   save 2 whole strawberries
low-fat aerosol cream

Just perfect for a sunny evening, we love the shortcake layer in this fruity trifle. Not to be confused with shortbread biscuits, shortcake is an American-style crumbly cake similar to a scone. You can even experiment with different fruity flavours – why not try swapping out the strawberry for raspberries instead? It'll still taste just like summer!

Weekly Indulgence

For the jelly layer, add the jelly crystals to a heatproof measuring jug and pour over the boiling water. Stir until the crystals have dissolved then add 140ml cold water. Stir again.

Split the sliced strawberries between the four serving dishes and top with the sugar-free jelly. Pop in the fridge until the jelly is set (at least 2 hours).

While the jelly sets, make the shortcakes. Preheat the oven to 200°C (fan 180°C/gas mark 6) and line a baking tray with greaseproof paper.

Sift the flour and baking powder into a mixing bowl. Add the reduced-fat spread and rub into the flour using your fingertips, until it resembles breadcrumbs. Stir in the granulated sweetener.

Pour in the milk and stir the mixture until it forms a soft dough. Lightly dust your work surface with a little extra flour and place the dough onto the surface.

Roll out the dough and use the circle cutter to cut four circles from the dough. Place each circle onto the lined baking tray. Pop into the preheated oven for 10 minutes or until the shortcakes are lightly golden. Remove from the tray, place onto a wire rack and leave to cool.

When the jelly is set, mix the Greek-style yoghurt and custard together in a small mixing bowl until just combined. You should still be able to see the Greek-style yoghurt swirled into the custard. Slice the shortcakes in half

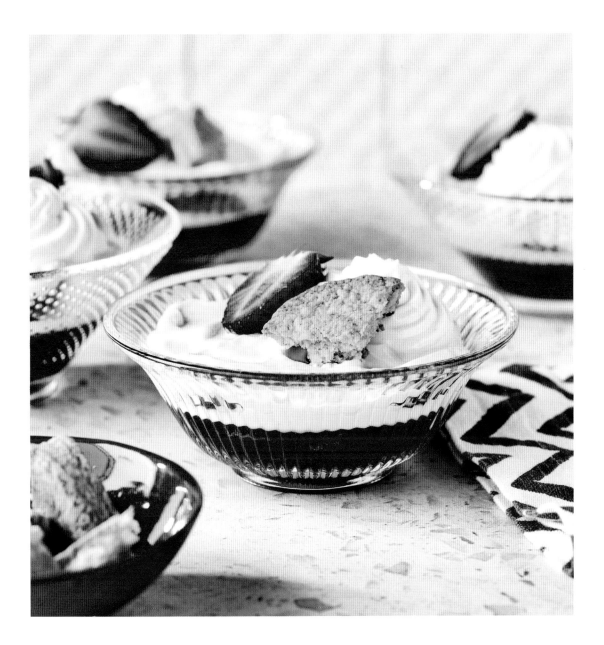

horizontally. Spoon some of the custard mixture on top of the jelly layer and top with one half of a shortcake.

Add some of the sliced strawberries on top of the shortcake, then top with the remaining custard and yoghurt mixture.

Cut the remaining shortcake halves in half again to make two pieces and slice the 2 whole strawberries in half.

Add a swirl of aerosol cream, the shortcake slices and half a strawberry to the top of each trifle.

MILLIONAIRE'S ICE CREAM

🕐 **15 MINS***   🗑 **NO COOK**   ✕ **SERVES 8**

*PLUS 8 HOURS FREEZING

PER SERVING:
156 KCAL / 17G CARBS

SPECIAL EQUIPMENT
2-litre freezer-proof container
Food processor or blender

1kg fat-free thick Greek-style
  yoghurt
6 tbsp low-calorie caramel
  syrup
3 tsp caramel flavouring
80g sugar-free creamy
  chewy toffees, chopped
  into small pieces
20g milk chocolate chips
5 reduced-fat Rich Tea
  biscuits, broken into small
  pieces

TIPS: Before starting, make sure you have room in your freezer for the freezer-proof container you are using. If making this on a hot day, chill your mixing bowl in the fridge before adding the blitzed semi-frozen yoghurt and place it back in the fridge between blitzing each batch. This will help to stop it from melting. Get the toffee pieces, chocolate chips and biscuit pieces ready in advance, so that you can fold them into the semi-frozen mixture without delay.

Imagine how nice an ice cream would be if it was loaded with Millionaire's Shortbread flavour! We've made the dream into a slimming-friendly reality with this rich and indulgent recipe. Loaded with toffee, biscuit and chocolate pieces, every scoop of this frozen showstopper is much lighter than it tastes, thanks to a few nifty swaps. Keep this cool, creamy treat handy in the freezer.

Everyday Light ──────────────────

Place the yoghurt into a mixing bowl and stir until smooth. Using a large spoon, fold in the caramel syrup and caramel flavouring, until evenly mixed.

Scrape into a 2-litre freezer-proof container and spread out evenly. Cover with a lid and place in the freezer for about 4 hours, or until solid.

After about 4 hours, remove the frozen yoghurt mixture from the freezer and leave for about 15 minutes, or until softened a little. Scoop out slightly softened chunks of yoghurt mixture, and place in a food processor or blender. Depending on the size of your food processor, you may need to do this in batches.

Blitz the slightly softened chunks of yoghurt mixture until smooth and creamy, and place in a medium mixing bowl. Working quickly, repeat with the remaining chunks. Continuing to work quickly, add the toffee pieces, chocolate chips and biscuit pieces to the blitzed frozen yoghurt mixture in the bowl.

Fold in using a large spoon until evenly combined. Don't allow the mixture to melt – it should still be semi-frozen. Scrape into the freezer-proof container and spread out.

Cover with a lid and freeze for about 4 hours, or until frozen throughout.

Remove from the freezer for about 15 minutes to soften a little before serving.

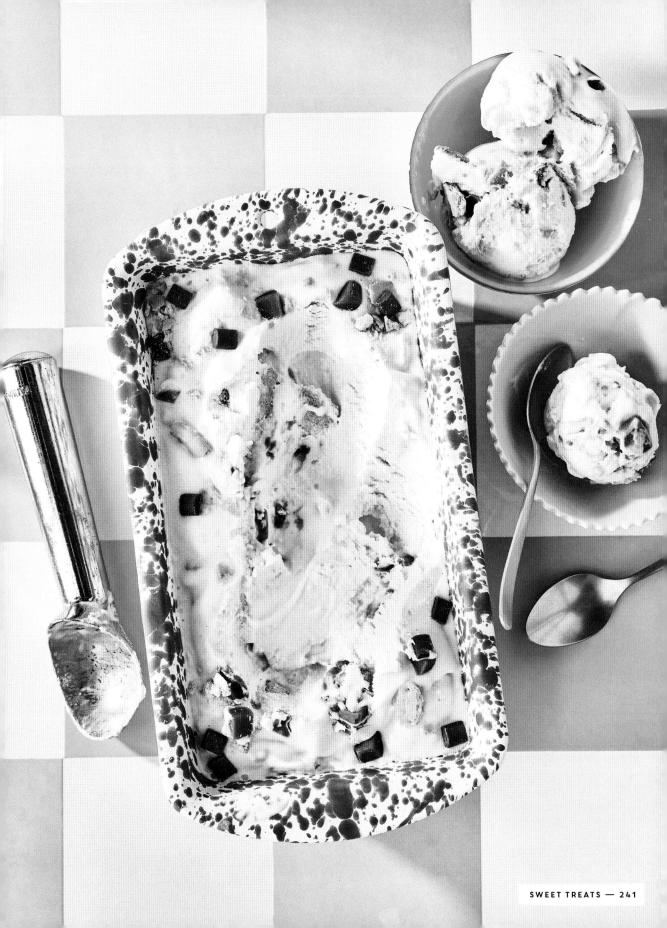

TROPICAL FRUIT FOOL

🕐 **20 MINS***   🗑 **NO COOK**   ✗ **SERVES 6**

*PLUS 30 MINS CHILLING

PER SERVING:
141 KCAL /12G CARBS

SPECIAL EQUIPMENT
Food processor or handheld stick blender
Electric whisk (useful but not essential)
6 x 200ml serving dishes

1 medium ripe mango, about 200g, peeled, stoned and diced
200g fresh ripe pineapple, peeled, cored, eyes removed and diced
grated zest of 1 small lime
2 tsp fresh lime juice
pinch of granulated sweetener (optional)
150ml light double cream alternative
150g fat-free Greek-style yoghurt

TO DECORATE
2 slices lime, halved

TO ACCOMPANY *(optional)*
6 sponge fingers (such as boudoir biscuits) (+ 27 kcal per finger)

You'd be foolish to say no to pudding with this creamy fruit dessert on the menu! We've stayed as true as possible to the traditional English Fruit Fool recipe, with a few handy swaps to keep things light. The trick's in using mangoes and pineapples at their ripest, so that those fruity puree swirls are bursting with yummy, tropical flavour!

Everyday Light

Place the mango and pineapple in a food processor and blitz until smooth (or you can use a stick blender).

Pour the fruit puree into a small mixing bowl and stir in the lime zest and lime juice. Taste the fruit puree and decide if it's sweet enough for your taste (this will depend on the natural sweetness of the fruit used). We found it was sweet enough, but you can add a little sweetener if you feel it needs it.

Place the light double cream alternative in a medium mixing bowl. Beat with an electric whisk until the cream makes soft peaks. Alternatively, beat with a balloon whisk, which will require more time and effort.

Place the yoghurt in the bowl with the softly whipped light double cream alternative. Fold in gently until just combined.

Add the fruit puree to the bowl and gently swirl into the yoghurt and light double cream alternative. Try not to mix too much, just a little so that swirls from the fruit puree and cream can still be seen.

Carefully spoon into individual serving dishes, retaining the swirled appearance as much as possible.

Chill for 30 minutes then decorate each with half a slice of lime. Serve alone or with a crisp biscuit of your choice.

SWAP THIS: You could swap the light double cream alternative for single cream, but don't forget to count the calories.

TIP: Beat the light double cream alternative until it reaches the soft peak stage, which will give the fool a light airy texture, but be careful not to overbeat, otherwise it will be too stiff to fold in with the yoghurt.

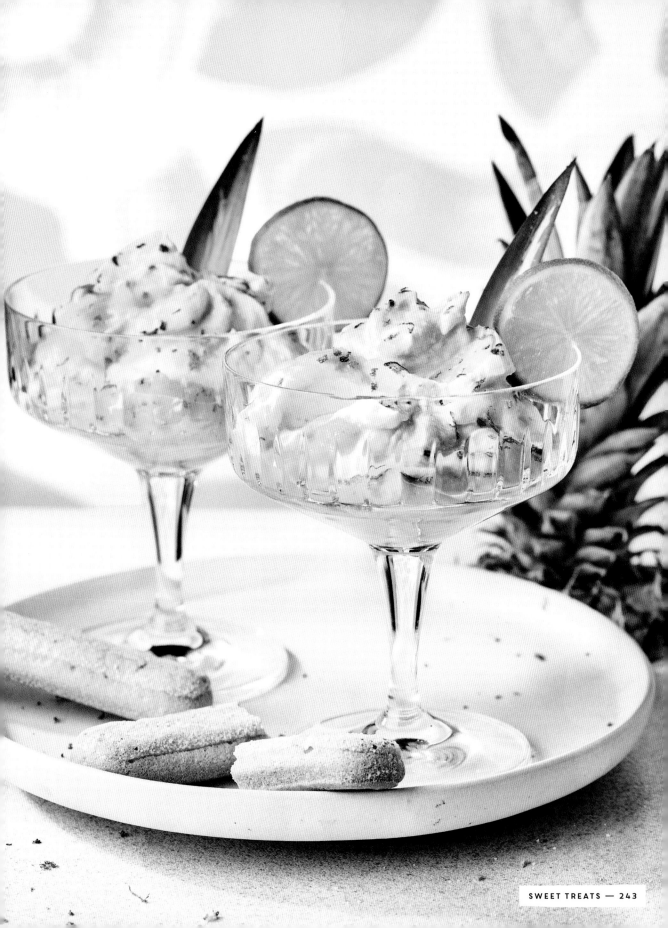

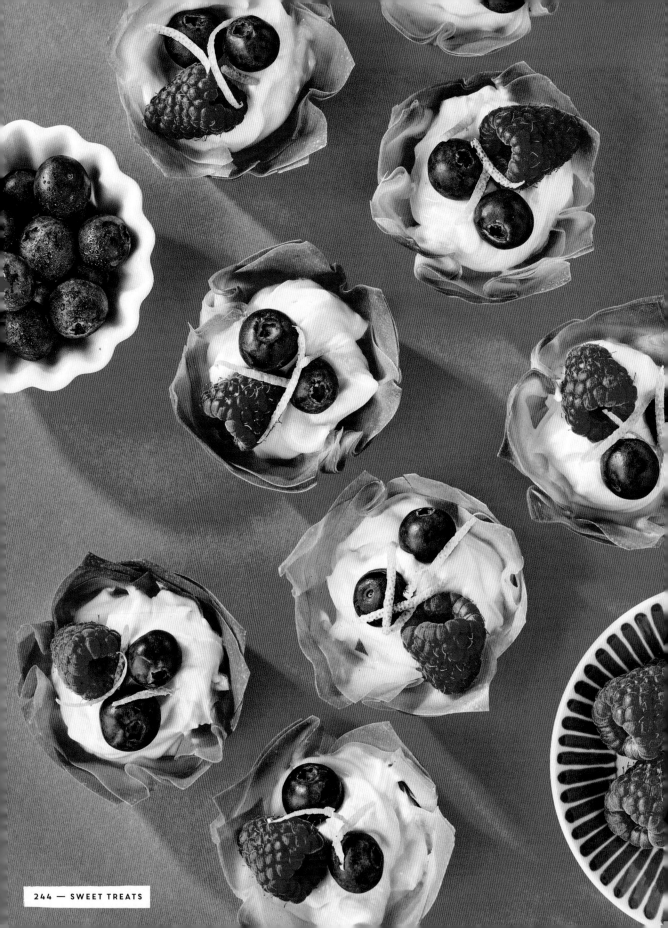

LEMON CHEESECAKE TARTS

🕐 12 MINS*   🗑 8 MINS   ✗ MAKES 8

*PLUS 10 MINS CHILLING

PER TART:
72 KCAL /10G CARBS

SPECIAL EQUIPMENT
12-hole muffin tin

low-calorie cooking spray,
  for greasing
1 sheet filo pastry, about 48g
1 tbsp skimmed milk
180g low-fat cream cheese
grated zest of 1 lemon
1 tbsp plus 1 tsp lemon curd
1 light digestive biscuit,
  crushed
8 raspberries
16 blueberries
pared lemon zest strips, to
  serve (optional)

These delicate Lemon Cheesecake Tarts are the perfect sweet yet citrusy addition to a cuppa. Made with crispy filo pastry, they have a creamy lemon cheesecake filling that'll pick you right up. Topped with berries and a drizzle of lemon curd for added pizzazz, they're almost as good to look at as they are to eat!

Everyday Light

Preheat the oven to 180°C (fan 160°C/gas mark 4) and lightly grease eight holes of the muffin tin with a little low-calorie cooking spray.

Place the sheet of filo pastry flat onto the work surface. Cut into 24 sections – they don't need to be perfect squares. Brush the first section with a little skimmed milk. Press into the first hole in the muffin tin, dry side down. Brush the next section and place on top of the first piece, then repeat with a third section of filo. Repeat with the other seven holes of the muffin tin. (There should be three pieces of filo per tart.)

Pop the tin into the oven for 8 minutes, until the pastry cases are golden brown and crisp. Leave to cool.

In a mixing bowl add the cream cheese, lemon zest and 1 tablespoon lemon curd. Mix until smooth and fully combined.

Once the pastry cases are cool, spoon the cream cheese mixture into each pastry case. Add a raspberry and two blueberries to the top of each tart.

Microwave the 1 teaspoon of lemon curd for a few seconds until runny. Sprinkle the crushed biscuit over the tarts and drizzle over the lemon curd. Pop into the fridge for 10 minutes to firm up and serve, garnished with lemon zest strips if you like.

MINCEMEAT SWIRLS

 10 MINS   **20 MINS**   ✗ **MAKES 16**

PER SWIRL:
96 KCAL /13G CARBS

SPECIAL EQUIPMENT
**Food processor or handheld
stick blender**

320g ready-rolled light puff
  pastry sheet
90g mincemeat
1 tbsp skimmed milk, for
  brushing
icing sugar, for dusting
  (optional)

These magical mincemeat swirls aren't just for Christmas!
To save on time and calories, we've used ready-rolled light
puff pastry and blitzed our mincemeat into a tasty paste
as it makes our festive-inspired filling go even further!
Delicious served fresh from the oven with a cuppa, they're
also handy to keep in the freezer until you've got the
hankering for a pastry treat.

Everyday Light

Preheat the oven to 200°C (fan 180°C/gas mark 6). Line a
baking tray with a sheet of non-stick baking paper.

Place the mincemeat in a food processor or use a stick
blender to blitz until it has a spreadable but coarse
consistency. Make sure there are no whole pieces of dried
fruit left.

Unroll the pastry sheet, leaving it on the greaseproof paper
packing and place on the work surface. Spread a thin layer
of the mincemeat paste evenly over the pastry, leaving a
1cm (½in) gap along one long edge.

Starting with the long edge without the 1cm (½in) gap, roll
it up, using the greaseproof paper packing to help you.
Keep rolling until you have made a 'Swiss Roll'. When you
have finished rolling the pastry up, make sure it is seam
side down.

Use a large serrated knife, such as a bread knife, to
carefully cut into 16 spiral shapes.

Place on the lined baking tray, leaving gaps between each.
Press the seam on each to ensure a good seal.

Brush the swirls with a little skimmed milk, then place in
the preheated oven for 15–20 minutes, until golden and
crisp. Watch carefully towards the end of cooking as
mincemeat can burn easily. Place on a wire rack to cool or
serve warm (but be careful as the mincemeat will be very
hot). Dust with icing sugar if you like.

TIPS: Blitzing the
mincemeat into a coarse
paste makes it easy to
roll the pastry swirls as it
wouldn't work as well with
whole pieces of dried fruit in
the mincemeat. If you find the
pastry difficult to slice, wrap
the roll up in the greaseproof
paper packaging and pop
back in the fridge to chill for
10 minutes. The pastry will
firm up and be easier to slice.

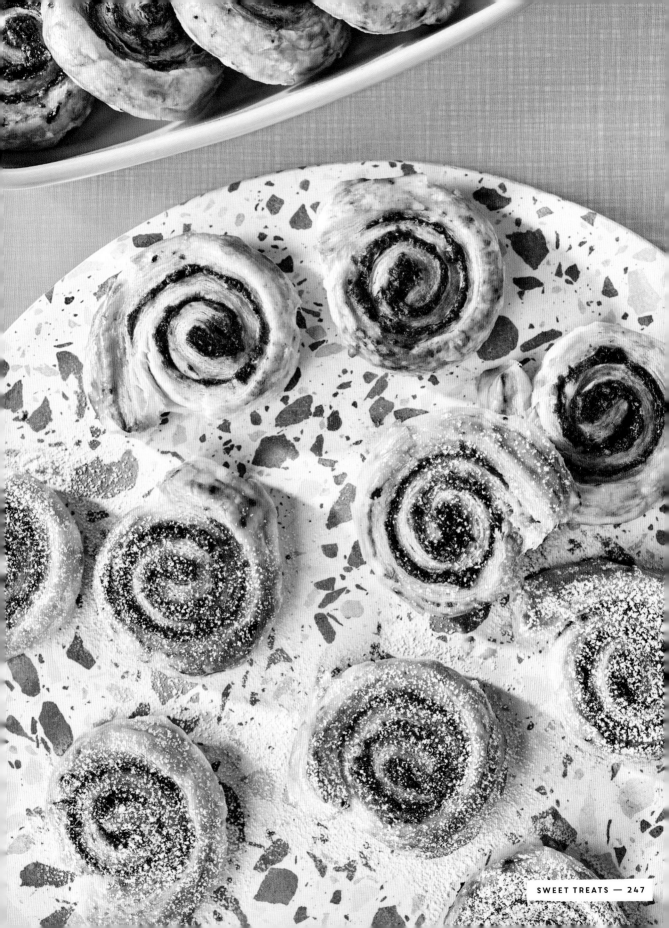

CARAMELISED BANANA YORKSHIRE PUDDING

🕐 **10 MINS** 🗑 **20 MINS** ✗ **SERVES 6**

PER SERVING:
166 KCAL / 17G CARBS

SPECIAL EQUIPMENT
6-hole muffin tin

low-calorie cooking spray
30g plain flour
2 medium eggs
75ml skimmed milk
pinch of salt

FOR THE FILLING
1 tbsp reduced-fat spread
2 tbsp maple syrup
¼ tsp ground cinnamon
2 medium bananas, peeled
  and sliced into 5mm
  (¼in)-thick slices
low-fat aerosol cream
  (optional)
6 pecan nuts, chopped

If you enjoy Yorkies only with your Sunday dinner, you're missing out! We've turned our classic, slimming-friendly Yorkshire Pudding recipe into a truly irresistible dessert. There's no sugar needed to make our sweet, syrupy caramel sauce, which helps keep the calories nice and low. Crunchy Yorkshire pudding, caramelised bananas and a sprinkle of pecans – what's not to like?

Everyday Light ─────────────────────

Preheat the oven to 210°C (fan 190°C/gas mark 6). Once the oven is hot, spray six holes of a muffin tin with low-calorie cooking spray and place into the oven. Heat the tray for 10 minutes to ensure the cooking spray is hot.

Meanwhile, add the flour, eggs, milk and salt to a mixing bowl. Beat with a balloon whisk until smooth. Leave to stand while the tray is heating up.

Pour the batter into a jug, then remove the hot tin from the oven. Carefully pour the batter into the muffin tin holes and return the tray to the oven.

After 10 minutes, without opening the oven door, turn the oven down to just under 200°C (fan 180°C/gas mark 6) and allow to cook for another 10 minutes.

While the puddings are cooking, add the reduced-fat spread to a frying pan and place over a low heat. Heat until the reduced-fat spread has melted. Add the maple syrup and cinnamon and stir until combined.

Add the sliced banana to the pan and cook for 2 minutes. Flip the slices over in the syrupy sauce to coat both sides. The bananas should have turned a lightly golden colour and begun to soften. Cook for a further 2 minutes.

When the puds are risen and nicely browned, remove from the oven. Carefully remove them from the tin and place on serving plates. Spoon over the bananas, drizzling over the syrupy sauce. Add a swirl of aerosol cream to each pud, if you like, and sprinkle over the chopped pecan nuts. Serve!

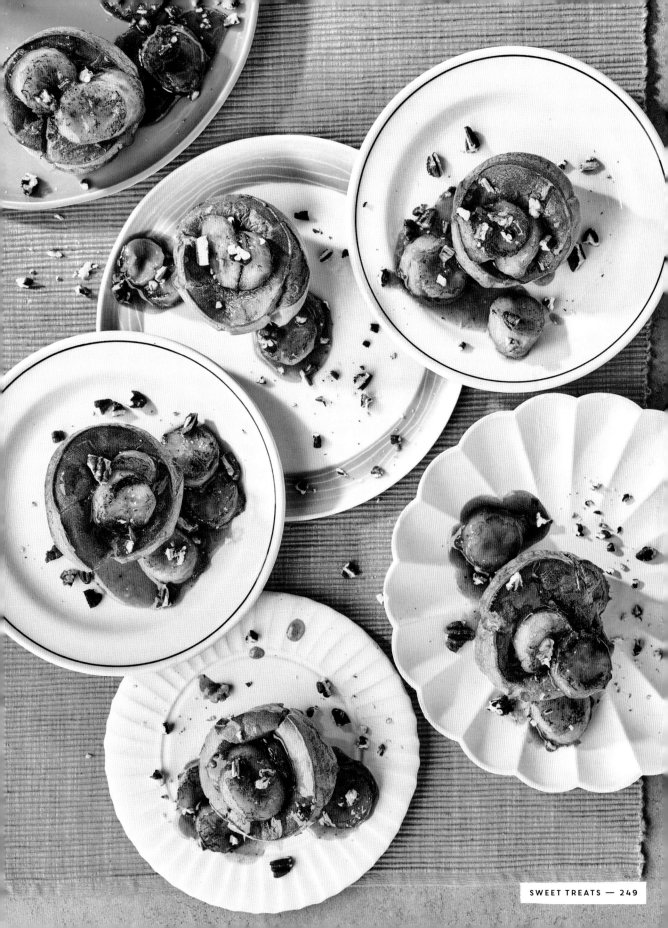

USE A
DF SPREAD

ST CLEMENT'S PUDDING
with CITRUS SAUCE

🕐 **20 MINS**   🗑 **VARIABLE** (SEE BELOW)   ✗ **SERVES 8**

PER SERVING:
295 KCAL / 40G CARBS

SPECIAL EQUIPMENT
1.2-litre ovenproof
pudding basin
Electric whisk (optional)
Ovenproof cooking string

FOR THE SPONGE PUDDING
125g reduced-fat spread, plus
  a little extra for greasing
125g self-raising flour
60g white granulated
  sweetener
60g caster sugar
2 medium eggs
1 tsp baking powder
2 tsp finely grated lemon zest
2 tsp finely grated orange zest

FOR THE TOP
2 tbsp low-calorie light syrup
1 tsp lemon juice
1 lemon slice, rind and pips
  removed
5 orange slices, rind and pips
  removed

FOR THE CITRUS SAUCE
juice of 2 lemons
juice of 1 orange
2 tbsp white granulated
  sweetener or caster sugar
3 tbsp cornflour

TO ACCOMPANY *(optional)*
Custard (from the Pinch
  of Nom website) (+ 58 kcal
  per portion)

We feel nostalgic just looking at this St Clement's Pudding! Made with oranges and lemons, this homely, retro pud has the perfect balance of sweet and sharp flavours. The silky citrus sauce is a heavenly match with the light sponge – we like to drizzle ours straight on top, or you can serve it in a jug and let everyone pour for themselves!

Special Occasion ─────────────────

OVEN METHOD
🗑 **45 MINS**

Preheat the oven to 180°C (fan 160°C/gas mark 4) and place a baking tray on the oven shelf. Grease the ovenproof pudding basin really well with reduced-fat spread. Cut out an 8cm (3in) disc of non-stick baking paper. Grease the disc of paper and place, greased side up, in the bottom of the pudding basin.

For the top, mix the light syrup with the lemon juice and pour on top of the greased paper disc. Place the lemon slice in the centre, on top of the syrup and arrange five orange slices around the lemon slice.

To make the sponge pudding, place the self-raising flour, reduced-fat spread, sweetener, caster sugar, eggs, baking powder, lemon zest and orange zest into a mixing bowl. Beat with an electric whisk for 1–2 minutes until you have a smooth cake batter. You can use a wooden spoon, but more effort will be needed.

Scrape the mixture into the prepared pudding basin, on top of the fruit and syrup, and level the surface if needed.

Make a lid for the pudding: cut out a 28cm (11in) disc of kitchen foil and a 28cm (11in) disc of non-stick baking paper. Place the foil disc on top of the non-stick paper disc to make a double layer. Make a double pleat, around 2cm (¾in) thick, across the width of the double-layered lid.

Place the foil and non-stick baking paper lid on top of the pudding and fold the edges down over the rim of the bowl.

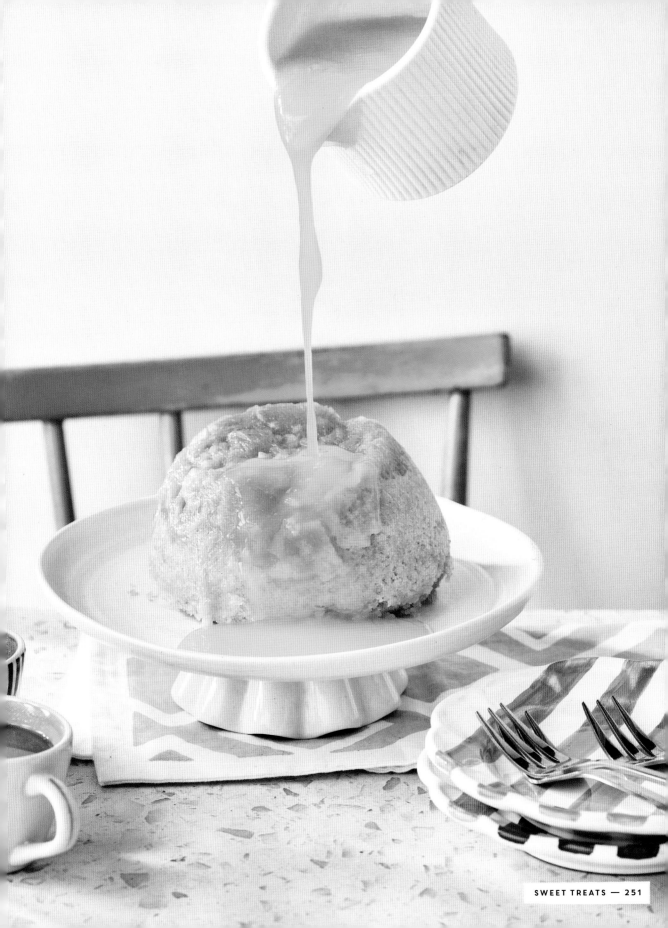

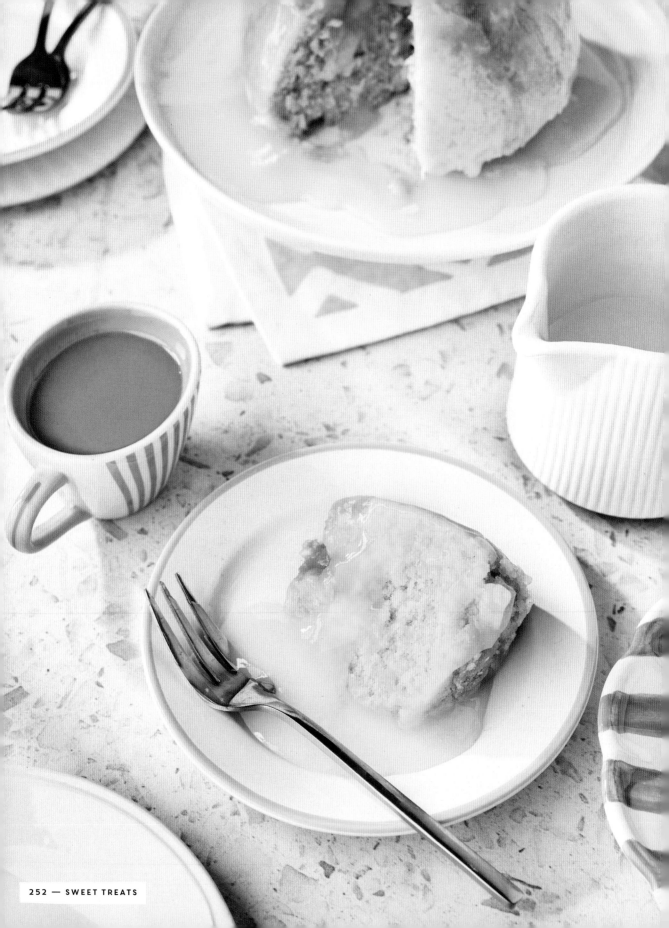

Tie cooking string around, just under the rim, to hold the lid in place.

Place the pudding basin on the preheated baking tray in the oven and cook for about 45 minutes. The pudding will be ready when it's risen, spongy and when a sharp knife inserted into the centre comes out clean. To check if it's cooked, snip the string, remove the lid and insert the knife. If you decide it needs a little longer, just put the lid back on (no need to tie with string again) and return to the oven for a few more minutes.

When the pudding is cooked, remove the lid, run a knife around the pudding to loosen it and carefully turn out onto a serving plate. Take care as the pudding will be very hot.

While the sponge is cooking, make the Citrus Sauce. Place the lemon juice and orange juice into a measuring jug and top up with water. You will need about 360ml water, but stop when you reach 500ml liquid in total. You may not need the full amount of water if your fruit is extra juicy. Pour the liquid into a medium saucepan and add the sweetener or sugar.

Place over a medium heat for 1–2 minutes, stirring until the sweetener or sugar has dissolved and the liquid is starting to steam. In a small bowl, mix the cornflour with 3 tablespoons of water until smooth. Stir the cornflour mixture into the saucepan and increase the heat a little so that the sauce begins to simmer.

Simmer uncovered for 4–5 minutes, stirring constantly with a wooden spoon or balloon whisk, until slightly thickened, smooth and glossy. We think a thinner sauce goes well with this pudding, but if you prefer it thicker, add a little more cornflour mixed with water until you reach the consistency you prefer.

Alternatively, you can cook the sauce in the microwave: place the lemon juice, orange juice, water, sweetener or sugar in a microwave-safe measuring jug. Stir, then microwave uncovered and on high for about 30 seconds. Stir until the sweetener or sugar

has dissolved. Mix the cornflour with 3 tablespoons of water until smooth, then stir into the liquid in the jug. Microwave, uncovered, for 4–5 minutes, stirring regularly, until slightly thickened, smooth and glossy.

Using a sieve, strain the hot sauce into a serving jug to remove any bits or stray pips. Pour some of the sauce over the hot pudding, or serve separately alongside with some custard, if you like.

MICROWAVE METHOD
13 MINS

Grease the ovenproof pudding basin really well with reduced-fat spread. Cut out an 8cm (3in) disc of non-stick baking paper. Grease the disc of paper and place, greased side up, in the bottom of the pudding basin.

For the top, mix the light syrup with the lemon juice and pour on top of the greased paper disc. Place the lemon slice in the centre, on top of the syrup and arrange five orange slices around the lemon slice.

To make the sponge pudding, place the self-raising flour, reduced-fat spread, sweetener, caster sugar, eggs, baking powder, lemon zest and orange zest into a mixing bowl. Beat with an electric whisk for 1–2 minutes until you have a smooth cake batter. You can use a wooden spoon, but more effort will be needed.

Scrape the mixture into the prepared pudding basin, on top of the fruit and syrup, and level the surface if needed. Loosely cover with cling film or a plate, making sure there is a small gap at the edge. Microwave on high for 6–6½ minutes. The pudding will be ready when risen, spongy and a knife inserted into the centre comes out clean.

Leave the pudding to stand for 4–5 minutes, then remove the covering. Run a round-bladed knife around the edge to loosen the pudding, then turn out onto a serving plate. Take care as the pudding will be very hot.

While the pudding is standing, make the sauce: place the lemon juice and orange juice into a measuring jug and top up with the water. You will need about 360ml water, but stop when you reach 500ml liquid in total. You may not need the full amount of water if your fruit is extra juicy. Pour the liquid into a medium saucepan and add the sweetener or sugar.

Place over a medium heat for 1–2 minutes, stirring until the sweetener or sugar has dissolved and the liquid is starting to steam. In a small bowl, mix the cornflour with the 3 tablespoons of water until smooth. Stir the cornflour mixture into the saucepan and increase the heat a little, so that the sauce begins to simmer.

Simmer uncovered for 4–5 minutes, stirring constantly with a wooden spoon or balloon whisk until slightly thickened, smooth and glossy. We think a thinner sauce goes well with the pudding, but if you prefer it thicker, add a little more cornflour mixed with water until you reach the consistency you prefer.

Alternatively, you can cook the sauce in the microwave (see how to do this in the Oven Method, page 253).

Using a sieve, strain the hot sauce into a serving jug to remove any bits or stray pips. Pour some of the sauce over the hot pudding, or serve separately alongside with some custard, if you like.

TIPS: Use white granulated sweetener that is the same weight and texture as sugar. We used Light Syrup made by Sweet Freedom. It's made from fruit extracts and contains 31% fewer calories than sugar, so it's a great way to reduce calories in this pudding. We cooked this recipe in an 800-watt microwave oven. Timings may vary a little depending on the power of your microwave oven and are a guide only.

SLOW-COOKER METHOD
🍲 1 HOUR 30 MINS–2 HOURS

SPECIAL EQUIPMENT
Slow cooker

Grease the ovenproof pudding basin really well with reduced-fat spread. Cut out an 8cm (3in) disc of non-stick baking paper. Grease the disc of paper and place, greased side up, in the bottom of the pudding basin.

For the top, mix the light syrup with the lemon juice and pour on top of the greased paper disc. Place the lemon slice in the centre, on top of the syrup and arrange five orange slices around the lemon slice.

To make the sponge pudding, place the self-raising flour, reduced-fat spread, sweetener, caster sugar, eggs, baking powder, lemon zest and orange zest into a mixing bowl. Beat with an electric whisk for 1–2 minutes until you have a smooth cake batter. You can use a wooden spoon, but more effort will be needed.

Scrape the mixture into the prepared pudding basin, on top of the fruit and syrup, and level the surface if needed.

Make a lid for the pudding: cut out a 28cm (11in) disc of kitchen foil and a 28cm (11in) disc of non-stick baking paper. Place the foil disc on top of the non-stick paper disc to make a double layer. Make a double pleat, around 2cm (¾in) thick, across the width of the double-layered lid.

Place the foil and non-stick baking paper lid on top of the pudding, and fold the edges down over the rim of the bowl. Tie cooking string around just under the rim, to hold the lid in place.

Place the pudding in the slow cooker and pour in boiling water to come halfway up the side of the pudding basin. Cook on high for 1½–1¾ hours. The pudding will be ready when it's risen, spongy and when a sharp knife inserted into the centre comes out clean. To check if it's cooked, carefully remove from the slow cooker, snip the string, remove the lid and insert the knife. If you decide it needs a little longer, just put the lid back on, tie with string and return to the slow cooker for a few more minutes.

When the pudding is cooked, remove the lid, run a knife around the pudding to loosen it and carefully turn out onto a serving plate. Take care as the pudding will be very hot.

Meanwhile, make the sauce: place the lemon juice and orange juice into a measuring jug and top up with water. You will need about 360ml water, but stop when you reach 500ml liquid in total. You may not need the full amount of water if your fruit is extra juicy. Pour the liquid into a medium saucepan and add the sweetener or sugar.

Place over a medium heat for 1–2 minutes, stirring, until the sweetener or sugar has dissolved and the liquid is starting to steam.

In a small bowl, mix the cornflour with 3 tablespoons of water until smooth. Stir the cornflour mixture into the saucepan and increase the heat a little, so that the sauce begins to simmer.

Simmer uncovered for 4–5 minutes, stirring constantly with a wooden spoon or balloon whisk, until slightly thickened, smooth and glossy. We think a thinner sauce goes well with this pudding, but if you prefer it thicker, add a little more cornflour mixed with water until you reach the consistency you prefer.

Alternatively, you can cook the sauce in the microwave (see how to do this in the Oven Method, page 253).

Using a sieve, strain the hot sauce into a serving jug to remove any bits or stray pips. Pour some of the sauce over the hot pudding, or serve separately alongside with some custard, if you like.

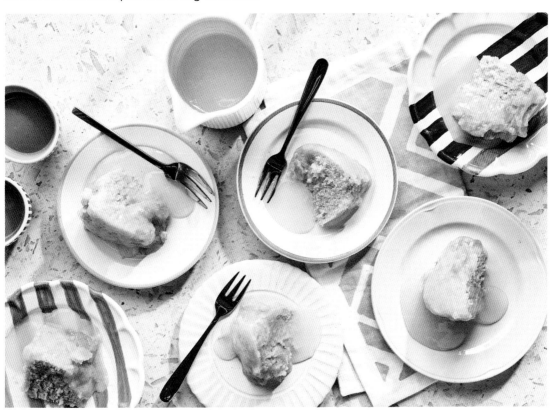

APPLE *and* CHERRY BAKES

🕐 **10 MINS**   🍲 **15 MINS**   🍴 **MAKES 6**

PER BAKE:
APPLE:
143 KCAL /25G CARBS
CHERRY:
158 KCAL /28G CARBS

FOR THE APPLE FILLING
250g Bramley apples, peeled, cored, and diced
2 tsp white granulated sweetener

FOR THE CHERRY FILLING
250g frozen cherries, defrosted, drained and juices reserved
2 tsp white granulated sweetener
2 tsp cornflour

FOR THE BAKES
6 soft sliced white or brown sandwich thins
1 medium egg, beaten
½ tsp white granulated sweetener

TO ACCOMPANY *(optional)*
300g fat-free Greek-style yoghurt (+ 27 kcal per 50g portion)

Can't stop thinking about your favourite bakery treats? We've got you covered with these fruit-filled baked delights. Okay, so they're not really pastry, but take a bite and you'll discover they're crispy on the outside, gooey and sweet on the inside, and just delicious. Whether you go for apple or cherry, these are a low-calorie way to indulge your sweet tooth.

Everyday Light ──────────────────────

To make the apple bakes, add the diced apple to a small saucepan. Add 3 tablespoons of water and 2 teaspoons white granulated sweetener and place the pan over a low heat. Cook for 5 minutes until the apple has softened.

To make the cherry bakes, add the drained cherries and 50ml of the reserved juices to a saucepan along with 2 teaspoons white granulated sweetener. In a small bowl, stir together the cornflour with 2 teaspoons of water until smooth. Stir the mixture into the cherries. Place over a low heat and simmer gently for 5 minutes until thick and glossy.

Line a large baking tray with a sheet of non-stick baking paper and preheat the oven to 180°C (fan 160°C/gas mark 4).

Divide the sandwich thins in half and lay out on a chopping board. Divide the apple or cherry filling into six portions and place a portion onto six of the bread halves, leaving a 1cm (½in) gap around the edge.

Brush beaten egg around the edge and place one of the remaining bread halves on top of the filling. Press the centre of the lid down gently with a flat hand, then press around the edges to seal. Use a fork to crimp the edges and seal well. Repeat with the remaining bakes.

Place the bakes on the lined baking tray and brush the tops with the remaining egg. Sprinkle over the remaining ½ teaspoon sweetener and bake for 10 minutes until golden brown.

Remove from the oven and place on a wire rack to cool. This will help stop the bases becoming soggy. Serve with Greek-style yoghurt, if liked.

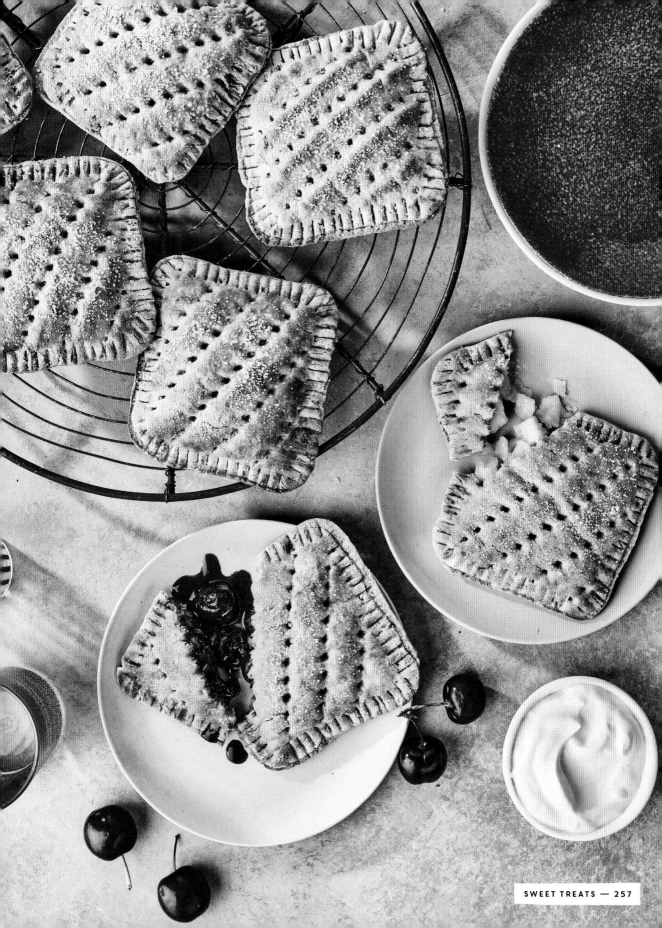

NUTELLA MOUSSE

🕐 **5 MINS***   🪣 **30 SECS**   ✕ **SERVES 4**

***PLUS 30 MINS CHILLING**

PER SERVING:
227 KCAL / 16G CARBS

SPECIAL EQUIPMENT
Electric hand whisk
4 x 125ml ramekin dishes

100ml light double cream
   alternative
80g Nutella hazelnut
   chocolate spread
100g fat-free Greek style
   yoghurt
½ tsp vanilla extract
½ Nutella B-ready wafer
   biscuit, roughly chopped

Why not sweeten up your evening with a slimming-friendly Nutella Mousse? By using reduced-fat cream alternative and fat-free Greek-style yoghurt, we've kept the calories low. As well as Nutella hazelnut chocolate spread, we've turned things up a notch with a crunchy topping of Nutella biscuit pieces too. Bound to be an instant hit, it's a good job it's so easy to make!

Everyday Light

Place the light double cream alternative in a medium mixing bowl. Whisk with an electric hand whisk, on high speed, for about 2 minutes until soft peaks are formed. Take care not to over-whisk the cream alternative, or it will become too stiff to fold in the remaining ingredients.

Place the Nutella spread in a small bowl and melt until completely smooth and runny. You can do this by heating in the microwave for about 30 seconds and stirring until completely runny, or by placing the small bowl in a slightly larger bowl containing boiling water, and stirring for about 2 minutes.

Place the yoghurt, melted Nutella spread and vanilla extract in the bowl with the whipped cream alternative. Fold in gently using a rubber spatula or large metal spoon, until completely combined. Take care not to knock the air out of the mixture.

Divide between the four ramekin dishes and sprinkle the Nutella biscuit pieces on top. Chill for about 30 minutes and serve.

SWAP THIS: You can swap the biscuits with a few chopped hazelnuts, if you don't mind the extra calories.

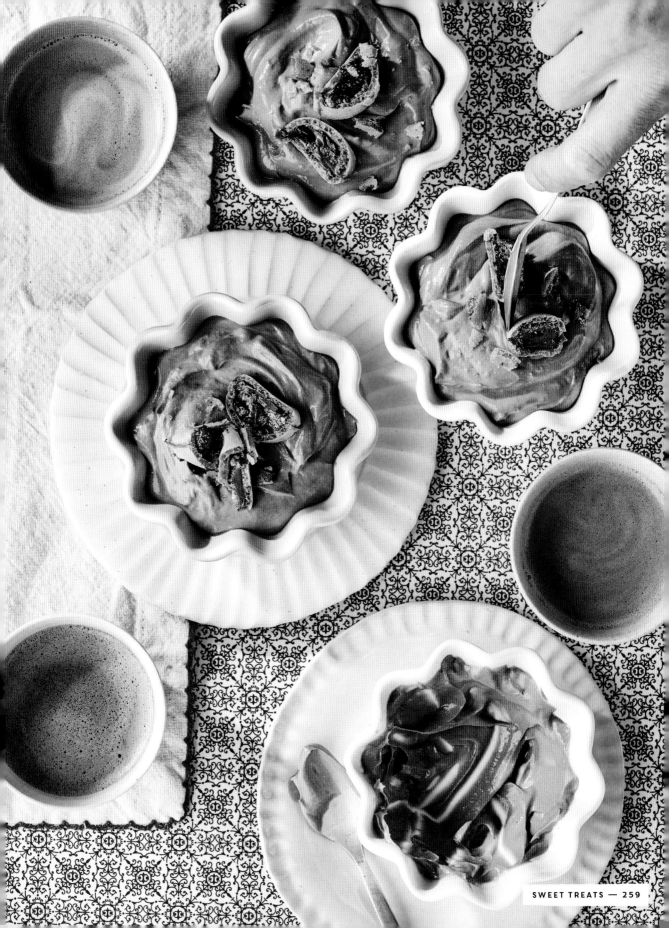

CHOCOLATE TOFFEE PUDDINGS

🕐 **10 MINS**   🗑 **10 MINS**   ✕ **SERVES 4**

PER SERVING:
215 KCAL / 25G CARBS

SPECIAL EQUIPMENT
4 x 125ml ramekin dishes or dariole moulds
Electric hand whisk

45g reduced-fat spread, plus a little extra for greasing
8 x sugar-free creamy chewy toffees (48g)
1 tsp light double cream alternative
45g self-raising flour
25g white granulated sweetener
15g cocoa powder
2 medium eggs
1 tsp vanilla extract
¼ tsp icing sugar, for dusting (optional)

TO ACCOMPANY *(optional)*
squirt of low-fat aerosol cream (+ 24 kcal per serving)

TIPS: We use a granulated sweetener that is crunchy and weighs like-for-like with sugar (not the powdered kind), Elmlea Light Double Cream alternative, and for the toffees, sugar-free chewy creamy toffees such as Werther's Original Sugar-free Creamy Toffees (not the hard butter candies).

Rich little chocolate puddings, with a sticky toffee twist! Sounds good, right? We've used a clever trick to keep these slimming friendly, and we're letting you in on the secret: we swapped out high-calorie caramel for sugar-free creamy toffees and it works like a dream! Try these dusted with icing sugar and still warm from the oven. Oh. My. Word!

Weekly Indulgence ——————————————

Preheat the oven to 160°C (fan 140°C/gas mark 3) and lightly grease the ramekin dishes or moulds with the little extra reduced-fat spread.

Place the toffees in a small microwave-safe bowl with the double cream alternative.

Pop in the microwave and cook on high for 10–20 seconds, stirring halfway through, until the toffees are partially melted. Remove from the microwave and continue to stir until completely melted and smooth. Set aside.

Put the reduced-fat spread, flour, sweetener, cocoa, eggs and vanilla extract in a medium bowl and beat together for 1–2 minutes with an electric hand whisk or a wooden spoon.

Divide the warm melted toffee mixture between the four ramekin dishes or moulds and allow to spread out over the bottom of each dish. Divide the cake mixture between the dishes, placing it on top of the toffee mixture.

Set the ramekin dishes on a baking tray and place in the preheated oven for 8–10 minutes, until risen and spongy. Take care not to overcook the puddings. Remove them from the oven when risen and spongy, but still a little wet on the top. Leave to stand for 5 minutes and the tops will dry out.

Serve in the ramekins or turn out onto serving plates. Dust with a little icing sugar and serve with a squirt of cream if you like.

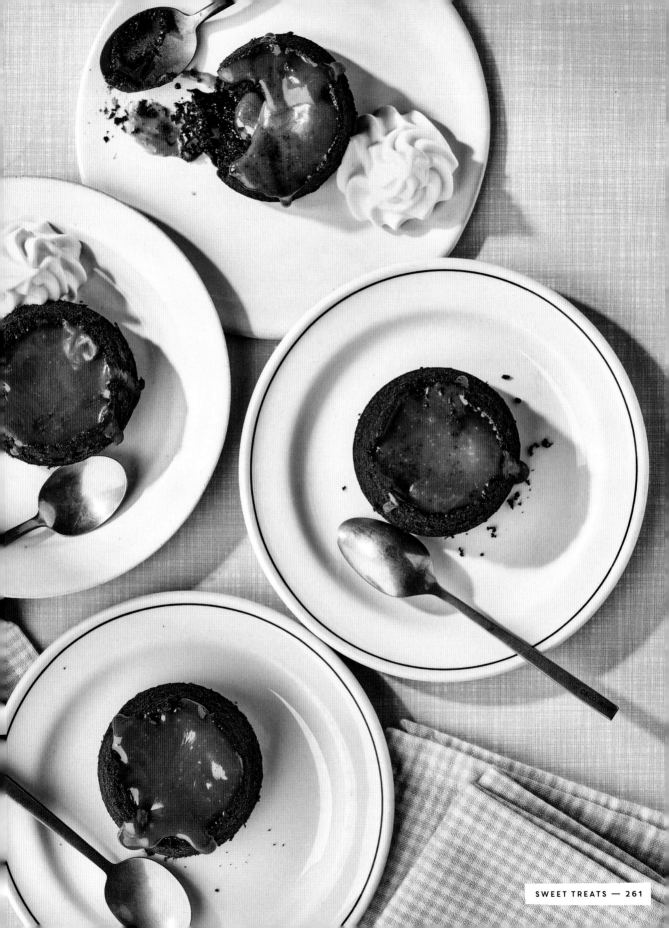

VEGGIE

FREEZE ME

GLUTEN FREE

USE GF BREAD
AND CHOCOLATE

BLUEBERRY *and* WHITE CHOCOLATE BREAD PUDDING

🕐 **5 MINS**   📦 **VARIABLE** (SEE BELOW)   ✗ **SERVES 4**

PER SERVING:
244 KCAL / 33G CARBS

6 slices lighter Danish white
  bread, about 160g total
70g blueberries
50g white chocolate, broken
  into squares
350ml skimmed milk
2 medium eggs
1 tsp white granulated
  sweetener
¼ tsp vanilla extract
grated zest of ½ lemon

TO ACCOMPANY *(optional)*
2 tbsp light single cream
  alternate (+ 35 kcal per
  serving)

We're going all retro with this one. You can't beat a good Bread Pudding, but you can give it a fruity new twist! This is the classic pud you know and love, only with a white chocolate custard and a sprinkling of plump, juicy blueberries. It's simple, satisfying and you can even make it in your slow cooker.

Weekly Indulgence

OVEN METHOD
📦 **30 MINS**

SPECIAL EQUIPMENT 25 x 16cm (10 x 6in) ovenproof dish

Preheat the oven to 190°C (fan 170°C/gas mark 5).

Slice the bread into triangles and arrange in the ovenproof dish in a single layer, overlapping the edges slightly. Dot the blueberries around the bread.

Add the white chocolate to a microwave-safe bowl and heat in 30-second bursts until fully melted. Pour in the milk, eggs, sweetener, vanilla and lemon zest and whisk together until smooth and combined.

Pour the milk mixture evenly over the bread slices. Pop the dish into the oven for 30 minutes until the custard has set and the bread has begun to brown and crisp around the edges. Serve with single cream, if using.

SLOW-COOKER METHOD
📦 **LOW: 2½–3 HOURS**
📦 **HIGH: 1 HOUR 30 MINS**

SPECIAL EQUIPMENT Slow cooker

Slice the bread into triangles and arrange into the bottom of the slow cooker pot, overlapping the edges slightly. Dot the blueberries around the bread.

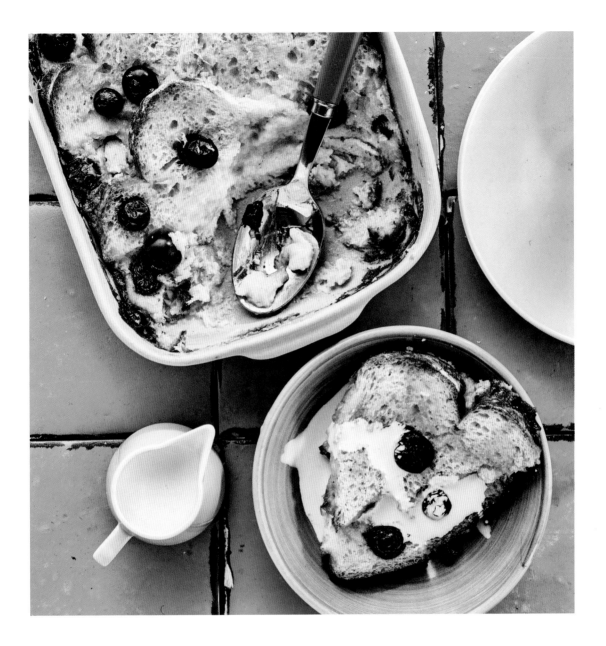

Add the white chocolate to a microwave-safe bowl and heat in 30-second bursts until fully melted. Pour in the milk, eggs, sweetener, vanilla and lemon zest and whisk together until smooth and combined.

Pour the milk mixture evenly over the bread slices.

Cover the slow cooker with the lid and cook on low for 2½–3 hours or high for 1 hour 30 minutes. The custard should be set and the bread will be beginning to brown and crisp around the edges. Serve with single cream, if using.

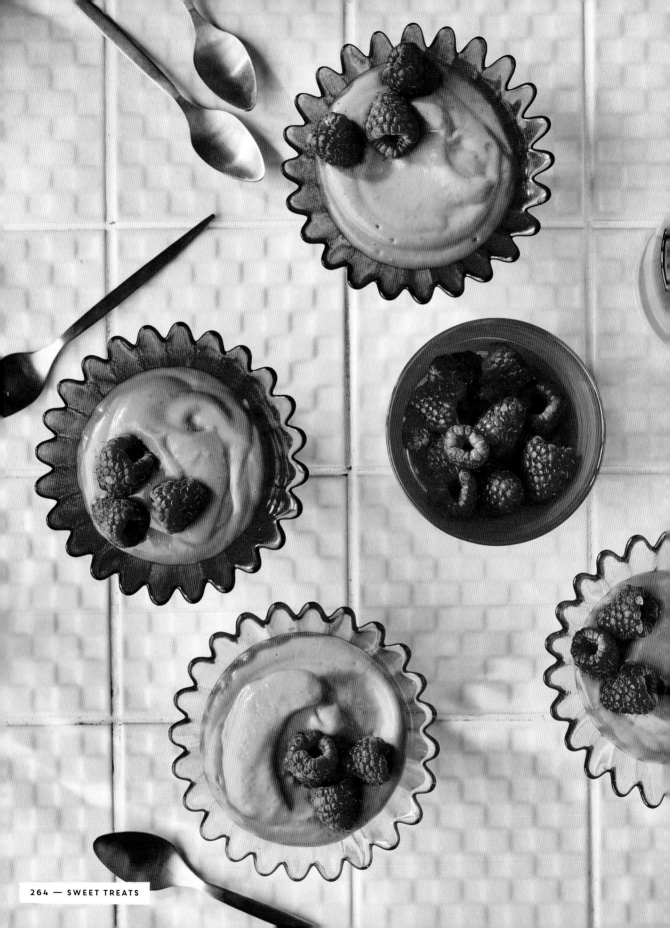

PINK RASPBERRY CUSTARD

🕐 **5 MINS**　🗑 **10 MINS**　✗ **SERVES 6**

DAIRY FREE

USE DF MILK ALTERNATIVE

GLUTEN FREE

PER SERVING:
157 KCAL / 23G CARBS

SPECIAL EQUIPMENT
Food processor or handheld stick blender

150g raspberries
3 medium egg yolks
3 tbsp cornflour
4 tbsp white granulated
　sweetener or sugar
500ml semi-skimmed milk
½ tsp vanilla extract
a few drops of pink food
　colouring (optional)

This pink custard brings back so many childhood memories for us. We used to have warm, pink custard poured over our puddings at school lunchtimes – usually on a Coconut and Jam Sponge or Jam Roly Poly, as an added treat. To give this one a fruitier, family-friendly twist, we've stirred in raspberries to enhance its natural pink colouring.

Weekly Indulgence

Puree the raspberries using a food processor or stick blender.

Place the raspberry puree in a sieve placed over a small bowl and push through with the back of a spoon to remove the seeds.

Scrape all the puree off the underside of the sieve into the bowl and discard the seeds.

Put the egg yolks, cornflour and sweetener or sugar in a large heatproof jug. Add 2 tablespoons of the milk and stir until smooth.

Pour the remaining milk into a medium saucepan and place over a medium heat. Heat until steaming hot, taking care not to let it burn or boil over.

Gradually pour the steaming-hot milk into the mixture in the jug, stirring with a wooden spoon or balloon whisk until completely blended.

Pour the mixture back into the saucepan and place over a medium heat. Cook the custard, stirring constantly with a wooden spoon or balloon whisk, for about 5 minutes, until there are a few small bubbles starting to appear on the surface and the custard has thickened.

As soon as the custard has thickened, remove it from the heat. Don't let the custard overheat or boil otherwise it may burn or split. Stir in the raspberry puree, vanilla extract and a few drops of pink food colouring (if using). Pour into a clean heatproof jug and serve warm with a dessert of your choice – we like it with raspberries.

SWAP THIS: If you wish to cut down on calories further, you could use skimmed milk instead of semi-skimmed, and adjust the calories accordingly. You could use dairy-free milk alternative if you prefer, and adjust the calories accordingly.

CHOCOLATE CHERRY
SHORTCAKE

🕐 **30 MINS**   🗑 **13 MINS**   🍴 **MAKES 9**

PER SERVING:
223 KCAL / 47G CARBS

FOR THE CHERRY FILLING
1 x 425g tin pitted black
   cherries in light syrup,
   drained, 50ml of syrup
   reserved
1–2 tsp white granulated
   sweetener (optional)
1 tsp cornflour

**FOR THE CHOCOLATE
SHORTCAKES**
200g self-raising flour, plus a
   little extra for dusting
25g cocoa powder
2 tsp baking powder
50g reduced-fat spread
100g white granulated
   sweetener
100ml semi-skimmed milk,
   plus extra if needed
½ tsp icing sugar, for dusting

FOR THE YOGHURT FILLING
100g fat-free Greek-style
   yoghurt
5g white granulated
   sweetener
4½ tsp low-calorie chocolate
   syrup, for drizzling (optional)

TIP: We use a granulated
sweetener that is crunchy
and weighs like-for-
like with sugar (not the
powdered kind).

Someone put the kettle on! This lovely treat can make
your morning cuppa feel more like afternoon tea. These
cherry-filled American-style shortcakes are less of a
biscuit and more like a soft, crumbly scone. Grab your
apron and get ready to show off your baking skills – your
friends and family are going to love them (if you can
bear to share them)!

Everyday Light ————————————————————————

Place the drained cherries and the reserved light syrup in a
small saucepan. Taste the cherries and syrup to see if they're
sweet enough for you. We found they didn't need sweetening,
but cherries can vary in sweetness, so you may wish to add a
teaspoon or two of white granulated sweetener at this point,
according to your taste.

In a small bowl, mix the cornflour with 1 teaspoon water
until smooth.

Place the saucepan of cherries and juice (and sweetener if
using), over a medium heat and stir in the cornflour mixture.
Simmer gently, stirring for about 3 minutes, until thickened and
glossy. The cherries should still be whole and glazed with a
small amount of sauce that's just enough to coat them.

Set aside and leave to cool while you make the shortcakes.

Preheat the oven to 200°C (fan 180°C/gas mark 6). Line a
baking tray with non-stick baking paper.

Sift the flour, cocoa and baking powder into a medium bowl
and stir to mix evenly.

Add the reduced-fat spread and rub it into the dry ingredients
using your fingertips, until the mixture resembles fine
breadcrumbs. Stir in the sweetener until well mixed.

Add the milk and, using a round-bladed knife, stir until a soft
dough is formed, adding another teaspoon or two of milk
if needed.

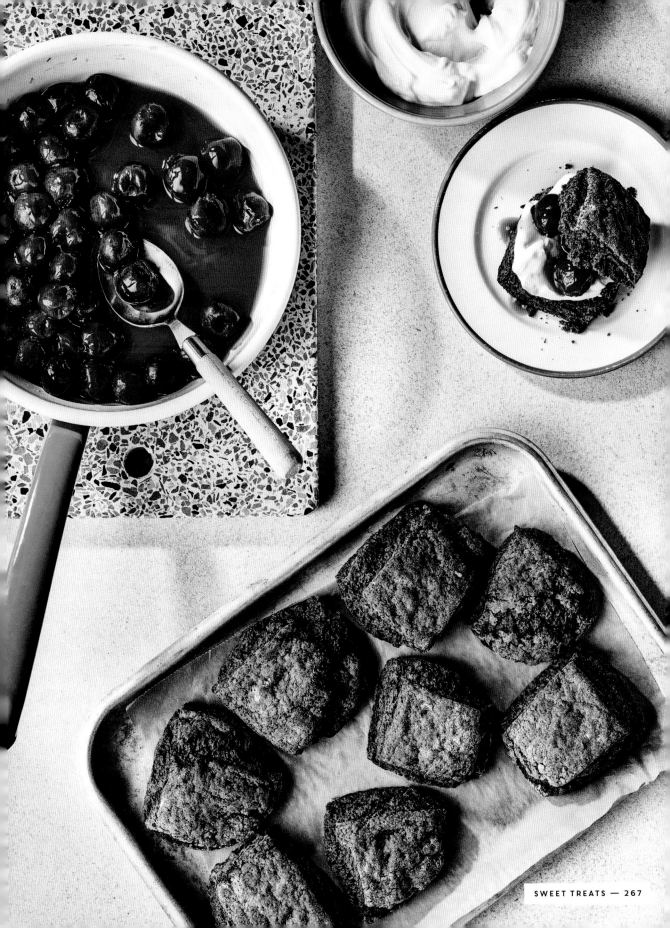

Form into a ball of dough, taking care not to over-handle, otherwise the dough may become tough.

Lightly dust a work surface with a little flour and turn the ball of dough out onto the surface. Roll the dough out into a square about 15 x 15cm (6 x 6in). Cut the dough into nine equal squares, each about 5cm (2in) across.

Place the squares on the lined baking tray, leaving space between them so they have room to rise properly. Place the baking tray into the preheated oven and bake for 10 minutes until risen. The shortcakes should sound hollow when tapped underneath.

Place on a wire rack and leave to cool.

To make the yoghurt filling, place the yoghurt in a small bowl and stir in the sweetener.

To assemble the shortcakes, use a serrated knife to slice the shortcakes in half horizontally. Place the bottom halves on a serving plate.

Divide the yoghurt filling between the shortcakes and spread out evenly. Spoon the cherry filling on top, dividing it equally as you go.

Drizzle ½ teaspoon low-calorie chocolate syrup over the yoghurt if you like, and place the shortcake lids on top and dust with a little icing sugar. Serve at once.

SWAP THIS: You can use about 200g of defrosted frozen cherries and 50ml of their juices instead of tinned cherries. Alternatively, halve pitted fresh cherries (without making the sauce), or any other soft fresh fruit of your choice, such as raspberries, and adjust the calories accordingly.

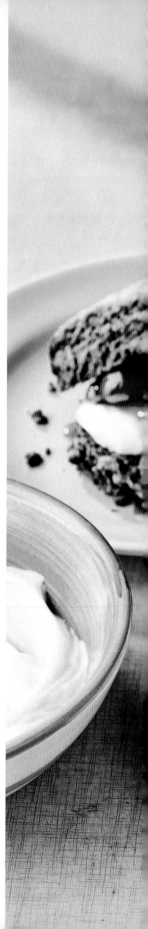

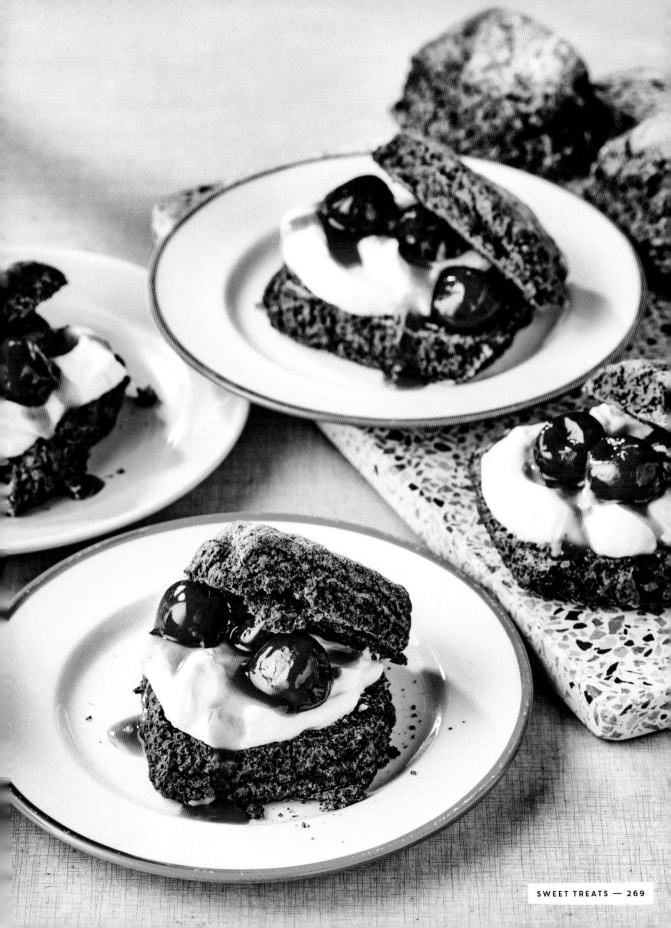

VEGGIE

USE VEGETARIAN
MARSHMALLOWS

**DAIRY
FREE**

USE DF MILK
AND AEROSOL
CREAM

**GLUTEN
FREE**

USE GF FLOUR
AND COOKIES

S'MORES PANCAKES

🕐 **5 MINS***   🗑 **8 MINS**   ✗ **SERVES 4**

*PLUS 30 MINS RESTING

PER SERVING:
289 KCAL /34G CARBS

50g plain flour
1 medium egg
150ml skimmed milk
low-calorie cooking spray
8 tsp chocolate spread
20g mini marshmallows
15g milk chocolate chips
4 sugar-free chocolate chip
  cookies, crumbled
low-fat aerosol cream

We've brought the popular campfire treat to the dessert table! We're talking melted chocolate, mini marshmallows, crumbled cookies – what a way to finish your meal. The trick to perfect pancakes is all in letting your batter rest, so don't be tempted to skip this step – good things come to those who wait!

Weekly Indulgence

Add the flour, egg and milk into a bowl or large jug, then whisk to a smooth batter. Set aside for 30 minutes to rest.

Place a medium frying pan over a medium heat and spray with low-calorie cooking spray.

When hot, pour a little of the batter into the pan and swirl until the bottom of the pan is coated. Cook the pancake for 1 minute until lightly golden-brown underneath, then carefully flip the pancake over and cook the other side. Remove to a plate and cover with foil. Repeat with the remaining batter. This should make four pancakes.

Add the chocolate spread to a small bowl and heat in the microwave for 30 seconds, until melted. Spread 1 teaspoon of chocolate spread onto the surface of each of the pancakes.

To the top right-hand corner of the pancake, add some mini marshmallows, chocolate chips and crushed biscuit. Fold the bottom half of the pancake over the top half and add more marshmallows, chocolate chips and crumbled cookie to the same quarter. Fold the left-hand side of the pancake over the top. You should now have a triangle-shaped, folded pancake.

Drizzle over the remaining chocolate spread and serve with a swirl of aerosol cream.

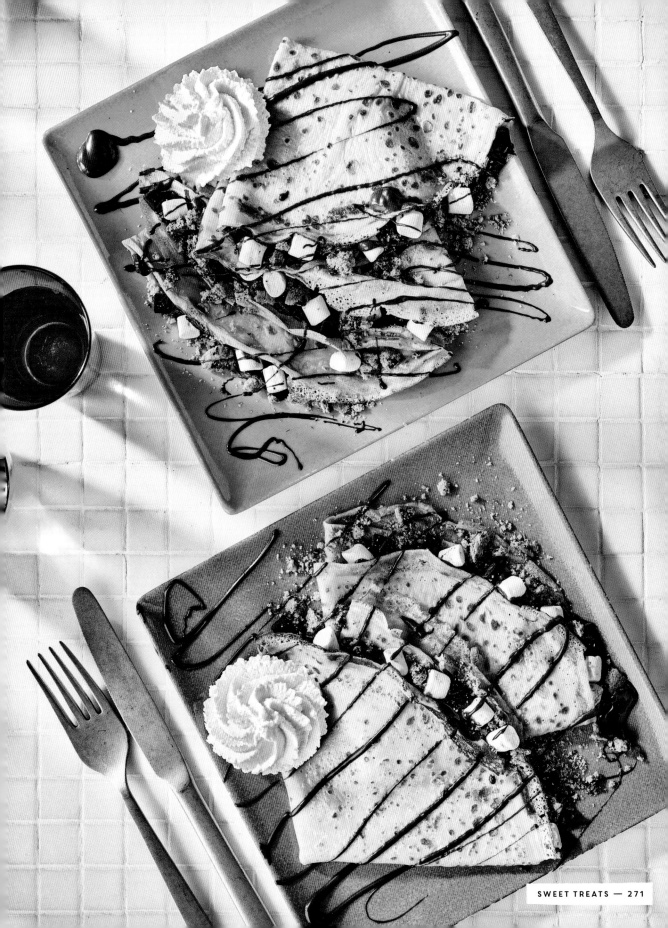

BANANA KATSU

🕐 **5 MINS**　　🗑 **VARIABLE** (SEE BELOW)　　✗ **SERVES 2**

PER SERVING:
174 KCAL / 29G CARBS

low-calorie cooking spray
20ml coconut dairy-free milk
  alternative
20g panko breadcrumbs
2 medium bananas,
  peeled and sliced in half
  lengthways
4 tbsp fat-free Greek-style
  yoghurt
3 tsp sugar-free salted
  caramel syrup

Craving something sweet? This fruity treat is speedy and slimming friendly; the very best combination. It might seem a little unusual, but you really CAN make this in your air fryer! The panko coating will crisp up nicely, with soft, sweet banana in the centre and a drizzle of sugar-free salted caramel syrup to finish. A simple, delightful dessert!

Everyday Light

HOB-TOP METHOD
🗑 **10 MINS**

Spray a frying pan with low-calorie cooking spray and set over a low to medium heat.

Pour the coconut milk alternative into a small bowl and the panko breadcrumbs into another bowl. Dip the banana into the milk and then into the panko, coating on all sides. Repeat with the other banana sections.

Add the bananas to the frying pan and fry for a minute. Flip the bananas and cook on the other side. Keep turning the banana, for about 10 minutes, until golden on all sides.

Stir the Greek-style yoghurt and 2 teaspoons salted caramel syrup together in a bowl. When the bananas are golden, serve with a dollop of the yoghurt and drizzle with the remaining syrup.

AIR-FRYER METHOD
🗑 **8 MINS**

SPECIAL EQUIPMENT　**Air fryer**

Preheat your air fryer to 180°C.

Pour the coconut milk alternative into a small bowl and the panko breadcrumbs into another bowl.

Dip the banana into the milk and then into the panko, coating on all sides. Repeat with the other banana sections. Add the bananas to the air fryer and spray with a little

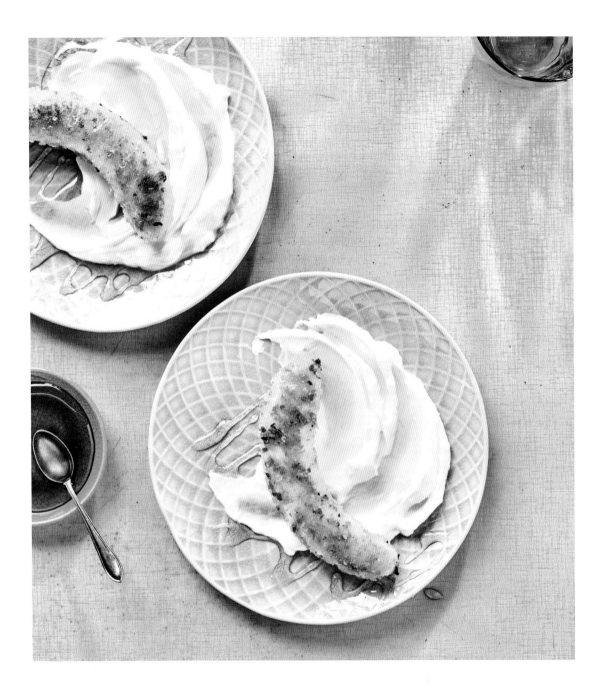

low-calorie cooking spray. Cook for 8 minutes, turning over halfway through until golden on all sides.

Stir the Greek-style yoghurt and 2 teaspoons salted caramel syrup together in a bowl. When the bananas are golden, serve with a dollop of the yoghurt and drizzle with the remaining syrup.

NUTRITIONAL INFO PER SERVING

Breakfast	ENERGY KJ/KCAL	FAT (G)	SATURATED FAT (G)	CARBS (G)	SUGAR (G)	FIBRE (G)	PROTEIN (G)
CREAMY STRAWBERRY FRENCH TOAST	828/196	4.5	1.4	28	7.3	1.6	10
HASSELBACK TOMATOES	721/172	6.4	3.9	9.8	9.1	3.2	14
CREAMY BACON AND MUSHROOM PANCAKES	1188/282	7.7	3.3	30	6.1	1.8	22
FRY-UP FRITTATA	1347/323	18	5.5	9.2	3.4	2.4	29
VIKING TOAST	1153/276	16	7.3	14	3	2.6	18
PUMPKIN SPICE SCONES	1025/244	7.7	2.9	35	3.9	1.8	7.3

FAKEAWAYS	ENERGY KJ/KCAL	FAT (G)	SATURATED FAT (G)	CARBS (G)	SUGAR (G)	FIBRE (G)	PROTEIN (G)
CHICKEN PICCATA	1123/265	2.5	0.7	31	7.1	2.8	27
CHANA MASALA	946/225	4.4	0.4	29	9.9	8.9	12
CHIPOTLE CHICKEN TAQUITOS	1954/464	13	5.2	52	14	5.3	31
TIKKA MASALA SALMON	1060/254	13	2.3	10	8.1	3.6	20
PERI-PERI CHICKEN WRAP	1266/300	3.8	0.8	47	24	6.3	16
CHILEAN-STYLE STEAK FRIES	1909/452	7.7	2.2	53	8.5	6.9	39
CARNE ASADA	1123/266	4.9	2.1	26	5.3	4	26
CHEESY NACHO BURGER	1921/458	17	5.5	39	5.6	5.9	33
PORK AND PINEAPPLE KEBABS	929/220	3.7	1.1	25	24	4.2	18
CHICKEN WITH YELLOW BEAN SAUCE	1678/400	6	1.1	26	14	4.7	27
STEAK AND PEPPER SKEWERS	1241/294	5.8	2.1	28	26	5	28
HARISSA CHILLI WITH CRISPY POTATOES	1653/392	5.9	1.6	38	11	10	41

FAKEAWAYS *Continued*	ENERGY KJ/KCAL	FAT (G)	SATURATED FAT (G)	CARBS (G)	SUGAR (G)	FIBRE (G)	PROTEIN (G)
CHICKEN AND CHEESE CURRY PIE	2113/501	11	5.9	49	12	7	48
SLOPPY JOE PIZZA	1243/295	7.5	3.5	30	9.6	5.3	23
TIKKA FISHCAKE WRAP	1026/243	3.2	1	29	3.8	4.2	22
STUFFED MEATBALL TORTILLA SKEWERS	1326/315	9.5	4.1	20	5.1	3.1	35
SPICY SPAGHETTI BOLOGNESE	2357/557	7.8	2.9	70	9	5.5	49
GARLIC AND GINGER CURRY	1350/320	7.1	1.8	16	12	3.2	45
PIZZA NACHOS	1232/295	15	2.6	32	3.4	2.5	6.4

STEWS *and* SOUPS	ENERGY KJ/KCAL	FAT (G)	SATURATED FAT (G)	CARBS (G)	SUGAR (G)	FIBRE (G)	PROTEIN (G)
GARLIC MUSHROOM SOUP	525/125	2.2	0.6	18	4.4	3.1	7.8
RAREBIT SOUP	1014/241	8.5	4.4	25	6.8	3.1	15
BUTTERNUT, BACON AND CHEDDAR SOUP	744/177	6.5	3	15	7.9	3.7	14
ROOT VEGETABLE CASSOULET	1020/242	2.3	0.4	39	13	12	9.9
DIJON CHICKEN AND DUMPLINGS	1433/340	7.9	1.5	33	5.8	3.4	34
CHICKEN GUMBO	824/195	3.2	0.6	13	10	5	26

BAKES, ROASTS AND ONE POTS	ENERGY KJ/KCAL	FAT (G)	SATURATED FAT (G)	CARBS (G)	SUGAR (G)	FIBRE (G)	PROTEIN (G)
BEEF OLIVES	1464/348	9.6	2.8	16	5.6	2.8	47
COTTAGE PIE WITH CHEESY CAULIFLOWER TOP	1793/427	14	7.2	21	13	6.3	53
OVEN-BAKED GARLIC CHICKEN AND RICE	1942/459	5.7	1.4	61	5.9	3	38
PESHAWARI-STYLE BAKED CHICKEN THIGHS	1464/349	13	2.7	19	16	4.3	36
MINESTRONE PASTA BAKE	894/212	4	1.7	30	8.2	6	10

BAKES, ROASTS AND ONE POTS *Continued*	ENERGY KJ/KCAL	FAT (G)	SATURATED FAT (G)	CARBS (G)	SUGAR (G)	FIBRE (G)	PROTEIN (G)
MINI CHICKEN KYIV BALLS	1389/333	20	6.6	17	1	1.4	21
STEAK AND KIDNEY PIE	1783/423	10	3.4	36	6.1	2.3	46
BAKED COD BALLS	1211/287	7.7	1.4	25	5.8	2.2	28
RAS EL HANOUT CHICKEN AND ORZO BAKE	2212/523	7	1.4	66	18	5.3	45
VEGAN BAKES	749/177	2.3	0.5	27	4	4.5	10
CRISPY HAM AND CHEESE NUGGETS	312/74	2.3	1.1	6.7	0.6	1	6.1
CRISPY TOFU NUGGETS	627/149	3.2	0.7	22	4.7	2.2	7.2
HERBY QUICHE WITH A POTATO CRUST	883/211	9.8	4.4	15	3.6	1.7	15
CREAMY VEGETABLE POT PIE	1657/397	24	13	32	5.5	3.8	11
PORK SCHNITZEL	860/204	6.3	2.1	6.6	0.5	0.5	30
SLOW-COOKED MEATBALLS IN TOMATO SAUCE	935/222	5.8	2.4	18	13	4.8	20
SPICED HADDOCK FISHCAKES	900/213	1.6	0.3	24	1.7	3.9	24
SALMON GRATIN	1716/408	14	4.3	44	7.5	4.4	25
CREAMY MAPLE AND BACON CHICKEN	1248/296	6	1.9	16	13	1.8	43
SPICY SALSA CANNELLONI	1277/303	7.1	3.1	30	12	5.9	26
CREAMY GARLIC MUSHROOM QUICHE	862/207	14	7	5.3	2.4	0.6	16
MEATBALL LASAGNE	1296/308	8.2	3.3	28	15	5	27
CREAMY BACON, ONION AND POTATOES	1122/266	5.7	1.8	27	8.8	3.9	24
NORMANDY-STYLE CHICKEN	1134/269	5.8	1.7	18	15	4.7	34
SOMERSET SAUSAGES	1489/356	15	4.8	26	13	7.2	23
CHICKEN SUPREME	951/225	5	1.8	8.8	5.8	1.2	36
CREAMY CAJUN-STYLE CHICKEN	943/224	4.3	1.6	14	10	4.1	30

BAKES, ROASTS AND ONE POTS *Continued*	ENERGY KJ/KCAL	FAT (G)	SATURATED FAT (G)	CARBS (G)	SUGAR (G)	FIBRE (G)	PROTEIN (G)
CHEESY MEATBALL PARMENTIER	2114/502	14	6.9	46	12	6.6	43
POULTRYMAN'S PIE	1652/391	5.1	1.6	42	13	8.7	40
SWEETCORN RISOTTO	1709/404	5.9	2.2	72	8.2	4.5	14

Snacks and SIDES	ENERGY KJ/KCAL	FAT (G)	SATURATED FAT (G)	CARBS (G)	SUGAR (G)	FIBRE (G)	PROTEIN (G)
CHICKEN TIKKA NAANWICH	1509/357	3.8	1.2	56	9.2	3.3	23
CHICKEN TIKKA PAKORAS	758/180	3.4	0.8	17	0.5	1.2	20
KEEMA NAAN PASTIES	1643/389	5.5	1.8	58	11	5.7	24
SALTED CARAMEL AND CHOCOLATE POPCORN BITES	289/69	2.8	1.5	9.9	3.8	0.6	0.7
POTATO PEEL CRISPS							
READY SALTED	190/45	0.5	0	9.1	0.5	1	1
SALT AND VINEGAR	194/46	0.5	0	9.2	0.5	1	1
CHEESE AND ONION	281/67	1.8	1	9.4	0.6	1	2.8
GREEK-STYLE BAKED BEANS	738/175	2.8	1.2	22	11	6.4	11
VEGETABLE SPRING ROLLS & SWEET CHILLI DIPPING SAUCE	480/114	1.8	0.4	20	4.2	1.4	3.3
GARLIC DOUGH BALLS	328/78	2.5	0.8	12	0	0.5	2.1
HONEY GARLIC POTATOES	834/197	0.5	0.1	41	7.2	4.6	4.6
CHEESY MARMITE MASH	1009/239	2.9	1.8	39	4.5	4	12
PEA AND BROCCOLI RICE	865/205	2	0.2	34	7.1	6.3	9
PIZZA PUFFS	769/184	8.8	4	20	1.9	1.8	4.9
CHEESE AND MARMITE SWIRLS	374/89	4.2	2	9.5	0.5	0.7	3.1
TUNA MELT TOASTS	773/184	5.8	3.2	13	2.6	2.6	19

Snacks and SIDES Continued	ENERGY KJ/KCAL	FAT (G)	SATURATED FAT (G)	CARBS (G)	SUGAR (G)	FIBRE (G)	PROTEIN (G)
GREEK-STYLE SPINACH AND RICE	948/224	1.8	0.5	43	3.1	2.7	7.6
CHICKPEA SALAD	1261/300	8	2.4	30	11	9.5	21
MEXICAN-STYLE STREET CORN SALAD	864/206	5.5	2.7	22	13	9.5	10
ROASTED SOY AND GINGER BROCCOLI	235/56	1.3	0.3	5	3.1	3.6	4.1
CHEESY GARLIC SWEET POTATO	801/190	5.1	3.1	27	8	3.1	7.8
ROASTED GARLIC MASH POTATO	1054/249	2.4	1.1	47	3.5	5	7.5

Sweet TREATS	ENERGY KJ/KCAL	FAT (G)	SATURATED FAT (G)	CARBS (G)	SUGAR (G)	FIBRE (G)	PROTEIN (G)
BANANA BREAD BROWNIES	535/128	4.5	1.7	20	4.1	1.1	3.5
BAKED PINEAPPLE CHEESECAKE	1132/270	11	5	31	15	1.1	12
SUMMER BERRY AND PROSECCO TIRAMISU	806/192	7.5	4.5	19	13	1.7	7.1
FROZEN PINEAPPLE WHIP	259/61	0.5	0.1	12	12	2.1	0.5
STRAWBERRY SHORTCAKE TRIFLES	1055/251	8.1	3.5	34	8.7	2.6	8.5
MILLIONAIRE'S ICE CREAM	658/156	3.3	1.6	17	6.7	0.5	14
TROPICAL FRUIT FOOL	587/141	8.9	5.3	12	9.8	0.6	3.6
LEMON CHEESECAKE TARTS	303/72	1.6	0.8	10	6	0.7	3.4
MINCEMEAT SWIRLS	401/96	3.8	1.7	13	4.1	0.8	1.8
CARAMELISED BANANA YORKSHIRE PUDDING	696/166	8.7	2.9	17	12	1	4.5
ST CLEMENT'S PUDDING WITH CITRUS SAUCE	1238/295	11	4.2	40	12	1.1	3.5
BAKES							
APPLE	605/143	4.4	0.5	25	4.8	1.4	5.2
CHERRY	669/158	4.4	0.5	28	7.5	1.8	5.6

Sweet TREATS *Continued*	ENERGY KJ/KCAL	FAT (G)	SATURATED FAT (G)	CARBS (G)	SUGAR (G)	FIBRE (G)	PROTEIN (G)
NUTELLA MOUSSE	943/227	16	7.4	15	15	0.6	4.7
CHOCOLATE TOFFEE PUDDINGS	898/215	11	3.8	25	0.5	0.9	5.6
BLUEBERRY AND WHITE CHOCOLATE BREAD PUDDING	1029/244	7.3	3.3	33	14	1.2	11
PINK RASPBERRY CUSTARD	662/157	4.4	1.7	23	5.7	1.9	4.7
CHOCOLATE CHERRY SHORTCAKE	941/223	3.4	1.1	47	7.6	1.6	4.6
S'MORES PANCAKES	1209/289	14	5.4	34	17	1.3	6.3
BANANA KATSU	738/174	1	0.4	29	22	1.6	11

INDEX

Page numbers in bold refer to illustrations.

ACKNOWLEDGEMENTS

As ever, we owe so many thank yous to so many people who work so hard to bring this book together. We really appreciate you all and can't thank you enough for the time and effort you put into making this book something we are hugely proud of.

We want to say a huge thank you firstly, to all of our followers on social media and all those who continue to make our recipes and let us know what you want next! We're so proud that Pinch of Nom has helped, and continues to help, so many people.

Thank you to our publisher Carole Tonkinson. To Martha Burley, Bríd Enright, Jodie Mullish, Sian Gardiner, Sarah Badhan and the rest of the team at Bluebird for helping us create this book and believing in Pinch of Nom throughout this journey. Major thanks also to our agent Clare Hulton for your unwavering support and guidance.

To Mike English for the amazing photos and to Kate Wesson for making our food look so, so good and to Octavia, Kristine and Jessica for all your assistance. Big thanks go out to Emma Wells, Nikki Dupin and Beth Free at Nic & Lou for making this book so beautiful!

We also want to thank our friends and family who have made this book possible.

Special thanks go to Laura Davis and Katie Mitchell for the endless hours you've put into this and for working so hard to get things right!

A huge thank you to our wonderful team of recipe developers who work tirelessly to help us bring these recipes to life : Lisa Allinson, Sharon Fitzpatrick and Holly Levell.

Massive thanks also go to Sophie Fryer, Hannah Cutting, Nick Nicolaou, Ellie Drinkwater and Laura Valentine for your writing and marketing support. To Cate Meadows and Jacob Lathbury for your creative and visual genius.

Additional thanks to Matthew Maney, Jessica Molyneux, Rubi Bourne, Vince Bourne and Cheryl Lloyd for supporting us and the business – we are so proud to work alongside you all.

To our wonderful moderators and online support team: thank you for all your hard work keeping the peace and for all your support.

Furry thanks to Mildred, Wanda, Ginger Cat, Freda and Brandi for the daily moments of joy.

And finally . . . Huge thanks go to Paul Allinson for your unwavering support. And to Cath Allinson who is never forgotten.

ABOUT THE AUTHORS

KATE and KAY

Founders of Pinch of Nom
www.pinchofnom.com

Kate and Kay Allinson owned a restaurant together on the Wirral, where Kate was head chef. Together they created the Pinch of Nom blog with the aim of teaching people how to cook. They began sharing healthy, slimming recipes and today Pinch of Nom is the UK's most visited food blog with an active and engaged online community of over 3 million followers.

Keep on track with the new

PINCH OF NOM FOOD PLANNER

PUBLISHING 2023